Principles of Neuroanatomy

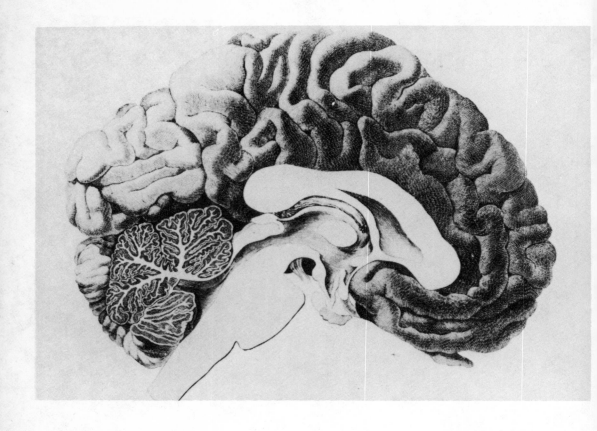

From an 18th century engraving of the medial aspect of the human brain prepared for Samuel Thomas Soemmerring, a famous German anatomist of the second half of the 18th century. He was particularly noted for the quality, accuracy, and art of illustrations drawn up under his direction. This figure is said to be the first correct picture of the sagittal aspect of the cerebral hemisphere. Moreover, it represents an effort to depict structure as it is seen in the living state, not in death. The picture captures the appearance of the fresh, unfixed human brain. (From E. Clarke and K. Dewhurst, *An Illustrated History of Brain Function*. University of California Press, Berkeley and Los Angeles, 1972)

Principles
of Neuroanatomy

JAY B. ANGEVINE, JR.
Professor of Anatomy
College of Medicine
University of Arizona, Tucson

CARL W. COTMAN
Professor of Psychobiology
Department of Psychobiology
University of California, Irvine

New York   Oxford
OXFORD UNIVERSITY PRESS
1981

Library of Congress Cataloging in Publication Data
Angevine, Jay B., Jr.
Principles of neuroanatomy.
Bibliography: p.
Includes index.
1. Neuroanatomy. I. Cotman, Carl W., joint author.
II. Title. [DNLM: 1. Nervous system—Anatomy and
histology. WL 101 A587p]
QM451.A53   611'.8   80-28228
ISBN 0-19-502885-6   ISBN 0-19-502886-4 (pbk.)

Printed in the United States of America

To Emeline, Spencer, Samuel, and Janice
and
Ann, Adrian, Danna, Daniel, and Cheryl

Preface

This book is written to provide an outlook on neuroanatomy for medical students, advanced undergraduates, and any others who desire some basic explanations of the fundamental principles of organization and plans of circuitry of the nervous system. A concise and convenient compilation of such generalizations should provide a useful supplement to the student's conventional neuroanatomy texts, a guidebook for anyone seeking a simple, integrated sampling of a complex subject, and even (we hope) a new view or a review for experts.

In neuroanatomy, basic principles are all too easily lost. Our goal is to distill from the seemingly endless detail the central facts, concepts, and principles of neural organization that make neuroanatomy the fundamental and enjoyable science of brain function that it is. Most, but certainly not all, of these principles have been known for many years, and are satisfying philosophically for their beauty of natural order. When brought out from the undergrowth of facts, they make neuroanatomy a meaningful topic where before it was mostly memory and mystery. The straightforward features reflected in the overall design of the nervous system give the student encouragement and a sense of purpose in learning the plethora of names and welter of pathways, from which at some point we know there can be no escape.

In our presentation, frequent analogies and comparisons are made with everyday matters. We try to carry over into our text certain informal qualities that come out when we are lecturing to medical and biology students. At these times, such rough-and-ready explanations of neural function are often the best ways to get the message across. Its informality notwithstanding, this book is as accurate as we can make it, contains what we believe are the most important concepts, and reflects our impressions of the latest outlooks of neuroscience.

A special effort has been made to provide an overview of the organization of neurotransmitter subsystems in the nervous system. This extremely important information is now an integral part of neuroanatomy. Our respective backgrounds in neuroanatomy and neurochemistry have encouraged us to combine our views of this exciting horizon on the brain.

This work grew out of a previous effort in which we collaborated on sections of an introductory psychobiology text, *Behavioral Neuroscience* (Academic Press, Inc., 1980). In presenting neuroanatomy at an elementary level for that text, we felt that an easy style provided an attractive view of neuroanatomy, one that encouraged the student to like the subject. Thus, we decided to undertake this book, striving for an overview, a light, clear style, and good illustrations. In places, we have retained sentences or expressions from Chapters 2 and 18 of the earlier book, because we found that we could not say certain things better or express ourselves more clearly.

We hope this book can be used for many years—as an adjunct to standard texts, as a checklist of basics for students and teachers, and as a primer for students and scientists from other fields. Last but not least, we think of all those people who ask so many questions about the brain. If they can find answers in this volume, or at least a new perspective that makes them glad they asked, we shall feel well repaid.

Acknowledgments

The authors wish to thank the various people who have helped in so many ways to make this book possible. Dr. Philip R. Weinstein (Chief, Division of Neurosurgery, University of Arizona College of Medicine) generously provided assistance and expertise in the preparation of Chapter 15. In addition we wish to thank Dr. Bryant Benson, Dr. David E. Blask, Dr. James Fallon, Mr. Craig A. Stockmeier, and Mr. Chris A. Leadem for helpful discussion on various aspects of the text. We are grateful to our illustrators, particularly Mrs. Maureen Killackey who did the drawings for most of the figures; Ms. Karin Fouts provided assistance with preparation of the last few figures. Janie Marshall, Toni Richardson, Maria Felix, and Anne Brown at the University of Arizona and Debbie Franks at the University of California, Irvine provided expert assistance in the typing of the material and Susanne Bathgate provided administrative assistance. We especially thank Mr. Jeffrey House for his very helpful editorial comments on the manuscript and members of the Oxford University Press staff, particularly Brenda Jones, for their concern and efficiency in the publication of the book. Finally we appreciate the support and encouragement of our wives and families during the many hours of work which went into the creation of our book.

Tucson, Arizona   J.B.A.
Irvine, California   C.W.C.
October 1980

Contents

Introduction, xiii

1. Basic Principles and Elements, 3
2. General Regions of the Nervous System, 14
3. The Auditory System, 54
4. The Vestibular System, 73
5. The Visual System, 87
6. The Somesthetic System, 115
7. The Olfactory System and Taste, 150
8. The Thalamus, 166
9. The Motor System, 185
10. The Spinal Cord, 210
11. The Reticular Formation and Core Mechanisms of Integration, 230
12. The Limbic System and Hypothalamus, 253
13. The Cerebral Cortex and the Lobes of the Brain, 284
14. The Chemical Coding of Neural Circuits, 314
15. The Circulation of the Brain and the Cerebrospinal Fluid, 354

Suggested References, 376
Index, 379

Introduction

The brain is a many-layered structure containing billions of neurons and countless numbers of neuronal connections, thousands of specialized regions, and dozens of functionally oriented subsystems. All these elements, moreover, have an interdependent scheme of organization. For example, sight is the special task of the visual system. Yet this system, like others, does not work alone. Its analyses of objects seen are combined at some point with information gathered by other sensory systems—the auditory and somesthetic (body sense) systems and perhaps the olfactory and gustatory ones as well. Perceptual meaning emerges as all this sensory information is pulled together, along with a plan for responding. The nervous system regulates the affairs of the body, plans and commands programs of response, and even initiates activity in the absence of sensory stimuli.

It is useful at this point to list nine obvious but crucially important attributes of the nervous system. We do this to begin with the "big picture." These simple, yet fundamental, principles provide a context for considering the design of individual subsystems as part of the whole.

1. The Ubiquity of the Nervous System

With over 100,000 miles of nerve fibers, the nervous system is nearly as extensive as the vascular system. Both systems pervade the body, and in fact are intimately related and interdependent. By means of nerve impulses and circulating hormones, respectively, the nervous and vascular systems integrate the activities of organs, protect them, enhance their performance

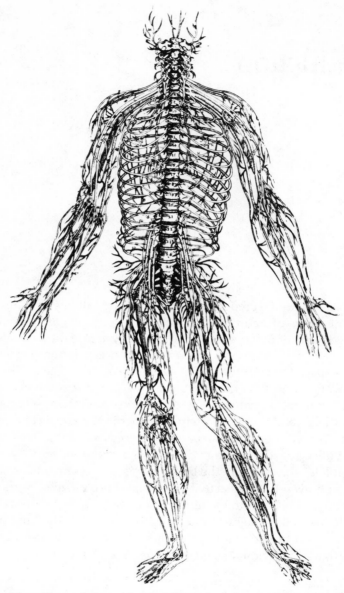

The Nerve Man. Through its widespread distribution, the nervous system pervades the body, attaining an almost global representation in its substance. This cardinal principle was recognized by the ancient anatomists, as this anatomically beautiful and highly accurate plate from Vesalius shows. This plate, as well as other plates showing the blood vessels, muscles, and bones, was designed by that master dissector to be cut out, glued to cardboard or other backing, and superimposed, so that his students could build up a three-dimensional picture of the body along with the intricate details of anatomy.

to meet stress or exercise demands, promote their growth, and maintain their healthy tone and vigor.

The central masses and myriad outreaching threads of the nervous system trace not only the external form of the body, but nearly every structure and feature in it (see accompanying figure). However, the density of nerve supply varies from place to place according to local tissue requirements. The degree of innervation in a body region signifies how large a role that region has in sending or receiving neural messages. In places liberally supplied with nerve endings (such as the cornea, lip, or bed of a nail), stimuli are almost always felt, and can be especially painful. In places not well supplied by nerve fibers (such as the thigh or buttocks), stimuli are less well discriminated, and when they lead to pain are often more easily tolerated. Similarly, muscles vary in the numbers of nerve fibers relative to muscle fibers; the higher this ratio, the more delicate the control of the muscle and the movements in which it is employed.

2. The Unity of the Nervous System

All parts of the nervous system are linked so that each part (at least potentially) can be in touch with every other. Some connections are quite direct, while others involve many intervening neurons. But although its circuitry is complex, the nervous system has total connectivity, thus offering body-wide communication.

A message from any body part enters the peripheral nervous system (PNS) and travels centrally over its network of branches until it reaches the brain or spinal cord, depending on where the message came from. Once inside the central nervous system (CNS), the message is analyzed there. How? By a process called integration, whereby central neurons combine and compare messages from many sources. In this process, some messages go to nearby points through local circuits, others to remote locations over long-distance lines. Ultimately, instructions are sent back to muscles and glands. Thus, though the transactions are often complex and unpredictable, activity in one part of the body can affect, through the agency of the nervous system, the activity of the other parts. Out of all these neural transactions comes a unified body, its parts working in harmony.

3. Centralization of the Nervous System

The term central nervous system is no coincidence. Indeed, the basic design plan of the nervous system is centralization. In delivering appropriate and all-encompassing responses, the nervous system generally does not allow for local transactions between body parts without involvement of the CNS. The system does not provide direct peripheral "hookups" over which, let us say, the index finger and thumb could hold a private conversation. Except for the passage of nerve impulses from one point along a nerve to another, incoming signals from one part of the body seldom reach another part directly, no matter how close that other part may be. Exceptions to this principle relate to local responses to painful stimuli. The swelling, reddening, and itching/burning feeling following irritation of the skin are associated with inward conduction of nerve impulses for short distances along a nerve fiber, and then outward conduction over a branch of that same fiber—along with release of substances related to tissue damage. This cutaneous "triple response" is either primitive or quite advanced.

But mainly, the signals that go out to body parts are not the same as the sensory messages that entered the CNS beforehand. On the contrary, such outgoing signals convey instructions drawn up by a multitude of central neurons in various brain regions. Some of these neurons not only monitor the incoming signals, but also keep track of others received simultaneously, earlier, or later from other parts of the body. And these multimodal neurons may be under directives from still other parts of the CNS itself, as to plans in the making. The result is a comprehensive analysis derived from a well-centralized organization.

4. Structural Specialization of the Nervous System

From the single neuron to the entire system, the nervous system displays structural and functional specialization. Sensory stimuli are processed by specialized subsystems (the visual system, auditory system, etc.). Less obvious are the special circuits for particular types of activities—eye movements, respiration, pain modulation, and affect, to cite just a few contrasting examples.

Structural specialization includes adaptations for speed of processing (as in a reflex), dependability (as in parallel processing and cellular redundancy), and peripheral feedback (as in closed-loop circuits). The neurons that carry out these functions are as structurally specialized as the subsystems themselves. In fact, neurons and their myriad connections are the foundation of specialization.

5. The Purposefulness of Neural Components

Each specialized component of the nervous system has a definite function, though we do not yet appreciate the task of each and every part. While the essential structural relationships—neurons, neuronal processes, synapses, and so forth—have been known for years, much of neuroanatomy is yet unknown. New information continues to emerge rapidly, particularly regarding the relationship of function to structure. Often, the maze of detail seems meaningless, and even bothersome at the time it is learned. Nevertheless, it has always turned out that each part of the nervous system has an important role, and thus understanding each part contributes to the understanding of the whole. Each neural component, therefore, is both necessary and functional.

6. Precision of the Nervous System

The vertebrate nervous system is accurately and reproducibly assembled. In animals of the same species and genetic background, the nervous system is virtually identical. There are marked variations between species, but the general properties and overall organization are sufficiently similar to develop generalizations, albeit careful and well considered ones. In man, there may be much more individual variation in brain structure, but still the common themes far exceed the differences.

Much of our knowledge of human neuroanatomy is derived from analysis of pathways and structures in other mammals and extrapolation of these findings to man. One of the great frontiers in modern science is to identify and understand in more detail the unique features of the human brain.

7. Plasticity of the Nervous System

Though reliable, the circuitry of the nervous system displays an inherent modifiability or plasticity. Abnormal visual experience early in development, for example, can produce remarkable changes in the synaptic organization of the visual cortex (Chap. 5). Such inherent plasticity probably permits the repair or fine tuning of circuits for certain changing functions—for example, depth perception must be recalibrated as the head

grows and interpupillary distance changes. Neuroanatomy is just beginning to identify the adaptive modifications of the nervous system which
occur with maturation and aging. Moreover, following injury, nerve fibers
(probably more than we realize) can sprout new connections and rearrange
old ones, not only in the periphery but in the CNS itself.

8. Chemical Coding of Neural Circuitry

Function is determined not only by a neuron's structure, integrative properties, and connections, but by the transmitter it delivers. This chemical
messenger may exert brief, focused effects or long-lasting, generalized
influences on the target nerve cell. All neural circuitry is chemically coded
(Chap. 14), and the new neuroanatomy is being written in terms of connections *and* transmitters.

9. Metabolic Demands of the Nervous System

An important aspect of neuroanatomy is the vasculature of the nervous
system, the set of vessels providing delivery of nutrients and removal of
waste products. As we might expect, the metabolic requirements of the
nervous system, in terms of substances needed and energy consumed, are
high relative to those of the total body. About a fifth of the oxygen that we
extract from each breath and a fifth of the calories (in the form of glucose)
that we ingest as food each day are the prodigious expenses we pay for the
ceaseless activity and readiness (with no need for warmup) of the system.
This constant and almost unvarying need for oxygen and glucose by the
nervous system (whether we are asleep or awake, relaxed or busy solving
problems) is met by a rich blood supply (see Chap. 15). In keeping with
these figures, the circulatory system brings about a fifth of the blood
pumped from the left ventricle directly to the brain, and it supplys additional amounts of blood to the spinal cord and all the craniospinal nerve
branches as well.

  This list of organizing principles is by no means complete, but it does call
attention to some remarkable attributes of the system. In this text, we shall
refer back to these basic principles, and point out others. All are worth
keeping in mind: they afford perspective and make the subject meaningful.

Principles of Neuroanatomy

Basic Principles
and Elements

1

Neurons

The design of the brain is in large measure the design of its constituent neurons (Fig. 1-1), although its supportive neuroglial cells probably have greater importance than we know. Neurons, truly remarkable cells, are the fundamental genetic, anatomical, functional, and trophic (nutritive or sustaining) units of the nervous system. These characteristics are the four tenets of the neuron doctrine, a once-controversial restatement of the cell theory applied to nervous tissue around the turn of the century.

One truth emerges more than any other: the variety of cell structure in the nervous tissue, central or peripheral, is far more complex than that seen in any other tissue. Whereas cells in other tissues, such as red blood cells, are highly redundant, nerve cells are highly individualized. In certain neural regions, they approach, or even attain, "zero redundancy." There are many specialized populations of neurons, and within a population single cells express their own individuality, both by their position in some circuit(s) and by their form. It is, above all, this neuronal specialization that gives the system its speed, fidelity, and flexibility as well as its integrative capacity.

In order to understand such complex cells as neurons, it helps to have some means of categorization. There are many classifications, and each has its limitations. Nonetheless, it is useful to distinguish two major classes: *projection neurons* with axons coursing between one region of the CNS and another, and *local-circuit neurons* with axons extending to other cells in the immediate vicinity.

3

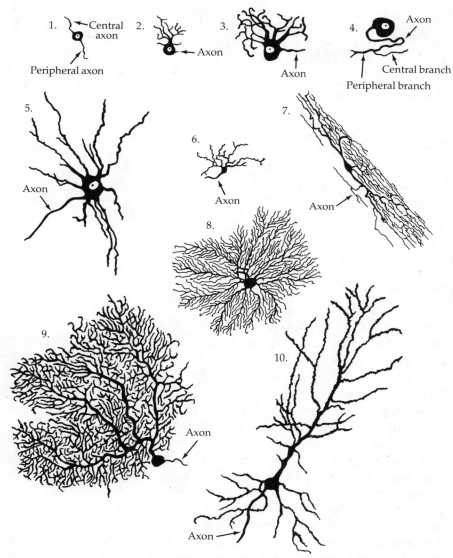

FIG. 1–1. *Neurons and neuronal variety.* Scaled drawings of neurons to illustrate their great diversity. (1) Bipolar neuron in nodose ganglion of vagus nerve. (2) Parasympathetic neuron. (3) Sympathetic neuron. (4) Pseudounipolar neuron of trigeminal ganglion. (5) Spinal motor neuron. (6) Small neuron in substantia gelatinosa of spinal trigeminal nucleus. (7) Spindle-shaped neuron from nucleus of tractus solitarius. (8) Cortical projection neuron in thalamus. (9) Purkinje cell from cerebellum. (10) Pyramidal cell from cerebral cortex. (Cells redrawn from S. Ramón y Cajal and also from C. Fox, Wayne State University)

Projection neurons and local-circuit neurons are not classified on the basis of cell size, length of axon or type of contact; it is only their role in either long-distance or local communication that separates them. A projection neuron is often large, with a long axon, and a local-circuit neuron is frequently small, with a short axon; but these features do not necessarily go together.

This scheme is different from, but not inconsistent with, the traditional one of sensory neurons, motor neurons, and interneurons (see below). It can be traced back to the concepts of early neuroanatomists. Faced with the astonishing richness of neuronal types in the CNS, the Italian histologist Camillo Golgi suggested late in the 19th century that nerve cells be classified according to the length of their processes. At about the same time in Spain, Ramón y Cajal similarly grouped all neurons into long-axon and short-axon cells. While the discoveries and thoughts of these scientists, and others of their time, are outside the scope of this book, many of their ideas are still with us today.

Projection Neurons and the Parts of Neurons

Most large neurons are projection neurons, and such big cells fit into the "classic" mold of a neuron: they have a long axon, a cell body, and dendrites emanating from that cell body. These cells are thus multipolar, have many synaptic endings on their dendritic tree, and send impulses to one or more places over their axon. Motor neurons, pyramidal cells in the cerebral cortex, and Purkinje cells in the cerebellar cortex are familiar examples.

The several major parts of a typical projection neuron are readily identifiable. The cell body is developmentally the earliest part of the neuron to arise, and it is the trophic part that maintains the life of the neuron and its often far-flung processes.

The dendrites form treelike arborizations, which are often marvelously elaborate; they are the primary receptive processes of the neuron. They afford contact points (synapses; see below) for the terminals of incoming nerve fibers (axons), and for other fibers passing by the dendrites to different destinations. They act as minicomputing centers to receive and integrate all the different inputs. In CNS neurons, dendrites originate from the cell body as one or more primary branches, which in turn branch and become finer and finer. Most nerve fibers arriving at dendrites terminate on spines — minute thorns of the dendrite's surface that serve as highly specialized ports of entry for afferent signals. As one might expect, the total cytoplasmic volume of the dendrites exceeds that of the cell body many times.

The axon projects to one or many targets, depending on the design of the circuit and how many branches (collaterals) the axon has. For neurons that communicate with many others, these collaterals can be numerous, extremely long, and/or complex in pattern of ramification. The specialized cell-to-cell junctions where neurons communicate with other nerve cells or with muscle are called *synapses*. The number of them in our CNS is unimaginable: 10^{14} is the best current estimate.

Most long axons are wrapped in *myelin*: specialized cells near the axon (Schwann cells in the PNS and oligodendroglia in the CNS) wrap part of their cytoplasm and plasmalemma around the axon many times, forming a spiraling, largely fatty membrane sheath around the conductile process. By forcing the nerve impulse to jump from one interspace between successive myelin segments to the next interspace (saltatory conduction), myelin greatly speeds up passage of the impulse, thus increasing the efficiency of the axon in its signaling function.

Axon terminals are specialized structures at the end of the axon, or at the ends of its fingerlike preterminal branches when they exist. It is from these terminals that transmitters are secreted. Axonal endings have a variety of shapes: bulbous, buttonlike (boutons terminaux), climbing-vine, rosette, and so forth. Similar structures are encountered along the course of certain axons (boutons en passant, or endings in passing). These variously shaped presynaptic terminals form synapses with similarly specialized postsynaptic regions of the target neuron, where the receptor sites for transmitters are located.

Local-Circuit Neurons and Their Importance

Local-circuit neurons (a type of interneuron) usually have short axons, or sometimes no axons at all (amacrine cells), as in the retina and olfactory bulb. They are involved in localized events within a functional group of cells, rather than transactions between separate groups. They are far more numerous than projection neurons in the mammalian CNS. For example, the cerebral cortex has about three times more local-circuit neurons than projection neurons. In the caudate nucleus, a large mass of forebrain neurons shaped like a fish with a long tapering tail, 95% of the neurons are local-circuit neurons.

Thus, local-circuit neurons are of great interest. We are just beginning to appreciate their roles. Their general structure has been known for many

years, but their functions are evasive because few methods exist for studying these cells. Many are too small, and there are just too many kinds to
count, let alone describe. Certain select examples, however, are fairly well
understood, and the analysis of these has cast some light on their functional significance. A well-studied local-circuit neuron is the basket cell of
the cerebellum, which will be described in Chapter 9.

Flexibility of the Parts of Neurons

The various parts of neurons are extremely adaptable. There are now
known to be many important exceptions to the classical definitions of the
principal processes of neurons. For example, certain regions of the axon
(normally thought of as conductile) may serve receptive functions: an axon
may receive input from other axons at the beginning (axon hillock) or near
the end (preterminal branches) of its course. In some cases dendrites (usually considered receptive) may conduct impulses swiftly along their length
—in a manner somewhat similar to an axon. And sometimes dendrites
may even act as effectors and transmit activity to other dendrites (in so-
called dendrodendritic synapses). It is helpful to regard the cytological
structure of neurons as flexible: virtually any part of a neuron can perform
any of the cell's communications functions, if special circumstances or
modes of cellular arrangement make it advantageous to the nervous system. The only invariant feature of a nerve cell is the location of its vital
center or trophic part: it is always the cell body, and if this perikaryon is
damaged severely enough, the rest of the neuron dies, no matter how
far-flung its dendrites and axon or how crucial its role in a circuit.

Design and Polarity of Neurons

Neurons are especially adapted for their situation in the overall circuitry of
the nervous system, and sometimes the functional significance is obvious
on first sight. Bipolar neurons, which can be considered projection neurons
(they sometimes signal over long distances), illustrate this point: the distal
process extends to the periphery, while the central process leads to the
brain. These cells are primitive but straightforward biological specializations of the columnar epithelial cells from which they seem to have
evolved. In the human nervous system they are found in the olfactory
mucous membrane, in the retina, and (slightly modified) in the auditory
and vestibular ganglia of the inner ear.

Another type of neuron has two opposing processes which shift about the cell body during development and combine into a single conductile process that divides a short distance away like the bars of the letter T. Such neurons are called "pseudounipolar" because in the embryonic condition they had two processes to begin with. This type of cell is found in the dorsal root ganglia of spinal nerves and in the sensory ganglia of all cranial nerves except the auditory/vestibular nerve just mentioned.

True unipolar neurons are rarely encountered in vertebrates, except in early embryonic stages. In invertebrates, however, they are the preeminent population, and hence constitute by far the greatest number of neurons on earth. The single process of a true unipolar neuron is remarkable: at certain points it receives and integrates like a dendrite, and at other points it conducts and transmits like an axon. We mention this feature of invertebrate neuroanatomy to underscore the flexibility of neuronal design and to point out a similarity with some vertebrate neurons. The distal branchlets of certain sensory neurons in vertebrates seem to act as such a combination dendrite/axon, in mediating the local responses to painful stimuli and tissue injury mentioned earlier. While some may view these versatile processes as "primitive" features generally found in "lower" animals, we see them as superbly efficient biologic specializations common to a wide range of living creatures.

In a functional scheme, bipolar and pseudounipolar neurons are classified as sensory neurons, in keeping with their usual sensory function. In vertebrates, however, multipolar neurons, such as the one illustrated in Figure 1-2, are the most common type, making up virtually all of the neurons of our CNS — motor neurons, pyramidal cells, basket cells, etc. Functionally, these staggering numbers of nerve cells (more than 10^{12}) fall into two groups: motor neurons, which project to muscles and glands, and interneurons, the myriad ones between sensory neurons and motor neurons. Since we shall encounter several kinds of multipolar neurons in the course of this book, suffice it to say here that the multipolar neuron is the "hallmark" of the vertebrate CNS. The integrative power of our nervous system is rooted in this efficient type of cell with richly branched dendrites, and communications in the brain and spinal cord and with the effector organs via long and short axons depend on such cells.

FIG. 1–2. *The processes of neurons.* (A) Multipolar neuron drawn by Deiters (1865). This is the first pictorial demonstration that one of the processes of a neuron is different physically and chemically from all of the others. At that time, this process was known as the axis cylinder, because it is the axis (hub) of the neuron; it is now called the axon. The other processes are called dendrites. Many of Deiters' observa-

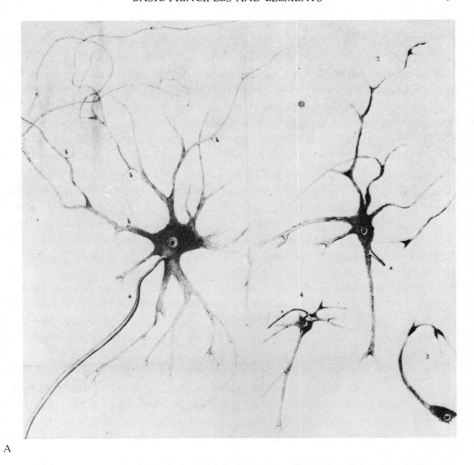

A

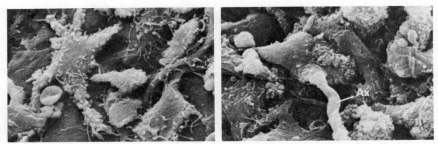

B

tions were made from neurons meticulously dissected out of the brain in the fresh state. (B) Scanning electron micrographs of multipolar neurons. Synaptic boutons, some of which have a segment of axon still attached, appear scattered over the surface of the cell body and dendrites. Ax, axon. (From R. G. Kessel and R. H. Kardon, *Tissues and Organs: A Text-Atlas of Scanning Electron Microsiopy*, W. A. Freeman, San Francisco, 1979)

Neuroglial Cells

These "nerve-glue" cells outnumber the trillion neurons five to ten times, and make up half the total volume of the CNS. Thus our neurons lie in a sea of glia. We shall only briefly mention these cells to afford perspective, leaving a more detailed account to other texts.

Neuroglia are not merely mechanically supportive cells, although they give neurons a lot of structural support. They are metabolically active elements that assist their companion cells, the neurons, in performing communicative and integrative functions. One type of glial cell, the oligodendrocyte (cell with few processes), makes and maintains myelin in the CNS (peripherally, myelin is formed by Schwann cells). Oligodendrocytes are also found closely apposed to neuronal cell bodies, apparently conveying materials to and from them in a manner similar to the satellite variety of Schwann cells encountered adjacent to perikarya in peripheral ganglia.

A larger, star-shaped glial cell is the astrocyte. In gray matter astrocytes have thick, sheetlike processes, while in white matter these extensions are fibrous and more delicate. Astrocytes provide structural support, convey nutrients, gases, and wastes between neurons and blood vessels (or between neurons and the cerebrospinal fluid), parcellate inputs to neurons and make repairs (scar tissue) after damage due to disease or trauma.

Microglia are small cells; their scanty perikarya give rise to branching, wavy processes with spinelike projections. They are said to be mesodermal in origin and to invade the CNS at the time the brain vasculature is elaborated. Normally, they are inactive, but when inflammatory or degenerative damage to the CNS occurs, they proliferate rapidly, as do certain meningeal and perivascular connective tissue cells. All these cells migrate toward the injury and turn into phagocytes, scavenging the debris.

Ependymal (meaning "upper garment") cells line the cavities of the upper regions of the CNS — the central canal of the spinal cord and the ventricles of the brain. A modified version of them lines the choroid plexuses, those convoluted grapevinelike structures in the ventricles where cerebrospinal fluid (CSF) is produced (see Chap. 10). These cells confine and help to form the CSF, which, among other roles, acts to support the weight of the CNS, to protect it from injury, and to provide a sort of kidneylike sump for the brain.

The Normal and Pathologic Significance of Neuroglia

In general, the neuroglial cells have been relatively neglected, due in part to the obvious attractiveness of neurons for study but also in some measure to the reluctance of many neuroscientists to confront the enormous numbers of glial cells and their enigmatic roles. We should keep in mind that in partitioning inputs to neurons, regulating ion concentrations in extraneuronal space, and providing high-energy compounds to neurons, the neuroglia may play a much greater role in the communications functions of the CNS than is now thought. And in neural development, we now know that the primitive ependymal and astrocytic cells of the CNS provide structural scaffoldings for migratory young neurons, systems of radially arranged processes or struts that guide nerve cells to their destinations. Unhappily, however, this major developmental assistance that the glia provide is offset by their vulnerability to disease later in life, or even at birth: the neuroglia are the chief source of neoplasms in the CNS. The study of such gliomas, as well as the varied responses of the neuroglia in cerebrovascular disease, CNS infections, and other types of neurological disorders, is a central subject of neuropathology.

General Concepts

The first determinant of neuronal function is structure. The position of the neuron in a circuit and the extent and geometry of its axon and dendrites specify what things a neuron will "listen to" and over which lines it will "talk." The PNS conveys signals from the environment (both external and internal) to the CNS. There, with flexibility, speed, and reliability, though not without metabolic cost, these reports are integrated and considered in relation to current and past events, including even the history of the species. A decision is made, a memory formed, or a response initiated for the PNS to carry out. Sometimes, we may achieve impressive performances, exceeding our own goals in a measure our brain had not foreseen.

Glossary

Cortex: an additional sheet of gray matter that lies outside the white matter in the cerebral hemispheres, roof of the midbrain, and cerebellum. In these "extra coats" of gray matter, the nerve cell bodies are arranged in distinct layers, and the inputs and outputs show an extremely orderly plan of organization.

Ganglion: a round or fusiform cluster of sensory nerve cell bodies in the peripheral nervous system (PNS) or of motor cell bodies in the autonomic nervous system (ANS), sheathed by connective tissue (epineurium). A ganglion usually discharges a wider range of functions than a nucleus. For example, the hypoglossal nucleus is restricted to supplying motor axons to the tongue muscles, whereas the trigeminal ganglion mediates several modes of cutaneous and deep sensation from the entire face, and the celiac ganglion distributes a wide variety of visceral motor fibers to splanchnic regions.

Gray matter: the core of the CNS, containing nerve cell bodies (somata, perikarya), their dendrites, and the proximal stretches of their axons (distally, the axons enter the surrounding white matter). Neuroglial cells and numerous blood vessels (especially capillaries) are also present.

Interneurons: also known as internuncial neurons, these comprise all neurons between the primary neuron and the motor neuron. The CNS contains an astronomical number of interneurons, and neuroanatomy is largely the study of interneurons. *Note:* A common mistake is to think an interneuron must be small. Many of them are, e.g., the granule cells of the cerebellar cortex. But many others are large: the Purkinje cells of the cerebellar cortex, the pyramidal cells in the cerebral cortex, and certain neurons in the brainstem reticular formation. The important thing about an interneuron is that it lies in the middle of the basic circuit plan: between pure sensory and motor neurons.

Motor neuron: the final neuron or "final common pathway" (Sherrington) through which neural activity passes to the effector organs (muscles and glands). Examples are the large anterior horn cells of the spinal gray matter and similar effector cells in the brainstem (e.g., in the nucleus of the hypoglossal nerve). Again, the number of motor neurons in relation to the total neuronal population is quite small: about 2 million or so. The visceral motor system, or so-called autonomic nervous system, has a serial arrangement of two small motor neurons — a preganglionic one with its cell body in some part of the CNS and a postganglionic one with its cell body in an autonomic ganglion.

Nucleus: a functional cluster of nerve cell bodies in gray matter (not to be confused with the nucleus of a cell). The dendrites and especially the axons of the cell bodies in a given nucleus may extend far beyond the arbitrary but accepted nuclear boundary. Some nuclei are spherical in three-dimensional form; others have a fusiform, cylindrical, or cushionlike configuration.

Primary neurons: the first neuron in the sequence of sensory information processing by the nervous system. Examples are the pseudounipolar neurons in the posterior (dorsal) root ganglia of spinal nerves and the sensory ganglia of certain cranial nerves (V, VII, IX, and X), as well as the bipolar cells in the olfactory mucosa (CN I) and the acoustic/vestibular ganglia (CN VIII). In relation to interneurons, their number is small (in the millions).

Tract: a bundle of myelinated or "unmyelinated" (poorly myelinated) axons in the white matter, running from one place to another — often over long distances. Where functions are known, tracts are given functional names (optic tract). Otherwise, descriptive terms (medial forebrain bundle) or binomial designations of origin/termination (corticospinal tract) are used.

White matter: immediately around the central gray, it contains axons of neurons whose cell bodies lie in the gray matter, in a region of cortex or in ganglia outside the CNS. The axons are of various caliber and degree of sheathing by myelin, a fatty substance that is glistening white in the fresh state. As in gray matter, neuroglia and blood vessels are additional constituents, but white matter contains fewer capillaries.

General Regions of the Nervous System

2

We have characterized the work of the nervous system in the Introduction and Chapter 1: Its service is the maintenance and successful performance of the body, and its product is human behavior. As we might expect, it has many functional subdivisions that we recognize as numerous, highly individualized structural components.

The Fundamental Parts of the Central Nervous System

If we remove the dense nerve branches of the peripheral nervous system (PNS), we can see the central trunk or central nervous system (CNS): the brain and spinal cord (Fig. 2-1). To understand these adult structures we must examine the fundamental subdivisions of the embryonic CNS (Fig. 2-2). There are five main parts of the brain, deriving from the five thin-

---

FIG. 2–1. *Overview of the CNS.* Visible in this lateral overview are the cerebrum, cerebellum, pons, and medulla oblongata. The medulla leads smoothly into the underlying spinal cord, the tip of which, indicated by the arrow, lies at the level between the first and second lumbar vertebrae in the small of the back.

The reason for the disparity in length between the vertebral column and spinal cord is that during embryonic development the axial mesoderm grows more rapidly and for a longer period of time than the caudal part of the neural tube. There are 31 pairs of spinal nerves: 8 cervical, 12 thoracic, 5 lumbar, 5 sacral, and one coccygeal. In exiting the vertebral column at their appropriate intervertebral foramina, the nerve roots become increasingly angulated at lower cord levels. (The respective levels of origin of the various groups of nerves are indicated; see Chap. 10 for details)

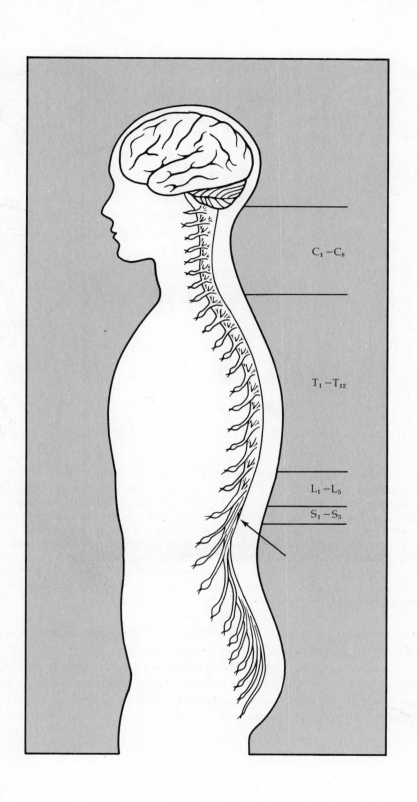

$C_1 - C_8$

$T_1 - T_{12}$

$L_1 - L_5$

$S_1 - S_5$

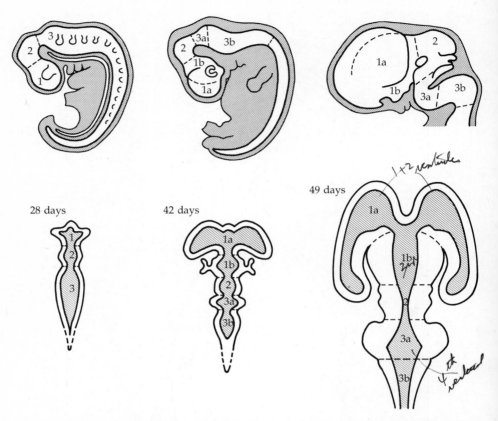

FIG. 2–2. *The basic subdivisions of the CNS.* By the time the embryo is one month old, the forebrain, midbrain, and hindbrain are clearly defined watery vesicles (here given numerical designations 1, 2, and 3). These fundamental chambers, separated by constrictions, lie at the cephalic end of the rapidly elongating neural tube, which has now folded shut from its primitive open condition throughout its length. Two weeks later, five vesicles are recognizable, because (as the numerical scheme 1a, 1b, 3a, and 3b indicates) the forebrain and hindbrain have undergone additional subdivision. The midbrain (2) does not become subdivided. The caudal part of the neural tube becomes the spinal cord. The main adult derivatives of the key components of the embryonic CNS are indicated in Table 2-1.

walled, fluid-filled vesicles that comprise it during development, and a sixth long, tubular component extending caudally, the spinal cord. All these hollow structures develop from the neural tube, originally part of the outer or ectodermal layer of the embryo. These subdivisions are of great importance in describing and studying the nervous system. Their Latin terms and English names are universally used in texts, research papers,

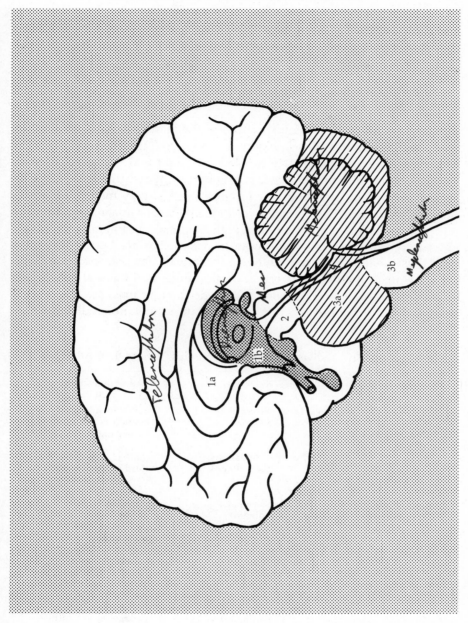

FIG. 2–3. *Adult derivatives of the brain vesicles.* Sagittal view of the adult brain to show what becomes of the five fundamental subdivisions of the embryonic brain (compare Fig. 2-2). Numerical scheme as on Fig. 2-2; diencephalon and metencephalon shaded to clarify boundaries.

and clinical accounts. Accordingly, we provide a picture of the adult brain that shows their application to its fully developed structure (Fig. 2-3 and Table 2-1).

The Cerebrum: Cerebral Hemispheres and Diencephalon

The largest and most striking structure in the mature nervous system derives chiefly from the telencephalon or "endbrain"; it is the cerebrum. The cerebrum is almost completely divided into right and left cerebral hemispheres, each consisting of a core region of gray matter (the basal ganglia), a mass of white matter, and an overlying sheet of gray matter that forms the cerebral cortex. The hemispheres look like mirror images, but they are not completely alike, at least not in higher animals and man. Each makes special contributions to overall brain function that are better developed than these abilities are on the other side. In man, for example, one hemisphere is instrumental in speech and calculation, and has a strong liaison with consciousness and deliberate, analytic thought process. The other is necessary for our appreciation of spatial relationships, nonverbal ideation,

Table 2-1. The Main Subdivisions of the Embryonic CNS and their Adult Fates

Three-vesicle stage	Five-vesicle stage	Adult derivatives
1. Prosencephalon (forebrain)	1a. Telencephalon (endbrain)	Cerebral hemispheres, lateral ventricles, basal ganglia
	1b. Diencephalon ('tweenbrain)	Thalamus, hypothalamus, third ventricle, optic nerves/tracts, retinae
2. Mesencephalon (midbrain)	2. Mesencephalon (midbrain)	Tectum (colliculi), cerebral aqueduct and peduncles, midbrain tegmentum
3. Rhombencephalon (hindbrain)	3a. Metencephalon (afterbrain)	Cerebellum, rostral fourth ventricle, pons, pontine tegmentum
	3b. Myelencephalon (cordbrain)	Medulla oblongata, caudal fourth ventricle, medullary tegmentum
4. Remaining caudal part of neural tube	4. Remaining caudal part of neural tube	Spinal cord (myel; from Greek, "marrow") and central canal

and holistic thinking. In both hemispheres, however, the degree of neural integrative function is profound. The analysis of environmental features and the selection of response patterns is carried out in the cerebral cortex to a degree of detail matched in few other places in the nervous system. The closest competitor would probably be the thalamus, which develops from the embryonic diencephalon or "betweenbrain." Lying deep within the cerebrum, the thalamus works hand-in-hand with the cerebral cortex in high sensory and motor functions.

The Cerebellum and Pons

Lower down the neuraxis is the cerebellum, part of the metencephalon, or "afterbrain." (The midbrain will be described later on). Its bulk is partly hidden by the overlying cerebral hemisphere. It is a bilobed mass with a median part (vermis) connecting the two hemispheres. The hemispheres are deeply fissurated in a remarkably parallel fashion, a characteristic resulting in closely opposed folds or folia covered by cortical gray matter. The cerebellum is a sort of computer; it regulates the rate, range, and force of movements. It works in concert with the cerebrum, as well as with the spinal cord and other structures. Unlike the cerebrum, it does not play a major role in conscious experience of sensation or in initiating willed movements. Without the cerebellum, we would probably still have most of our sensations — our conscious ones, at least. But its loss would seriously impair the dexterity and smooth execution of our movements (particularly the skilled movements of our distal extremities), noticeably diminish our strength and muscular tone, and upset our posture and equilibrium.

Below the cerebellum is the pons, another part of the metencephalon. It is a bridge of nerve fibers which crosses the midline. It seems to bind the cerebellum to the brainstem, much as one would strap a backpack around one's waist. But the pons is not just holding two parts of the brain together. It is a key link between the cerebrum and cerebellum. A massive cable emanates from the pons through which the motor region of one cerebral hemisphere "plugs in" to the contralateral cerebellar computer. This crossed link in the cerebrocerebellar connection forms the middle cerebellar peduncle; its presence is essential if volitional movements are to be carried out in a coordinated, flowing, and well-directed manner. Immediately caudal to it lies the inferior cerebellar peduncle, over which information from the spinal cord and other structures in the medulla oblongata is brought to the cerebellum. Rostral to the middle peduncle is the superior cerebellar peduncle; through it, cerebellar output is distributed to various motor control centers in the brainstem.

The Medulla Oblongata

Protruding caudally from the pons, the medulla oblongata (myelencephalon or "cordbrain") tapers smoothly into the spinal cord below. Like many brain regions, it has an importance out of proportion to its size. Although scarcely larger in diameter than a fountain pen, it is crucial to survival. Even small injury to it leads to devastating, if not fatal, consequences. Through it run tracts of nerve fibers, long cables over which the brain and cord communicate in performing different functions. Within the medulla lie nuclei (clusters of neurons) that initiate and regulate vital activities — breathing, swallowing, regulation of heart rate and caliber of smaller blood vessels, waking and sleeping, and other critical life functions. Moreover, certain medullary neurons have broad powers, exercised through chemical neurotransmitters and pervasive connections, over general levels of activity in the entire neuraxis. Thus, consciousness and alertness depend on the upward influences of the medulla, while the readiness and coordination of spinal reflexes for posture, locomotion, and visceral control rely on its downward activity.

The Spinal Cord

The lowermost part of the central nervous system is the spinal cord. Through its treelike roots, the many pairs of spinal nerves, bodily sensations enter the CNS. By means of its ascending tracts, sensory messages flow up to the overlying brain. Along certain high-speed descending tracts, commands from the brain, including the brainstem and cerebral cortex, flash down to spinal motor centers — to motor neurons (see Chaps. 9 and 10) or to local interneurons in their vicinity. These interneurons regulate the motor neurons, and also integrate their activity from one level to another and across the midline. Although such intrinsic spinal neurons are closely supervised by the brain, they accomplish the swift and complex spinal reflexes in an efficient manner on their own, sometimes playing out movement "programs" (such as walking or running) as if from a tape deck.

The Peripheral Nervous System

There must be a way to relate central nervous activity to the rest of the body. The PNS provides all the neural routes over which sensations can reach the brain and spinal cord and by which, in response, motor commands can affect the muscles and glands. As we shall see later, however, the vascular and endocrine systems provide other routes over which the CNS can exert its almost global effects on the body.

The PNS comprises the long, branched system of cranial and spinal nerves. The spinal nerves are remarkably similar, affording a segmental pattern of motor and sensory innervation for the entire body. This pattern of innervation is clarified by human embryology, specifically the formation of the somites, or body segments, and the outgrowth of the limb buds. In contrast, the cranial nerves are distinctive; no two pairs are exactly alike. Owing to the complex anatomy of the head and neck and the presence of the organs of special sense (eye, ear, and nose), these nerves show great variety and functional specialization. They must be considered individually (see Table 2-2).

The Lateral Aspect of the Brain

Looking more closely at the lateral aspect of the brain (Fig. 2-4), we see that the cerebrum is highly convoluted. Its rumpled surface is thrown up into many hills (or gyri) and criss-crossed by numerous valleys (or sulci). Here and there, deeper infoldings, canyons called fissures, provide major boundaries for the lobes of a cerebral hemisphere (see Chap. 13). The lateral fissure (of Sylvius) and central sulcus (fissure of Rolando) are the most prominent.

Such folding enormously increases the cerebral surface area and, thereby, the surface–volume ratio. Over two-thirds of this surface lies hidden in the many involutions, and those territories that can be seen are even larger than they appear to be, due to the arched profile of the con- volutions. What is the advantage of all this surface area? How do certain mammals — ungulates, carnivores, and especially man and fellow pri- mates, elephants, and cetaceans (whales, porpoises, and dolphins) — with so much of it differ from those with a smooth cerebrum — mice, rats, rabbits, and so many other vertebrates?

The answer to these questions is that all this surface provides room for a great amount of cerebral cortex. This recent, crowning gift has been be- stowed, in overt form at least, only upon mammals, and in abundance only on a select few. In reptiles and birds, the equivalent neuronal components seem to be there, but lie buried in the forebrain, in the basal ganglia. The cerebral cortex is the latest of what we believe were three great steps in the evolution of the nervous system. This process of refinement has taken place over eons of phylogenesis in innumerable kinds of animals. The first

Table 2-2. Names, Components, Constituent Neurons, and Functions of Cranial Nerves

Nerve	Name	Components	Location of cell bodies	Functions
I	Olfactory	SVA	Bipolar cells in nasal mucosa	Olfaction
II	Optic	SSA	Ganglion cells of retina	Vision
III	Oculomotor	GSE	Principal oculomotor nucleus	Vertical and inward ocular movements; elevation of lid
			Accessory oculomotor nucleus (nucleus of Edinger-Westphal)	Pupillary constriction and accommodation of lens
IV	Trochlear	GSE		
V	Trigeminal	SVE	Motor nucleus of nerve V	Chewing; tensing ear drum
		GSA	Trigeminal ganglion	Anterior cranial sensation (face, nose, mouth, dura)
			Mesencephalic nucleus of V (primary sensory neurons)	Stretch input from chewing muscles; pressure from teeth
VI	Abducens	GSE	Abducens nucleus	Outward eye movement
VII	Facial	SVE	Facial nucleus	Facial expression; tensing stapes
		GVE	Superior salivatory nucleus	Lacrimation and salivation
		GVA	Geniculate ganglion	Nasal and palatal sensation
		SVA	Geniculate ganglion	Taste (anterior two-thirds of tongue)
		GSA	Geniculate ganglion	Sensation from external ear
VIII	Vestibulocochlear	SSA	Vestibular and spiral ganglia	Sense of stability; hearing
IX	Glossopharyngeal	SVE	Nucleus ambiguus	Swallowing movements
		GVE	Inferior salivatory nucleus	Salivation
		GVA	Petrosal ganglion	Pharyngeal sensation
		SVA	Petrosal ganglion	Taste (posterior third of tongue)
		GSA	Superior ganglion	Sensation of skin behind ear
X	Vagus	SVE	Nucleus ambiguus	Swallowing and phonation
		GVE	Dorsal motor nucleus of X	Regulating visceral motility
		GVA	Nodosal ganglion	General visceral sensation
		SVA	Nodosal ganglion	Taste (epiglottis)
		GSA	Jugular ganglion	Sensation of skin behind ear
XI	Spinal accessory	SVE	Nucleus ambiguus	Laryngeal movements
		GSE	Spinal accessory nucleus	Head and shoulder movements
XII	Hypoglossal	GSE	Hypoglossal nucleus	Tongue movements

*GSA general somatic afferent; GSE general somatic efferent; GVA general visceral afferent; GVE general visceral efferent; SSA special somatic afferent; SVA special visceral afferent; SVE special visceral efferent.

Note: Input from stretch receptors in the extraocular and facial muscles may be mediated by cells in the trigeminal ganglion, and similar input from lingual muscles by inconstant ganglion cells along the hypoglossal rootlets.

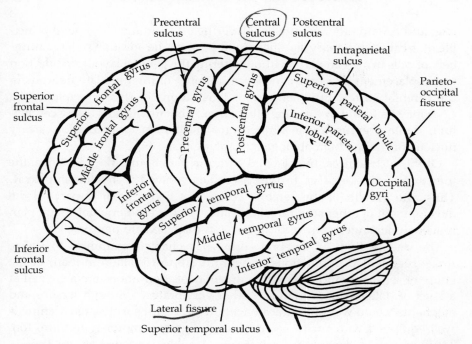

FIG. 2–4. *Cerebral landmarks.* Sulci and gyri on the lateral aspect of the left cerebral hemisphere. The landmarks illustrated here represent the most important infoldings or convolutions of the lateral cerebral surface. Of these, the central sulcus and lateral fissure are very important; they provide major boundaries for delineating the lobes of the cerebral hemisphere.

step was probably the origin of neurons, modified epithelial (surface) cells that could respond to changes in the environment. The second was likely the alignment of these neurons into three categories — sensory, motor, and intermediate, the last for analysis of stimuli and integration of responses. The coming of mammals, in which the incomparably connected cortex and its enormous number of intermediate neurons appeared, is thought to have been the third step. Although this last advance took place relatively recently, it was profound in its implications. Quiet and slow as all these advances may have been, they were true revolutions in the format of nervous systems. And evolution seems to be still at work where the design of the human brain is concerned. We will see examples of such adaptive remodeling when we consider the somesthetic pathways (Chap. 6) and limbic system (Chap. 12).

The biological process of folding a sheet of cells into hills and valleys of cortex unquestionably reaches its most extensive degree in the cerebrum of man and certain other mammals. Nevertheless, folding is a general principle of great evolutionary significance. It permits the addition of large numbers of cells in a given place without altering the general layout. In addition to the placement of a vastly increased number of intermediate neurons in the cerebral cortex, other important illustrations of this principle in the CNS may be found in the cerebellar cortex, dentate nucleus of the cerebellum, dentate gyrus of the hippocampal formation, and inferior olivary nucleus of the medulla oblongata, to name just a few.

Of these structures, the cerebral cortex is paramount in importance; the four areas mentioned as further examples evolved in relationship to it. Thus, the growth of the cerebral cortex has had a great impact on the development of other structures, even though the fundamental circuit plan remains unchanged: sensory, motor, and intermediate neurons.

The deeply fissured cerebral cortex has enabled mammals to utilize huge, regimented populations of neurons (10 to 15 billion in man) in the study of sensation and elaboration of behavior. Sensations are analyzed at a level of detail seldom found in other vertebrates, although whales and elephants, could we communicate with them, might surprise us. Mammals well-equipped with cortex seem to have a greater motor repertoire, too. They appear to draw more selectively, flexibly, and directly on the resources of different brain regions than do other vertebrates.

The Sagittal Aspect of the Brain

A comprehensive view of the brain can be obtained if we cut it down the middle into halves with a sharp knife (Fig. 2-5). The cerebral hemispheres are almost completely separate to begin with, but the underlying brain structures are largely continuous across the midline, and therefore must be sliced apart. Hence the midsagittal surface we see after bisecting the brain is mostly artificial; only that of the cerebral cortex facing the midline is present in the living brain. Nevertheless, this surface is instructive. We can see the entire neuraxis at once and all its parts in natural order from top to bottom; when Figs. 2-2 through 2-5 are compared, we see how these parts fall into the five major brain subdivisions. The view we get is one that almost everyone recognizes immediately as a picture of the human brain.

Gray Matter and White Matter

All parts of the CNS display two fundamental and contrasting substances: gray matter and white matter (Fig. 2-6). Nerve cell bodies and their im-

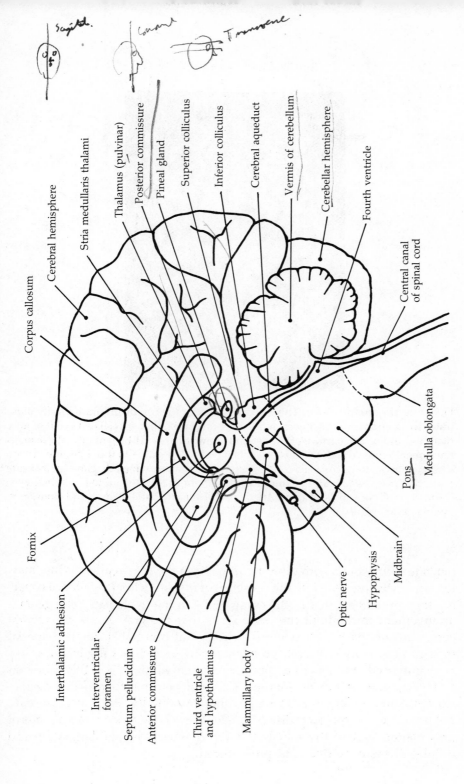

Sagittal.   Coronal.   Transverse.

Corpus callosum

Cerebral hemisphere

Stria medullaris thalami

Thalamus (pulvinar)

Posterior commissure

Pineal gland

Superior colliculus

Inferior colliculus

Cerebral aqueduct

Vermis of cerebellum

Cerebellar hemisphere

Fourth ventricle

Central canal
of spinal cord

Medulla oblongata

Pons

Midbrain

Hypophysis

Optic nerve

Mammillary body

Third ventricle
and hypothalamus

Anterior commissure

Septum pellucidum

Interventricular
foramen

Interthalamic adhesion

Fornix

FIG. 2–5. *The divided brain.* Human brain in the sagittal plane to illustrate major landmarks and relationships.

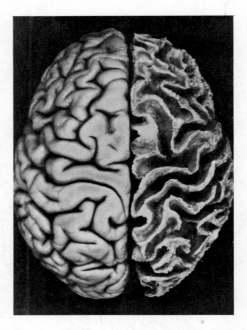

FIG. 2–6. *The cerebral cortex*. This superior view of the cerebrum dramatically illustrates the amount and thickness of the cerebral cortex, that special extra coat of gray matter found on the surface of the cerebral hemispheres. The meninges of the brain have been removed, but the cortex is intact on the left side. On the right, it has been dissected away to uncover the underlying white matter, which displays an intricate pattern of ridges and leaflets extending up into the core of the various cerebral gyri. (From E. Ludwig and J. Klingler, *Atlas Cerebri Humani*. Little, Brown and Company, Boston, 1959, plate 1)

mediate connections with other neurons form the gray matter. White matter can be distinguished by the presence of myelin, a lipid substance covering the nerve fibers that is glistening white in the fresh state. The general arrangement throughout the neuraxis is that the gray forms the central core, surrounded by the white (Fig. 2-7). But cerebral cortex is a special type of gray matter. Its cell populations are astronomically large, as we have indicated, and its cell bodies are regimented: they lie neatly arranged in layers, one on top of another. Cerebral neurons themselves display extraordinary variety in size, shape, and connectivity. Such attributes are not unique to the cerebral cortex. Indeed, they characterize other regions of gray matter, such as the spinal gray. But nowhere else are lamination and cellular diversity so clear and pronounced.

The border between gray and white matter is especially clear in the cerebellum (see Frontispiece), as seen in sagittal section; it follows a distinctive curvilinear pattern with the neatness of a draftsman's ruling pen. This gray matter is the cerebellar cortex, an extra coating of neurons that, as in the cerebrum, has developed outside the white. In such superficial sheets of gray matter, neurons and their connections may be more easily arranged in orderly layers to discharge different functions than would be possible amidst the welter of fibers that wind their separate and devious ways through the brainstem.

The Corpus Callosum

Perhaps the most prominent structure in the midsagittal aspect of the human brain is the corpus callosum, a large, curved structure in the center of the cerebral hemisphere resembling an overturned canoe. Its name means "hard-body," a designation that arose because this bridge of millions of nerve fibers between the two hemispheres offered resistance to the probing fingers of ancient anatomists. Through the corpus callosum, axons transfer information from the cortex of one hemisphere to that of the other. These communications are important, because, as stated earlier, each cerebral hemisphere is very specialized in its functional role.

The Limbic Lobe

A wide belt of cortex girdles the corpus callosum; it forms the limbic lobe. "Limbic" means "border," in this case the borderland of the cortex and the brainstem. The limbic lobe, comprising the cingulate and parahippocampal gyri, provides much of the brain's emotional machinery. It is important for stable, purposeful behavior. Beneath the callosum, the wall of the hemisphere is so thin that the cerebral cortex and underlying white matter cannot be distinguished. Instead, an almost translucent partition, the septum pellucidum, covers a large cavity, the lateral ventricle, that is visible in Fig. 2-7. (Recall from Fig. 2-2 that the brain is hollow, developing embryonically from a simple tube.) Anteriorly, this partition thickens to form the septal area: its cell clusters negotiate transactions between the limbic lobe and brainstem important to behavior, visceral functions, and neuroendocrine activities.

A massive cable, the fornix, curves downward under the corpus callosum and plunges into the hypothalamus, conveying messages in both directions. It is a major link between the forebrain and midbrain.

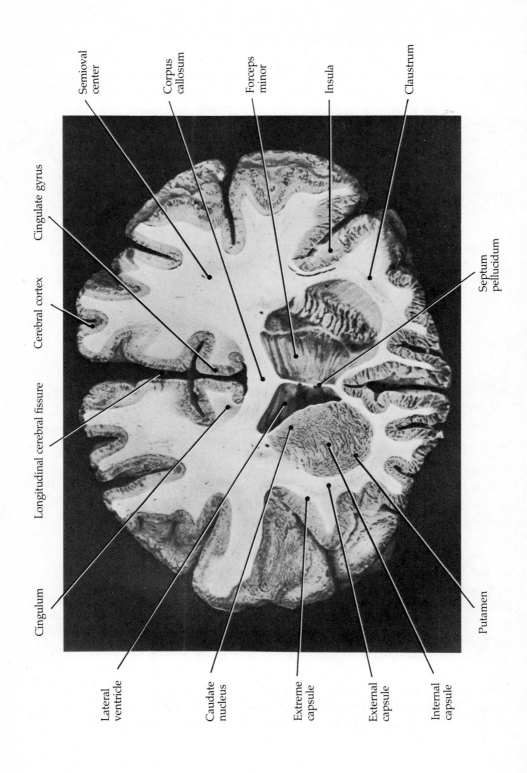

Semioval center

Corpus callosum

Forceps minor

Insula

Claustrum

Cingulate gyrus

Cerebral cortex

Septum pellucidum

Longitudinal cerebral fissure

Cingulum

Lateral ventricle

Caudate nucleus

Extreme capsule

External capsule

Internal capsule

Putamen

The Visual Cortex

In the occipital lobe, the calcarine (spurlike) sulcus branches, like a fork in a canyon, from the deep parieto-occipital fissure and runs toward the occipital pole. On the banks of this deep cleft, the visual world is analyzed. The lower and upper halves of the visual field shared by both eyes (Chap. 5) are mapped out along the upper and lower margins of this sulcus, respectively.

The Thalamus and Hypothalamus

At the center of each half of the forebrain lies the thalamus, derived from the diencephalon or "'tweenbrain." It is a large ovoid mass of gray matter with the larger end facing posteriorly. The two thalami are usually in contact with one another by way of a small adhesion across the midline.* The name thalamus means "inner chamber"; long ago it was thought to be a cavity supplying "animal spirits" to the optic nerve. In reality, the two thalami form the greatly thickened walls of a cavity, the third ventricle, filled with cerebrospinal fluid (see below and also Chap. 15). But the intimate association with the optic nerve is a good hint of one of the chief functions of the thalamus. It is the great sensory portal to the cerebral cortex. Sensations are scrutinized here, before passing to the cortex for further study.

*While the term "thalamus" is usually used to designate one of the two thalami, it is sometimes employed in a more general way — to refer to both thalami collectively in a functional context. The same thing may be said for the hypothalamus.

FIG. 2–7. *Coronal section of the human frontal lobes.* The central cavities (lateral ventricles) of the cerebrum (partially divided by the longitudinal cerebral fissure) are surrounded by concentric zones of inner gray matter, outer white matter, and superficial gray matter (cerebral cortex). The inner gray is represented by the putamen and caudate nucleus (scooped out by dissection on the right). The white matter is a mass of myelinated axons (semioval center). It includes association fibers (cingulum; external and extreme capsules) interconnecting the various gyri of each hemisphere. Commissural fibers (corpus callosum; laterally coursing fibers visible as forceps minor) interconnect various regions of the two hemispheres. Projection fibers (internal capsule) interconnect the cortex with subcortical structures. The cerebral cortex covers the crown of each gyrus (such as the cingulate) and dips down into each sulcus, forming an extensive, uninterrupted curving band, the cortical ribbon, on the surface of the brain. (From E. Ludwig and J. Klinger, *Atlas Cerebri Humani.* Little, Brown and Company, Boston, 1959, plate 62)

Beneath the thalamus is the hypothalamus, a tiny region weighing only four grams of the brain's 1400 g total. It encloses numerous small cell clusters that regulate many vital functions — visceral, neuroendocrine, and metabolic activities; temperature regulation; the sleep-wakefulness cycle; and the outward (emotional) expression of internal states.

The Midbrain

A slender cylinder, the midbrain or mesencephalon, extends between the thalamic region and the pons. The midbrain is about the size of a broomstick in diameter, and its plan of organization is little changed from its original tubular condition in the developing brain. It is in essence a pipe connecting the hindbrain (pons and medulla oblongata) with the forebrain. But it has as obvious significance as our neck does to our head! Numerous tracts pass up and down the midbrain, some of them coming from the spinal cord, others from the cerebral cortex. Even a minute injury here, such as a pinpoint hemorrhage (Chap. 15), can have serious results. Major trauma will almost certainly lead to coma, if not to death.

In the roof of the midbrain tectum lie two pairs of small but important mounds of gray matter, the superior and inferior colliculi. One of each pair is seen in sagittal section (see Fig. 2-5), and internally they show a cortical plan of organization. The superior and inferior colliculi analyze visual and auditory signals, respectively, and are essential for certain reflex responses to sights and sounds. Furthermore, they play major roles in elaborating visual and auditory responses. Beneath them, in the floor of the midbrain (in what is called the tegmentum), are motor neurons that mediate eye movements and constrict the size of the pupils. Here also lies the most rostral part of the brainstem reticular formation, an interwoven arrangement of gray and white matter that forms a long, continuous cylindrical core to the midbrain, pons, and medulla. It exerts extremely important facilitating and inhibitory effects on sensory and motor neuron activity (see Chap. 11). Within the reticular formation, two large masses of neurons are found: a rounded, highly vascularized aggregate, the red nucleus, and an underlying pigmented region, the substantia nigra. Both are important in motor control. At the base of the midbrain, the paired crura cerebri (or pedes pedunculi) provide routes for fascicles of cortical fibers down to the pons, medulla, and spinal cord; only one crus cerebri (or pes pedunculi) would appear in the sagittally cut brain.

The Cavities of the Brain

The brain retains the hollow character it had as part of the embryonic neural tube (Fig. 2-2). Each embryonic subdivision has its own chamber, filled with watery fluid. Thus, the two paired telencephalic vesicles each have a large cavity that ultimately becomes the lateral ventricle of a cerebral hemisphere (Fig. 2-8). Superior, posterior, and inferior horns of each lateral ventricle depart in their respective directions from a common antrum and lead into the frontal, occipital, and temporal lobes of the hemisphere, respectively. Within each ventricle is the choroid plexus, a long, highly convoluted stringy structure, resembling a mass of grapes on a vine. It secretes the cerebrospinal fluid (CSF).

The single, median cavity of the embryonic diencephalon becomes the adult third ventricle. A small, tubular channel, the interventricular foramen (of Monro) runs ventromedially from the superior horn of each lateral ventricle down into this narrow, slitlike chamber between the two bulging halves of the thalamus. The choroid plexuses of the two lateral ventricles pass through this aperture and continue posteriorly as the paired choroid plexuses of the third ventricle, coming to an end just rostral to the midbrain.

A narrow channel, the cerebral aqueduct (of Sylvius), is all that remains of the tubular cavity of the embryonic mesencephalon in the adult. It has no choroid plexus, and hence serves only as a conduit that drains the cerebrospinal fluid in the third ventricle down to lower regions. If obstructed or overly narrowed (stenosed), as is sometimes the case in the newborn infant, the entire ventricular system above this point will be congested with CSF, producing the most common form of congenital hydrocephalus ("water on the brain"). Such a serious condition can often be effectively alleviated by neurosurgical placement of a shunt tube leading to the subarachnoid space surrounding the brain, thus bypassing the choked aqueduct.

The cavities of the embryonic metencephalon and myelencephalon are not sharply demarcated, sharing instead the diamondlike shape of the rhomboid fossa of the original hindbrain. This single, large cavity becomes the fourth ventricle of the pons and medulla oblongata. Its floor contains various motor and sensory nuclei of cranial nerves, embedded in the underlying tegmental core of the brainstem.

The roof of the fourth ventricle is formed by the cerebellum and, more posteriorly, by a transparent windowlike region or "skylight" called a tela

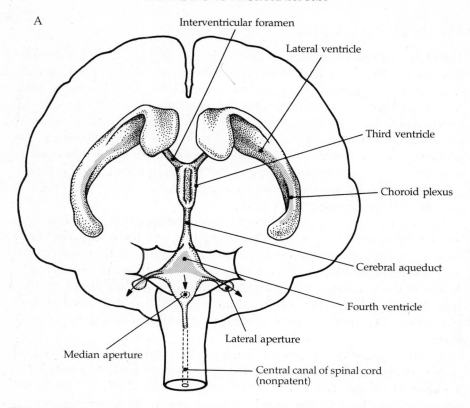

FIG. 2–8. *The brain ventricles.* (A) Frontal view in which the brain has been rendered as if transparent. The two telencephalic lateral ventricles, one in each cerebral hemisphere, communicate with the diencephalic third ventricle through the interventricular foramina (of Monro). The narrow cerebral aqueduct leads down to the rhombencephalic fourth ventricle, surmounted by the cerebellum and underlain by the pons and medulla oblongata. Three tiny apertures, a median foramen (of Magendie) and two lateral foramina (of Luschka), permit the escape of cerebrospinal fluid (CSF) into the subarachnoid space and its various cisterns.

choroidea. In this region, the brain wall is extremely thin, and hence the vascular pia mater investing the brain lies immediately outside the ependymal cells that line the ventricular cavity. A choroid plexus is formed at such locations by the invagination of the pia by the adjoining pial blood vessels (see Fig. 2-8). In the case of the fourth ventricle, the tela choroidea and its pendant choroid plexus are easy to see. A similar but less obvious arrangement is found in the roof of the third ventricle and along almost the entire curvature of the superior and inferior horns of the lateral ventricle. In all of these places, the brain wall is exceptionally thin and susceptible to

B

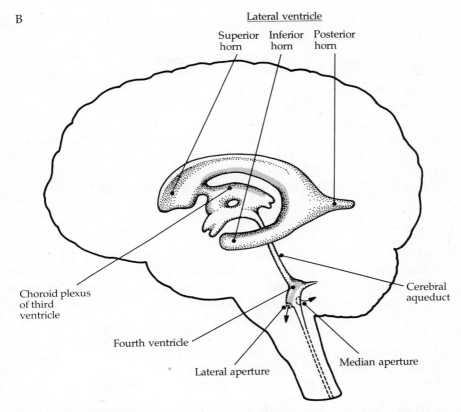

(B)The choroid plexuses (locations shaded) of the lateral, third, and fourth ventricles produce the CSF. The fluid flows out of the foramina of the fourth ventricle into
the subarachnoid space: between the innermost membrane of the brain (pia mater)
and the surrounding arachnoid (spidery) membrane.

trauma, essentially a pial-ependymal membrane where pial vessels invagi-
nate to form a choroid plexus.

At the peak of the tentlike fourth ventricle is a tiny median aperture
(foramen of Magendie) and at the two lateral corners of the ventricle are
two lateral apertures (foramina of Luschka). Through these three small
openings, the accumulated CSF produced by all three sets of choroid
plexuses (in the lateral, third, and fourth ventricles) escapes into the subarachnoid space that surrounds and protects the brain and spinal cord
(Chap. 15). Once inside this space, the fluid protects and buoys up the
CNS and is eventually resorbed into the bloodstream through arachnoidal
granulations that empty into the venous sinuses of the outermost brain

membrane, the dura mater, as well as through similar structures along the dorsal roots of spinal nerves. CSF pooled in the lumbar cistern, an enlarged region or reservoir at the caudal and of the subarachnoid space, may be withdrawn by lumbar puncture, a valuable investigative technique in neurologic diagnosis. Less frequently (because of the obvious danger to the underlying medulla oblongata), the cerebellomedullary cistern (cisterna magna) may be tapped for this purpose.

A common form of acquired hydrocephalus may occur if the three tiny orifices of the fourth ventricle are occluded. Such a problem may result from inflammation of the meninges (meningitis) and subsequent formation of adhesions that block the outlets for CSF from the ventricular system.

The Dissected Brain

A lateral view of a dissected brain (Fig. 2-9) reveals a surprisingly ordered and beautiful internal topography: gracefully sculptured masses of gray matter, curling ribbons of white. The cerebral cortex is sharply defined; it crowns each gyrus and forms the banks of the fissures and sulci. In the underlying white matter, myriad nerve fibers follow obviously prescribed routes from place to place — from gyrus to gyrus, from lobe to lobe, from one hemisphere to another, and from cerebral cortex to underlying brainstem structures.

The Basal Ganglia

A conspicuous deep mass of gray matter is the caudate nucleus. It is so named because its tapering bulk curls around into the temporal lobe, like the tail of a minnow. Its shape conforms to the curvature of the lateral ventricle (see above) in which it lies. Lateral to the caudate nucleus lies an even larger mass of gray matter, the putamen (a "shell" which covers deeper structures).

FIG. 2–9. *Long-distance circuits of the brain.* Photograph of the lateral aspect of a dissected left side of the brain to show the course of some long fiber tracts. Two major functional axes are prominent: the visual axis sweeps horizontally from optic nerve to the occipital pole (via optic radiation), while the corticospinal axis (pyramidal tract) plunges vertically from the cerebral cortex to reach, through an "in-parallel" arrangement of fibers, almost every important subcortical structure, including the spinal cord. (From E. Ludwig and J. Klinger, *Atlas Cerebri Humani.* Little, Brown and Company, Boston, 1959, plate 23)

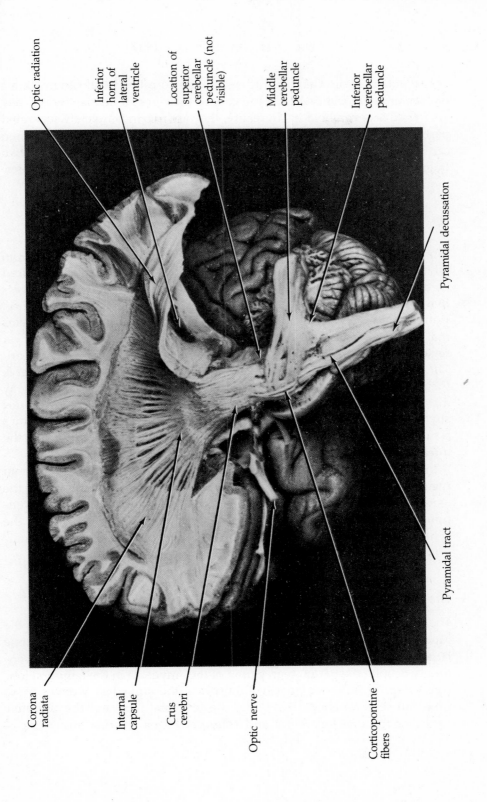

Optic radiation

Inferior horn of lateral ventricle

Location of superior cerebellar peduncle (not visible)

Middle cerebellar peduncle

Inferior cerebellar peduncle

Pyramidal decussation

Corona radiata

Internal capsule

Crus cerebri

Optic nerve

Corticopontine fibers

Pyramidal tract

The putamen and caudate nucleus are the so-called basal ganglia, huge masses of nerve cell bodies in the core of the cerebral hemispheres. They are joined at several places. In reality, they are two incompletely separated parts of a larger mass of deep gray matter. Together, the caudate/putamen can be thought of as a giant boulder partially split by weathering into two fragments, which are of unequal size and dissimilar shape. The outer, more bulky part is the putamen, the inner curved piece the caudate.

The Internal Capsule

The cleft between the putamen and caudate, the "crack in the rock" from which so many radiating fibers seem to sprout, has indeed been produced by a kind of a weathering — a slow but inexorable evolutionary process that probably started soon after the cerebral cortex made its appearance. With the passage of time and continued elaboration of the cortex, it seems that an ever-increasing number of fibers running from the cortex to lower regions of the CNS began to "split" the obstacle of the basal ganglia apart. The head and extreme tip of the tail of the caudate still strongly preserve their unity with the putamen, but elsewhere only jagged strands of gray matter remain between the two. The fibers that enter or leave the cortex stream up and down between these narrow bridges, and these fibers form a compact zone of white matter around the underlying thalamus called the internal capsule.

In its direct fiber connections (see Chaps. 9 and 10) with other brain regions and with the spinal cord, the cerebral cortex thus interrupts the anatomical continuity of the basal ganglia. Nevertheless, the cortex continues to work closely with the deeper gray on matters relating to the synthesis, execution, and monitoring of movements. The cortex also interacts with the cerebellum in these matters.

The Amygdala

The amygdala ("almond") is another basal ganglion, closely related to the caudate and putamen. In many vertebrates, the three structures form one large complex. Indeed, in the human brain, they maintain obvious continuity despite the partial segregation of the amygdala in the temporal lobe (see Chap. 9). Like its larger counterparts, the amygdala receives input from the cerebral cortex (including the temporal lobe and the primitive cortex of the olfactory bulb) and connects to many other structures —

especially the hypothalamus. As to the functions of the amygdala, we are less certain. Its activity seems closely related to internal needs of the body — visceral demands — and to their outward expression or gratification in movement and posture.

Association, Commissural, and Projection Fibers

Beneath the cerebral cortex, short association fibers loop from one gyrus to another. Longer association fibers sweep through the white matter like huge cables; the major ones are identified in Fig. 2-10. Some axons, commissural fibers, enter the corpus callosum to link part of both hemispheres instead of different regions of one hemisphere. Others, projection fibers, leave the hemisphere and travel to other CNS structures; many go all the way down to the spinal cord (Fig. 2-9).

Behind the putamen, a broad fan of fibers unfolds, first curling forward into the temporal lobe and then looping back again, as if with a flourish, to sweep broadly and gracefully to the occipital pole. This is the visual radiation; it carries messages that have reached the thalamus from the retina via the optic nerve and tract to the site of ultimate analysis, the visual cortex.

The Cerebellar Peduncles

The fiber interconnections of the cerebrum and cerebellum mentioned earlier are obvious in the dissection shown in Fig. 2-9; here we can see how reciprocal these affiliations are. Descending axons from the cerebral cortex end within the pons as corticopontine fibers. There they meet pontocerebellar fibers which run across the midline and extend laterally into the cerebellum as the middle cerebellar peduncle. It is also called the brachium pontis or "arm of the pons." In this manner, fibers from virtually every cortical region of a cerebral hemisphere pass messages to pontine fibers, which in turn convey them to the cortex of the opposite cerebellar hemisphere.

In the acute angle behind the middle peduncle, the inferior cerebellar peduncle may be seen, curving up and backward from the medulla. Because it looks like a slack rope, it is often called the restiform or "ropelike" body. It brings additional input from the cerebral cortex, which in this case arrives via the contralateral inferior olivary nucleus. It also brings in messages from the spinal cord: reports of stretches and tensions on muscles and tendons, respectively. Such information is essential if the cerebellar

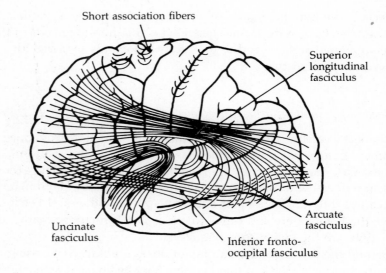

Short association fibers

Superior
longitudinal
fasciculus

Uncinate
fasciculus

Arcuate
fasciculus

Inferior fronto-
occipital fasciculus

A

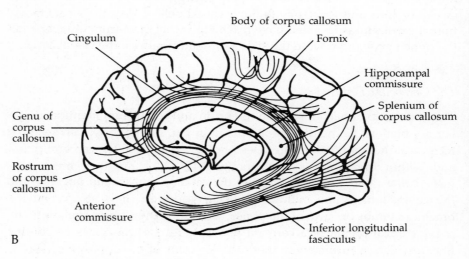

Body of corpus callosum

Cingulum

Fornix

Hippocampal
commissure

Genu of
corpus
callosum

Splenium of
corpus callosum

Rostrum
of corpus
callosum

Anterior
commissure

Inferior longitudinal
fasciculus

B

FIG. 2–10. *Integrating fiber systems of the cerebral hemispheres.* (A) Association fibers shown schematically against the lateral aspect of the left cerebral hemisphere. The many interconnecting routes in the white matter of the hemisphere range from extremely thick, long, and heterogeneous systems (e.g., the superior longitudinal fasciculus, which runs from pole to pole) to slender, short, and limited connections (the short association fibers looping from one gyrus to the next). The origins and terminations of the larger bundles have been charted in only the most rudimentary way for the human brain; they appear to be organized in an extremely precise manner.

computer is to refine posture and movement. Both aspects of motor control are demanding and unremitting tasks, even though standing still seems easier than moving about.

Thus the cerebellum "listens" to the cerebral cortex above and the spinal cord below. Its "answers" — how to employ muscles at any moment — are dispatched through the superior cerebellar peduncle, or brachium conjunctivum. This "crossed arm" runs to the thalamus, from which messages ultimately pass back to the same cerebral hemisphere in which this long-range conversation began in the first place. This time, however, the signals are focused on a very important strip of cortical gray just anterior to the central sulcus: the motor cortex.

The Cranial Nerves

The Distinctive Nature of the Olfactory and Optic Nerves

Two of the twelve cranial nerves have had strong evolutionary effects on the design and role of the forebrain. One is the olfactory nerve (Cranial Nerve I or CN I) that conveys the primordial sense of smell. When the brain is removed from the skull, the tiny, short filaments that comprise the "nerve" break or tear off in the ethmoid bone, which the fibers penetrate in their inward course from the nose. The broken stumps of these filaments, a fine stubble on the olfactory bulb, are all that remains of the olfactory nerve in the usual postmortem brain specimen. What is often mistaken for the nerve is the olfactory tract, which conveys olfactory sensations to other central analyzer regions.

The optic nerve (CN II) is a thick cable of over a million nerve fibers leading in from the retina, which is itself part of the brain. As an important initial step in integrating visual information, half of its fibers cross the midline at the optic chiasm, thus passing messages from one eye to both sides of the brain. Like the olfactory tract, it is really not a nerve. The optic fibers which might (at least conceptually) correspond to those of a

---

(B) Association and commissural fibers shown against the medial aspect of the right cerebral hemisphere. As in (A), both long and short association systems are visible. One of the long routes, the cingulum, offers major circuits for the limbic system. The commissural fibers are like association fibers, but cross the midline. They travel in the anterior commissure, corpus callosum, and a posterior region of the fornix (the hippocampal commissure).

peripheral nerve elsewhere in the nervous system are tiny, extremely short, and inwardly directed processes of unusual neurons (bipolar cells) that lie entirely within the retina. The retinal bipolar cells cannot generate nerve impulses (action potentials) of their own, and hence the fibers in the optic "nerve" are those of large retinal projection neurons (retinal ganglion cells).

Instead of having true cranial nerves to bring in sensory nerve impulses, the olfactory and optic components of the brain are themselves located near the surface of the body, monitoring the activities of special olfactory epithelial cells within the nasal cavity or of photosensitive elements in the retina, respectively. Thus, in gathering smells and sights, our brain, imprisoned in the bony cavity of the skull, comes as close to the outside world as it ever gets.

The Remaining Cranial Nerves and Their Functional Components

The other ten cranial nerves, as we have mentioned earlier, are quite distinctive; no two pairs are alike. In overview, we can group them in certain broad categories, leaving details to Table 2-2 and other textbooks. Let us look first at those nerves in which we find motor fibers, and then take another look at where sensory axons travel to the brain.

Three cranial nerves, the oculomotor (III), trochlear (IV), and abducens (VI), are purely motor. They act mainly to turn the eyeball in different directions — to provide for searching movements and smooth pursuit of visualized objects. A similar nerve is the hypoglossal (XII), which mediates movements of the tongue. Still another, the spinal accessory (XI), brings about turning of the head to the opposite side, and assists in elevating the shoulders. Except for visceral motor fibers in CN III (see below), all five of these nerves are classified as "somatic efferent," i.e., they convey motor impulses to somatic (somite-derived) skeletal muscle. Their neurons of origin are thus the brain's equivalents of spinal somatic motor neurons. Instead of forming a continuous column of nerve cells, however, as at spinal levels, cranial somatic motor cell bodies are collected in various separate clusters or nuclei (see Table 2-2).

Four cranial nerves, the trigeminal (V), facial (VII), glossopharyngeal (IX), and vagus (X), also innervate skeletal muscle, in this case those muscles involved in chewing, facial expression, swallowing, and phonation, among other actions. These motor fibers are categorized as "branchial efferent," because the target muscles derive embryologically from branchial arch mesoderm, not from the somites as above. We would like to call these nerve fibers "special somatic efferent" (which is what they are), but they are conventionally termed "special visceral efferent," because they travel, at least in part, to visceral structures — the pharynx and larynx. These four cranial nerves are more complex than the others; they are mixed, containing sensory as well as motor fibers (see Table 2-2).

Visceral motor fibers pass outward as a distinct subset of fibers, a functional component, in four cranial nerves, all of which are mentioned above in other contexts: the oculomotor, facial, glossopharyngeal, and vagus. These so-called "general visceral efferent" fiber components mediate constriction of the pupil, lacrimation, salivation, and a wide range of important effects on the thoracic and abdominal viscera, including inhibitory influences on the heart. Collectively, this group comprises the cranial outflow of the parasympathetic division of the autonomic nervous system (see below).

Summing up this overview so far, we see that there are three groups of cranial nerves according to motor components: somatic, branchial, and visceral. On the sensory side, we find four groupings because the two obvious categories, visceral and somatic, are each broken down into "general" and "special" subdivisions. Except for CN VIII, all the nerves in these four groups were mentioned above.

"General visceral" afferents are those emanating from the mucous membranes and deeper structures of the oral cavity, pharynx, larynx, and other structures in the thorax and abdomen. "Special visceral" afferents convey gustatory information from taste buds on the tongue and epiglottis. By this time, the reader may be growing weary of such classification; fortunately, all these visceral sensory fibers (general and special) enter the medulla oblongata through only three nerves, the facial, glossopharyngeal, and vagus, and distribute to only slightly different regions of one sensory nucleus in the medulla: the nucleus of the solitary tract.

The Autonomic Nervous System

Integrating the work of the vital organs — the heart, lungs, and blood vessels; the digestive and urogenital systems; and all their associated glands — and bringing all this internal commotion into line with outward body activities are tasks of almost unimaginable complexity. As might be expected, the autonomic nervous system (ANS) which innervates the vital organs and regulates their function, is like a spiderweb in the detail of its many connections. In overview, however, it has a startlingly simple plan.

The Tandem Design of the ANS: Two Motor Neurons in Series

As conventionally defined, the ANS is a purely motor system, a seemingly autonomous organization of miniature motor neurons in the brainstem and spinal cord that, through a maze of extremely fine fibers, controls numerous structures — from the pupils of the eyes to the urinary and anal sphincters. A curious feature is that the many motor fibers of the centrally located effector cells of the ANS do not run directly to smooth or cardiac muscle, as those of motor neurons do to striated skeletal muscle. Instead, they travel indirectly — they pass to another group of small motor neurons outside the CNS en route to their myriad targets (see Fig. 2-11). These subordinate motor cells are found in autonomic ganglia that lie either close to the neuraxis or far away in the wall of the particular target organ. They are functionally characterized as "postganglionic" autonomic neurons, while the neurons in the CNS are "preganglionic."

Unlike the bipolar or pseudounipolar cells in sensory ganglia that pass news along without integrating messages, autonomic ganglion cells are multipolar, and receive several inputs. These characteristics suggest that they act as final integrators of centrally driven activity, which they then distribute over delicate plexuses of interlacing axonal threads throughout the substance and walls of solid and hollow organs. Although almost never studied in neuroanatomy courses in detail, these peripheral autonomic innervations have been beautifully delineated in specialized monographs. Views of the intricate and sometime strange appearance of the ANS are not unlike glimpses of life in the ocean's depths. And like the ocean's depths, this network deep within the body's organs is not without a bit of mystery.

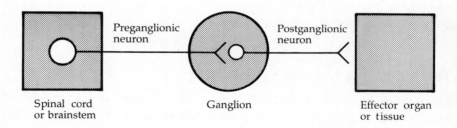

FIG. 2–11. *The visceral nervous system.* Fundamental plan of the autonomic nervous system. Small "preganglionic" motor neurons located in the spinal cord or brainstem innervate effector cells located in autonomic ganglia; these "postganglionic" neurons in turn act on target organs or tissues.

Visceral Sensations and the Limbic System

Sensations from the viscera are frequently (but not always) unpleasant, and sometimes compelling. They may demand response. Such sensations eventually reach the limbic system and hypothalamus, which then draw up appropriate and appropriately scheduled plans of action that are ultimately mediated through both neural and endocrine agencies and over a broad time scale — from instant protective reflexes to long-term hormonal adjustments, perhaps even to lifelong patterns of activity (see Chap. 12).

The Sympathetic and Parasympathetic Divisions of the ANS

Neural influences are delivered to target tissues in the viscera by one of the two main subsystems of the ANS — the sympathetic and parasympathetic divisions, anatomically referred to as the thoracolumbar and craniosacral divisions, respectively (Figs. 2-12 and 2-13). The postganglionic cell bodies of the sympathetic division lie in a continuous chain along the spinal cord, whereas those of the parasympathetic division lie chiefly in intramural ganglia, i.e., in or near the walls of the target organs.

Keeping a Common-Sense Perspective on the ANS

At one time, this visceral department of the nervous system, the one that looks after the internal activities or "house-keeping chores" of the body, was thought to have largely its own way, unsupervised by the corporate brain. Hence the origin of the term "autonomic nervous system." Even today, this curious term is used to encompass all the small visceral motor neurons in the nervous system, either in the CNS or in peripheral ganglia, that play upon the slowly contracting, smooth muscles that massage organ and vessel walls, or upon that tireless pump, the heart, most important of all muscles.

There is, to be sure, some measure of autonomy in the ANS. Its ganglion cells with their skimpy looking dendritic trees seem to require few central instructions, and whatever these cells do, much of the smooth muscle (and all of the cardiac) keeps on contracting, regulatory impulses or not. But the concept of a truly autonomic or independent part of the nervous system goes against a principle set forth in the Introduction. There we said that the nervous system pervades the body, and that it has unity. The ANS certainly does pervade the body, as Figs. 2-12, 2-13 and 2-14 show. But its classical definition as a more or less separate and autonomous visceral

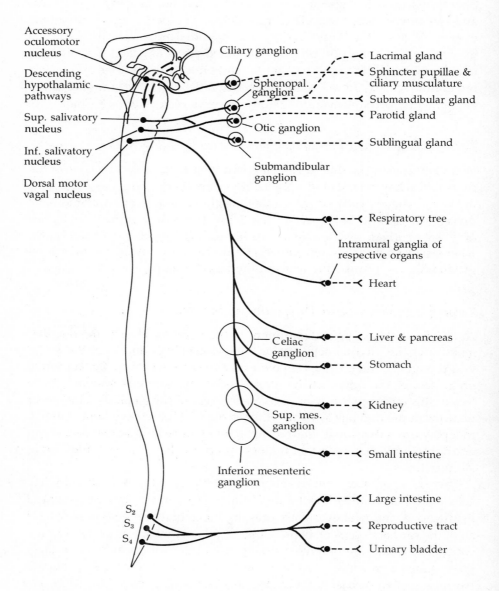

FIG. 2–12. *The parasympathetic division of the ANS.* Diagrammatic representation. (Modified from F. H. Netter, *The Ciba Collection of Medical Illustrations.* Volume I, Nervous System. Ciba Pharmaceutical Products, Summit, N.J., 1953)

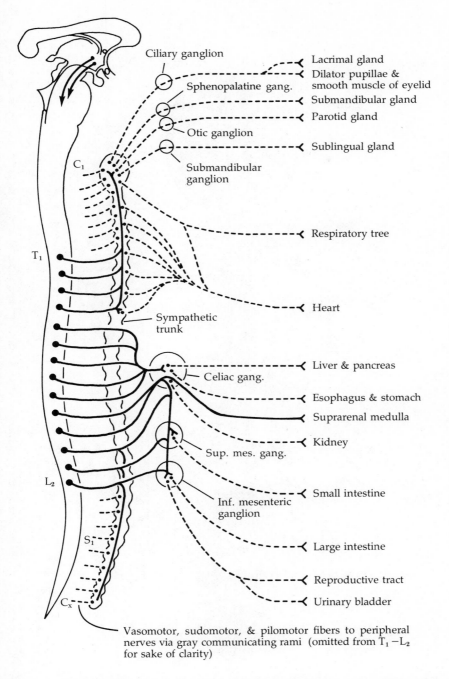

Ciliary ganglion

Sphenopalatine gang.

Otic ganglion

Submandibular
ganglion

C₁

T₁

Sympathetic
trunk

Celiac gang.

Sup. mes. gang.

L₂

Inf. mesenteric
ganglion

S₁

Cₓ

Lacrimal gland
Dilator pupillae &
smooth muscle of eyelid
Submandibular gland
Parotid gland
Sublingual gland

Respiratory tree

Heart

Liver & pancreas

Esophagus & stomach
Suprarenal medulla
Kidney

Small intestine

Large intestine

Reproductive tract
Urinary bladder

Vasomotor, sudomotor, & pilomotor fibers to peripheral
nerves via gray communicating rami (omitted from T₁–L₂
for sake of clarity)

FIG. 2–13. *The sympathetic division of the ANS.* Diagrammatic representation. (Modified from F. H. Netter, *The Ciba Collection of Medical Illustrations.* Volume I, Nervous System. Ciba Pharmaceutical Products, Summit, New Jersey, 1953)

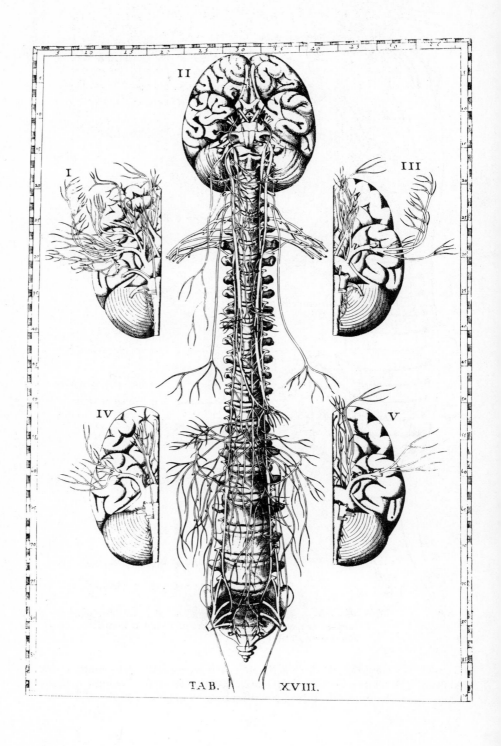

II

I   III

IV   V

TAB.   XVIII.

motor system runs counter to the unity of the nervous system. The reality is quite the reverse; the ANS, like the CNS, exhibits learned responses and, surprisingly, can be classically conditioned, as recent experiments with biofeedback show. We, then, can resolve the contradictions of general organizing principles posed by the ANS very simply — just by remembering that the term "autonomic nervous system" is a misnomer.

We know from everyday experience that visceral activities are regulated in a harmonious manner. Moreover, visceral and somatic functions are usually (not always) brought together in comprehensive strategies of response, and such viscerosomatic teamwork is accomplished by many structures of the CNS — the spinal cord, the brainstem reticular formation, and especially the limbic system and hypothalamus. The performances of many respiratory and digestive activities provide eloquent, familiar examples of total body function. Moreover, visceral sensations intrude deeply at times upon our thoughts and feelings. And, once activated or conditioned, the ANS can play a critical role in determining human decisionmaking and responses. Not surprisingly, psychologists, psychiatrists, and criminologists accord it high importance in their studies of normal, abnormal, and criminal behavior.

The way to get around the misleading concept of self-rule that sticks to the term "autonomic nervous system" is to use it for purely descriptive purposes: to designate all the visceral motor pathways (each having two motor neurons in tandem) that leave the CNS from upper midbrain to sacral cord. But we must remember that visceral organs have sensory fibers as well as motor ones, and that their activities are integrated and regulated by the CNS. Although visceral sensory pathways are extremely

---

FIG. 2–14. *The intricacy of visceral innervation.* Engraving prepared in 1552 by Bartholomaeus Eustachius, an Italian anatomist and physician (Eustachian tube), showing the base of the brain and the sympathetic nervous system as he understood it from his dissections. Today we know much more of its structure and function, but this excellent anatomist captured its essential features and labyrinthine complexity in an unforgettable manner. It should be noted, however, that the sympathetic chain is incorrectly shown arising from the base of the brain, and there are a number of other errors (including curious, intestinelike cerebral gyri).

The scales along three sides of the plate were supposed to bring out relationships between nature and mathematics and between life and geometry that were believed important in the 16th century. Furthermore, this ingenious system facilitated reference to specific structures, as do the marginal scales on a road map, obviating labels on the figure itself. (From Eustachius, B., *Tabulae Anatomicae*, ed. by Lancisi. F. Gonzagae, Rome, 1714; reprinted 1968 by Editrice Parnago, Modena, Italy)

difficult to follow with contemporary neuroanatomical methods, many visceral sensory fibers are well known (in the vagus nerve, for example). And there are clear-cut visceral sensory nuclei in the spinal cord and brainstem (such as the nucleus of the tractus solitarius) where the body's internal messages are received by the CNS.

General Concepts

We have seen that the nervous system has three distinct yet interconnected divisions (PNS, CNS, and ANS), and that each division has many specialized and interconnected parts: nerves and ganglia, tracts and nuclei, cortical formations and basal ganglia, ganglionic chains, and visceral plexuses. Despite the complexities and peculiarities of regional functions, harmonious interdependence usually takes precedence over local neuronal activity. Local needs and demands are usually met in the context of the total needs of the body, not only for the moment but over long periods, extending to a lifetime.

As we have begun to show, each part of the nervous system is made up of cellular units — neurons and neuroglial cells — and their fibrous processes — axons, dendrites, and neuroglial processes (collectively termed the neuropil). These elements of the nervous system generate, transfer, and integrate neural activity. They themselves are highly individualized and specifically designed for their functions. In order to fully appreciate the design and basic plan of the nervous system, we must approach the system more closely and examine the cells in action in its various subsystems.

Glossary

Amygdala: an almond-shaped complex of nuclei beneath the anteromedial surface of the temporal lobe; a component of the limbic system

Association fibers: cortical fibers which interconnect areas of the same cerebral hemisphere.

Autonomic ganglia: clusters of neurons outside the CNS which receive central input and project to various target organs and tissues.

Basal ganglia: large masses of gray matter in the core of the cerebral hemispheres; essentially very large nuclei involved in motor control.

Brainstem: the central, axial part or "fuselage" of the brain; anatomically, all parts of the brain except the cerebral and cerebellar cortices — the basal

ganglia, diencephalon, midbrain, pons, and medulla oblongata; in common medical practice, only the last three structures.

Caudate nucleus: one of the basal ganglia; lies medial to the putamen and
has a curved tail which follows the curvature of the lateral ventricle.

Central lobe: the hidden lateral part of the cerebral hemisphere, over-
grown by the frontal, parietal, and temporal lobes; the original lateral surface of the embryonic telencephalic vesicle.

Central sulcus: an important infolding of the lateral cerebral surface which
descends obliquely forward from the superior margin of the hemisphere;
the boundary between the parietal and frontal lobes.

Cerebellar peduncles: three pairs of massive fiber tracts (middle, superior,
and inferior) which link the cerebellum to the underlying brainstem; in a
dissected brain, as distinct as cables.

Cerebellum: the large, bihemispheric, and transversely fissurated "little
brain" overlying the pons and medulla oblongata; important to motor
coordination.

Cerebral cortex: a superficial sheet of gray matter covering the surface of
the cerebral hemispheres; subdivided into six layers and organized in
myriad functional columns.

Cerebral hemisphere: somewhat less than half the cerebrum as bisected by
the longitudinal cerebral fissure; includes cerebral cortex, half of the
semioval center and corpus callosum, basal ganglia, and a lateral ventricle,
but not the diencephalon, around which it grew as one of the two telencephalic vesicles. Segregated by fissures and sulci into six lobes (frontal,
parietal, occipital, temporal, central, and limbic).

Cerebrum: the large, uppermost part of the brain; consists of two fissurated cerebral hemispheres, interconnected by the corpus callosum, plus
the underlying diencephalon.

Choroid plexuses: long, convoluted structures, resembling strings of tiny
grapes, in the lateral, third, and fourth ventricles of the brain; secrete
cerebrospinal fluid (CSF).

Cingulate gyrus: the superior limb of the limbic lobe, arching medially to
the frontal and parietal lobes.

Commissural fibers: association axons which run across the midline from
one cerebral hemisphere to the other (via the anterior commissure, corpus
callosum, or hippocampal commissure).

Corona radiata: the broad fan of cerebral projection fibers protruding from
the curved edge of the internal capsule; includes thalamic axons running to

the cortex and cortical efferent fibers descending to various subcortical destinations.

Corpus callosum (hard body):   an extensive, massive bridge of fibers between the two cerebral hemispheres; shaped in midsagittal aspect like an over-turned canoe.

Cranial nerves: twelve highly specialized peripheral nerves that carry sensory signals to the brain and/or motor impulses to diverse structures (see Table 2-2).

Diencephalon ("betweenbrain"):   the second uppermost of the five embryonic brain vesicles; the epithalamus, thalamus, hypothalamus, third ventricle, optic nerves/tracts, retinas.

Fissures: classically, very deep infoldings of the cerebral hemisphere which indent the wall of the lateral ventricle (e.g., calcarine fissure; compare sulci.)

Fornix: a massive, cablelike tract which provides a major two-way link between forebrain and midbrain; a major input/output connection of the limbic system.

Frontal lobe: the most anterior cerebral lobe, including the motor cortex and an extensive prefrontal area (frontal pole).

Gyri: ridgelike convolutions of the cerebral cortex, each containing an inner core of white matter.

Hypothalamus: a diencephalic region located beneath the thalamus; regulates vital bodily functions by neural and neuroendocrine means.

Inferior colliculus: a large mound of neurons in the roof of the midbrain; involved in feature analysis of sounds and localization of sounds in binaural space.

Internal capsule: a broad, compact fiber band, V-shaped in horizontal section, bordered medially by the thalamus and caudate nucleus and laterally by the lenticular nucleus; extends upward into the corona radiata.

Lateral fissure: a deep, lateral fossa resulting from the embryonic downward and forward growth of the temporal lobe beneath the other cortical lobes; most prominent landmark of the cerebral hemisphere.

Limbic lobe: the most medial lobe of the cerebral hemisphere, facing the midline; comprises the cingulate and parahippocampal gyri and forms a border zone around the corpus callosum and subjacent brainstem.

Limbic system: an arbitrary collection of numerous brain areas (including the hypothalamus, hippocampus, limbic lobe, septal area, and habenula) that are richly interconnected with the limbic lobe; important to visceral activity and emotional behavior.

Medulla oblongata: the most caudal part of the hindbrain, indispensable to vital functions (breathing, swallowing, etc.); various fiber tracts run up and down through it. Tapers almost imperceptibly into the spinal cord.

Mesencephalon ("midbrain"): the third of the five embryonic brain vesicles; a tubular region of the CNS between the thalamus and pons, comprising the tectum, cerebral aqueduct, midbrain tegmentum, and crura cerebri.

Metencephalon ("afterbrain"): the fourth of the five embryonic brain vesicles; a region of the CNS between the midbrain and medulla oblongata, comprising the fourth ventricle, pontine tegmentum, and base of the pons.

Motor neurons: the final neurons in the chain of nerve cells within the CNS; generate and convey command signals via their axons in peripheral nerves to skeletal muscles and glands.

Myelencephalon ("cordbrain"): the fifth and most caudal of the five embryonic brain vesicles, resembling the spinal cord (myel); the medulla oblongata of the adult brain.

Occipital lobe: the most posterior cerebral lobe, including the visual cortex on the banks of the calcarine fissure.

Parahippocampal gyrus: the inferior limb of the limbic lobe, in the temporal lobe; lies next to the hidden gyrus called the hippocampus.

Parasympathetic nervous system: one of the two divisions of the autonomic nervous system; preganglionic cell bodies lie in four nuclei of the brainstem and three sacral segments of the spinal cord, while postganglionic cell bodies lie (usually) in the wall of their peripheral targets.

Parietal lobe: the part of the cerebral hemisphere between the frontal, temporal, and occipital lobes; includes the somatosensory cortex on the posterior bank of the central sulcus.

Pons: the region of the brainstem between the midbrain and medulla oblongata; comprises the fourth ventricle, pontine tegmentum, and base of the pons. The cerebellum, to which it is connected, is an outgrowth of it.

Primary sensory neurons: the initial neurons in the chain of nerve cells of the nervous system; cell bodies lie in sensory (dorsal root) ganglia, axons bifurcate into distal and proximal branches, leading to receptors and the CNS, respectively.

Projection fibers: cortical fibers which lead to, or come from, subcortical structures; in a broader context, fibers which convey impulses between structures at different levels of the CNS (such as spinocerebellar, cerebellothalamic, nigrostriatal, rubrospinal, etc.).

Putamen ("shell"):   one of the basal ganglia; lies lateral to the caudate nucleus, with which it is connected by bridges of gray matter.

Reticular formation: a continuum of nerve cell bodies, axons, and dendrites forming the midbrain, pontine, and medullary tegmentum; the central core of the brainstem, involved in virtually all aspects of brain activity.

Secondary sensory neurons: groups of internuncial neurons in the CNS which receive the proximal branches of axons of primary sensory neurons.

Semioval center: the elongate mass of white matter within the cerebral hemisphere; contains association, commissural, and projection fibers.

Septal area: a group of nuclei in the medial wall of the cerebral hemisphere, in the triangular region between the fornix and corpus callosum; superiorly, thins out into a chiefly glial sheet, the septum pellucidum.

Spinal cord: a thin, curving cylinder of nervous tissue (about 43–45 cm in length) coursing downward from the medulla oblongata to the tip of the CNS at the level of the upper lumbar spine; receives sensory input from the body periphery and provides motor output to the skeletal muscles.

Sulci: cerebral infoldings that, although distinct, do not indent the ventricle wall (e.g., central sulcus; *Fissure*); "fissure" and "sulcus" are frequently used interchangeably.

Superior colliculus: a large mound of neurons in the roof of the midbrain; involved in orientation to visual stimuli and control of eye movements.

Sympathetic nervous system: one of the two divisions of the autonomic nervous system; preganglionic cell bodies lie in the intermediolateral cell column of the thoracolumbar spinal cord, while postganglionic cell bodies lie either in the sympathetic chain ganglia alongside the cord or in collateral ganglia (e.g., the celiac ganglion or "solar plexus").

Tectum (roof):   the part of the midbrain posterior to the cerebral aqueduct; includes the superior and inferior colliculi.

Tegmentum: a continuous, elongated mass of gray matter extending from the upper midbrain down through the pons to the lower medulla oblongata; forms the floor of the fourth ventricle; (see reticular formation).

Telencephalon ("endbrain"):   the first and uppermost of the five embryonic brain vesicles; the cerebral hemispheres of the adult brain, including the cerebral cortex, lateral ventricles, and basal ganglia.

Temporal lobe: the most inferior cerebral lobe, including the auditory cortex on the inferior bank of the lateral cerebral fissure.

Thalamus ("inner chamber"): an egg-shaped mass of neurons in the diencephalon which serves as sensory portal to the cerebral cortex and a vital, integrative link in numerous motor and limbic circuits.

Ventricles: the five chambers of the brain; the two lateral ventricles, third ventricle, and fourth ventricle (the latter connected by the cerebral aqueduct), derived from the five cavities, or hollows, of the embryonic encephalon.

The Auditory
System

The auditory system detects and analyzes sounds in the environment, while its silent partner, the vestibular system, gives us information about body position. Such assignments are complex tasks indeed, and are really part of the larger task of gathering critical environmental information. Every moment, we receive and respond to many stimuli — sounds, sights, physical contacts, smells and tastes, as well as sensations of our body's movements and postures. Our six sensory subsystems (auditory, visual, somesthetic, olfactory, gustatory, and vestibular) are constantly "on line," monitoring these stimuli and feeding the news into the brain for integration and response. Although these inputs are multitudinuous and widespread, the responses are unified and focal. We gather many stimuli, but as a result we may make only one move — run away, for example. Thus, although it is convenient to discuss the sensory subsystems separately, we emphasize that the brain considers them all together.

Sounds and their Meaning

The physical characteristics of pure sounds are their frequency and intensity. Sounds are pressure waves in the air (rarefactions and compressions) with a given frequency (cps) and amplitude (decibels). Our perception of their frequency is called pitch, that of their amplitude is loudness. In real life, pure sounds are broken into patterns, and all but the most elementary sounds are a blend of many frequencies.

The task of the auditory system is to provide the brain with information on these features of sounds. We hear them, locate them, and relate our perceptions of them to present circumstances and past experiences. We know, as wild animals know, that certain sounds have special significance and portent: an unfamiliar noise, a snapping twig, a metallic click . . . . Even for man, the perception and analysis of sounds can mean survival, and the design of the auditory system as a superb network for general alertness and quick response expresses that high value.

The Inner Ear

The basic structures of the ear are shown in Figure 3-1. The ear is sub-divided into the external ear, comprising the auricle and ear canal; the middle ear, consisting of a cavity and three enclosed ossicles, the eustachian tube, and the tympanic or "drum" membrane; and the internal or

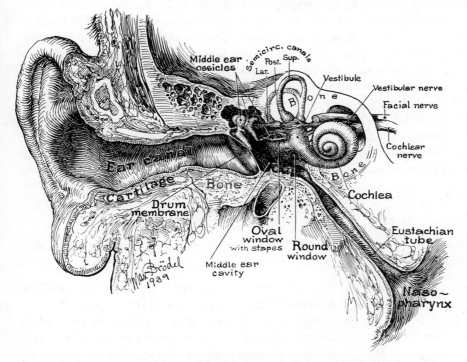

FIG. 3–1. *The human ear.* Basic structures of the ear, as drawn by Max Brödel, the famed medical illustrator at Johns Hopkins in the 1930's. Brödel was Director of the Department of Art as Applied to Medicine, the first academic department of its type. He revolutionized medical illustration, and his pioneer work is widely recognized. (From M. Brödel, in Malone, Guild and Crowe, *Three Unpublished Drawings of the Human Ear.* W. B. Saunders, Philadelphia, 1946)

inner ear, which includes the cochlea and vestibule, as well as the semicircular canals.

The inner ear is a structure that pinches off from the surface of the body during embryonic development and submerges to form a small, buried sac of highly specialized, ingrown "skin" (ectoderm). In this membranous sac the organ of hearing develops, along with that of equilibration and orientation in space (see Chap. 4). Leading from this sac is the auditory or vestibulocochlear nerve (CN VIII). Unlike other cranial nerves, this short nerve lies entirely within the skull. The outside world has tunneled in, as it were, to meet it.

Auditory Receptors

Betraying their common origin, the receptors in all the labyrinthine compartments and tunnels of this complex little chamber are remarkably alike: columnar cells that resemble certain sensory elements of invertebrates. They lack the long axonal processes and signaling properties of true neurons. They are really not neurons, but specialized epithelial cells that perform nervous functions. By movement of minute hairs (long, highly specialized microvillous processes) bristling from their free borders, they detect vibrations in the thin, watery fluid (endolymph) that fills these compartments and bathes their walls. The precise form of stimulus thought to excite these hair cells is deflection, or bending, of the microvilli toward the single (and probably nonmotile) kinocilium present on each cell.

How Sounds are Detected: Mechanical Energy Translations and Transduction

The major steps in sound detection are illustrated in sequence (Fig. 3-2) and are as follows:

(A) Air-borne vibrations collected in the ear canal (external auditory meatus) set up vibrations in the tympanic membrane or "ear drum."
(B) Vibrations of the tympanic membrane are transmitted by the middle ear ossicles (malleus, incus, and stapes) to the inner ear, where they impinge on the cochlea at the oval window. The ossicles are three tiny, articulated bones which, together with the tympanic membrane, effectively transfer sound wave energy from the air inwardly to the fluids in the cochlea and cochlear duct.
(C) The cochlea is a spiral-shaped bony chamber of graduated diameter; it resembles a snail shell, and has 2½ turns. It contains an ingenious and extremely delicate receptor system that converts the foregoing

mechanical vibrations to nerve impulses. The cochlea is filled with the watery perilymph, and it has three thin membranes stretched from wall to wall along its length. Sound waves thus lead, indirectly but most efficiently, to vibrations of the perilymph, and these in turn to vibrations of the membranes.

(D) The hair cells rest upon the basilar membrane, the lowermost of the three partitions. Collectively, these hair cells and their supporting elements comprise the organ of Corti, an obviously "shaky arrangement" of various types of epithelial cells (some of them bizarre in shape) extending the length of the cochlear duct. The microvilli or stereocilia of the hair cells are embedded in (or at least in contact with) another, thicker and stiffer sheet above them: the tectorial membrane.

A third membrane (Reissner's) lies above the tectorial membrane; it forms the roof of the cochlear duct, the floor of which is a complex of the organ of Corti, basilar membrane, and adjoining shelves of bone and connective tissue (not shown in the figure).

When the perilymph in the cochlea and the endolymph in the cochlear duct vibrate in resonance, the entire organ of Corti (including the tectorial membrane) moves up and down on the basilar membrane as if it rested on a waterbed. The vibratory movements of the basilar and tectorial membranes relative to one another set up a kind of shearing or displacement effect — much like that which occurs between the pages of a telephone book when it is flexed along its length. Such action deflects the stereocilia. When so disturbed, the hair cells (compare Fig. 3-3) generate electrical potentials.

In some manner, hair cells translate the mechanical energy of deflection of their microvilli into a voltage change across their cell membranes. These auditory receptors, therefore, convert sound energy into electrical energy. Such energy conversion is called transduction; it is a general principle of sensory information gathering by the nervous system. In various ways, receptors in all sensory subsystems transduce a particular kind of energy perturbation in the environment (external or internal) into the official language of the brain: electrical signals.

Tonotopy of the Auditory System

Sounds of different frequencies are picked up by the auditory receptive mechanism in a progressive spatial sequence in the organ of Corti along the length of the cochlear duct. Sound waves of a given frequency induce vibrations of the basilar membrane, the breadth of which varies along the

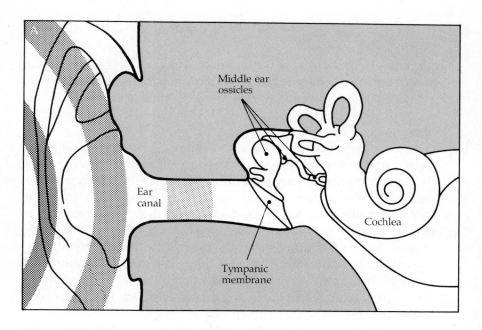

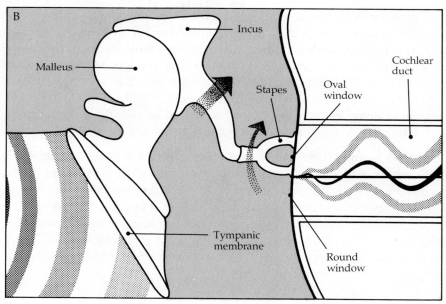

FIG. 3–2. *Auditory mechanisms.* Processes involved in sound transduction.

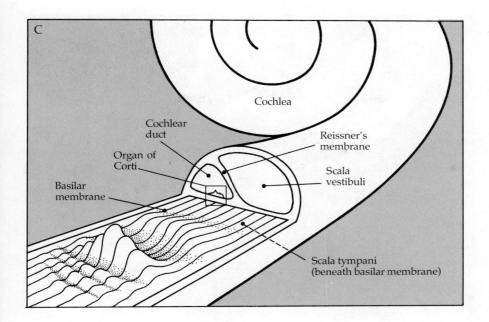

C

Cochlea

Cochlear
duct

Reissner's
membrane

Organ of
Corti

Scala
vestibuli

Basilar
membrane

Scala tympani
(beneath basilar membrane)

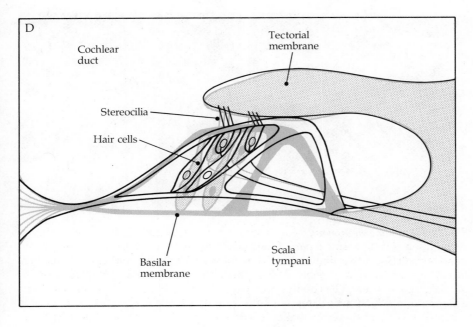

D

Cochlear
duct

Tectorial
membrane

Stereocilia

Hair cells

Basilar
membrane

Scala
tympani

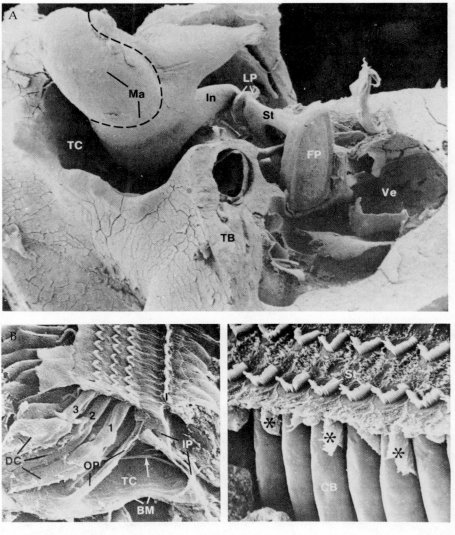

FIG. 3–3. *Scanning electron micrographs showing several parts of the ear.* (A) A fractured preparation encompassing a part of the middle ear cavity (TC), the underlying temporal bone (TB), and vestibule (Ve) of the inner ear. The three ossicles (malleus, Ma; incus, In; stapes, St) are visible. The footplate (FP) of the stapes is flattened on its medial surface where it lies on the oval window. The other end of the stapes forms a depression which articulates with the rounded lenticular process (LP) of the incus. The body of the incus makes a saddle-shaped facet (dashed lines) where it articulates with the head of the malleus. (From H. Engstrom and B. Engstrom, *Acta Otolaryngol.* 83:65-70, 1977, Almqvist and Wiksell Periodical Co. as reproduced in

several turns of the duct. The basilar membrane is widest at the blind end of the cochlea (its apex) and narrowest at the end near the ear ossicles (its base). In the exact same order, the frequency spectrum of response is precisely laid out from bass to treble clef (Fig. 3-4). This orderly, successive arrangement is called tonotopic organization, or tonotopy. While a long region of the basilar membrane may vibrate with a given sound tone or frequency, there will be a place of maximum vibration for that frequency, and another place alongside which will vibrate maximally for the next higher or lower frequency. Along its length, then, there is a gradation of frequency responsiveness in the cochlea, much like the gradation among the strings of various length that stretch across a piano sounding board.

The selective stimulation of hair cells, at a particular place along the basilar membrane by a sound of a particular frequency, in turn activates particular primary sensory neurons. By monitoring the activity of certain incoming nerve fibers, the brain can then tell which part of the basilar membrane is vibrating maximally and, accordingly, what frequency the sound has.

Frequency receives careful handling at all levels. Tonotopic organization does not stop at the receptor level; the neurons of the various auditory nuclei and the stacking of their axons in auditory tracts also show it to varying degrees. Elements that handle the lowest tones may lie in one part, those concerned with a slightly higher frequency will be immediately alongside, and so forth. At higher levels of the system, some tonotopy may be lost, or perhaps blurred. But in general the CNS seems to preserve this "frequency map" of the highly ordered receptive surface of the cochlear duct. Such topographical representation is a form of neural coding, a means for passing specific information to the CNS called place coding.

R. G. Kessel and R. H. Kardon, *Tissues and Organs: A Text-Atlas of Scanning Electron Microscopy*, W. H. Freeman, San Francisco, 1979)
(B) The organ of Corti in radial view. The basilar membrane (BM) forms the floor of the tunnel of Corti (TCQ). Several nerve fibers (arrow) traverse the tunnel between the inner (IP) and outer (OP) pillar cells. The sterocilia associated with the three rows of outer hair cells (1,2,3) are shown. The tectorial membrane has been fractured away in this tissue preparation. DC, Deiter's cells; I, inner hair cells. (From H. Engstrom and B. Engstrom, *Acta Otolaryngol.* 83:65-70, 1977, Almqvist and Wiksell; as reproduced in R. G. Kessel and R. H. Kardon, *Tissues and Organs: A Text Atlas of Scanning Electron Microscopy*, W. H. Freeman, San Francisco, 1979)
(C) The cell bodies (CB) and sterocilia (St) of the second row of outer hair cells. (From R. G. Kessel and R. H. Kardon, *Tissues and Organs: A Text-Atlas of Scanning Electron Microscopy*, W. H. Freeman, San Francisco, 1979)

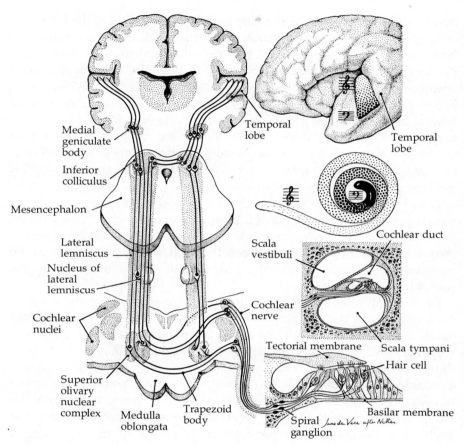

FIG. 3–4. *Auditory pathways.* Principal ascending auditory connections and their tonotopic organization in man. In the cochlea, a continuous gradation of frequencies proceeds inward, from high tones (indicated by treble clef) at the base (near the oval and round windows) to low tones (bass clef) at the apex (helicotrema). In the cortex, a similar tonal representation proceeds mediolaterally along the superior temporal plane from the insular margin to the transverse temporal gyri. (Modified from a painting by F. Netter, Ciba Collection, 1953 and included in *The Life of Mammals* by J. Z. Young, Oxford University Press, New York and London, 1957)

Place Coding – A Basic Theme

Place coding of information along neuronal pathways, sensory or otherwise, is an important principle, a consequence of the purposefulness of neural components and precision of the CNS. We shall see place coding again and again, in all sensory subsystems. A given fiber, or group of fibers, carries stimuli from a given sensory receptor, or set of receptors, to the brain or spinal cord, as the case may be. The spatial pattern of activation of receptors — along the cochlear duct, on the retina or elsewhere — is preserved in the spatial pattern of activation in all components of the sensory subsystem, and ultimately in the cortex. Thus, in auditory cortex there is a frequency map (along with other maps relating to binaural space, etc.), in visual cortex there are maps of the two retinae and their responses to objects seen, and in somatosensory cortex there are maps of the body surface according to various submodalities (pain, touch, etc.) and combinations of such submodes of body sensation. By monitoring such place-coded lines of information, the CNS can study over and over again the events recorded by particular receptors, interpret them in an increasingly critical manner, and keep some record of them for future comparison. At successful levels of analysis, stimuli are mapped, integrated, remapped, and integrated again — until, finally, evaluation of environmental phenomena and purposeful behavior result. In order to analyze and retrieve information, the brain keeps messages organized meticulously.

Central Circuitry

The auditory pathway is intricate, with many way stations. The incoming signals travel a great distance, from the inner ear through perhaps two to five intervening brainstem nuclei up to the thalamus and auditory cortex. Modulatory impulses, moreover, pass back down again through most or all these stations, right on out to the inner ear. Refer back to Figure 3-4 for an overview of the major ascending pathways.

Ascending Pathways

The primary sensory neurons are bipolar cells whose cell bodies lie in the spiral ganglion within the bony cochlea. These cells transmit the signals from the cochlea to the central neurons of the dorsal and ventral cochlear nuclei. The peripheral and central processes of the primary neurons are quite short. The peripheral processes lead outward, to the cochlear duct. There, in that delicate, convoluted inner chamber, they divide into finger-like branches that make intimate contact with a group of hair cells, "grasping" them in a variety of ways. After appropriate auditory stimuli, vibration-induced voltage changes in the hair cell membranes and subsequent electrical potentials at the tips of the fine nerve branches bring about the discharge of nerve impulses (action potentials) in the outer pro-

cesses. These impulses pass inward, over the cell bodies and central processes of the bipolar cells into the brain, where secondary sensory neurons
receive, integrate, and pass along the information to additional cell groupings — ultimately, to the cerebral cortex.

The Cochlear Nuclei. The secondary neurons are grouped in the dorsal and
ventral cochlear nuclei of the medulla (refer to Fig. 3-4). These cell clusters
receive the same messages through terminal branches of eighth nerve fibers, but process these messages in different ways. As in most other nuclei
of the auditory pathway, the neuronal population is heterogeneous.
Within both nuclei lie a complex variety of neurons, whose axons diverge
toward many destinations.

Beyond these initial way stations, the auditory system has many other
subcortical nuclei. It has been pointed out that the system is organized in a
combined "in-series, in-parallel" arrangement. Some fibers may run to a
nucleus located next door; others may bypass that nearby place and
synapse farther along the pathway.

In the cochlear nuclei, the peripheral tonotopic localization is retained
and, once again, laid out in an orderly fashion. The base of the cochlea is
represented dorsally and the apex ventrally, and individual cells respond
only over a narrow frequency range. Proceeding up the pathway, some
amount of tonotopic representation of frequency seems to be present at
each way station of the auditory system, although the details and degree of
clarity differ from place to place.

It is obvious that unilateral loss of the bipolar cells of the cochlear nerve,
or of the secondary sensory neurons in both cochlear nuclei due to some
vascular accident, would be tantamount to functional loss of the ear on that
side. These first- and second-order elements, which report the news or
pass the assignment on to other cells, respectively, are indispensable. But
above and beyond their levels, the auditory system puts so many neurons
in the brainstem to work on sound analysis that hearing losses from brain
damage will be bilateral and only partial. Unless the lesions are on both
sides and symmetrical, the functional deficits will probably not be very
obvious.

The superior olive and trapezoid nuclei. The next level of analysis takes place
in the superior olivary-trapezoid nuclear complex of the pontine tegmentum (the brainstem core of gray matter). This intricate region contains
several smaller nuclei, and receives bilateral input from the cochlear nuclei.

The superior olivary nuclei are believed to be particularly important in sound localization. Sounds originating off to one side of us reach our two ears at different times. It appears that (depending on the frequency) these differences in time of arrival or in intensity of sounds between the two ears are registered differentially in certain of the superior olivary nuclei. These signals are further processed and analyzed at higher centers.

Fibers from the superior olivary-trapezoid complex stream upward through the lateral lemniscus, terminating on its interstitial neurons (located in two small nuclei within the tract) in many instances. These fibers ascend through both sides of the brainstem reticular formation (and make many connections there en route), but the majority cross the midline in the trapezoid body. Directly or indirectly, the lemniscal fibers finally reach the inferior colliculus, a major integrating and modulating terminal of the auditory pathway.

The inferior colliculus and medial geniculate nucleus. The inferior colliculus is also involved in sound localization. As judged from changes in their firing rates, many of its neurons are exquisitely sensitive to the timing of afferent volleys reaching the two ears. These cells are so precisely specialized and wired up as to provide a neural map of our auditory environment. Thus, extrapersonal auditory space is transformed into intrapersonal brain space. As emphasized above, the time lag, however slight, in the arrival of sounds to the two ears provides essential information for sound localization. By integrative processes yet unknown, the brain performs an impressive, truly mathematical time–space transformation of auditory stimuli in the course of registering sounds in the world about us.

An important connection of the inferior colliculus is its arm or brachium that runs upward to the medial geniculate body of the thalamus, (see Fig. 5-5 for a view of this nucleus). Here the information is mapped and studied again, and the resulting pattern of neural activity is sent to the auditory cortex (Heschl's gyrus, Brodmann's area 41) on the superior temporal plane (Fig. 3-4).

The inferior colliculus and medial geniculate are not just large rounded cell clusters, "basketballs" crammed with neurons as most diagrams suggest. Instead, they are complex organizations of diversified and specialized cells and fibers arranged in a cortical manner (i.e., functional columns positioned vertically to the surface). Nor are these midbrain and thalamic way stations mere "relays" in the long route to conscious auditory experience. They are key communication centers, wherein ascending and descending influences are combined to good analytic purpose. Their functional importance correspondingly enhances feature extraction — even to the point of suppressing irrelevant information. In any part of the CNS, what goes in is never what comes out. This axiom holds true for single neurons and clusters of them. Wherever neurons handle information, integration takes place.

The auditory cortex. The primary auditory cortex receives its input primarily from the medial geniculate. As noted previously, frequency is probably represented in a tonotopic pattern, but most information on this subject comes from laboratory animals, and some of that is conflicting. We know very little about the human auditory cortex. In cats and monkeys, many cortical neurons have frequency responses as sharply limited as those of subcortical neurons, but others are more broadly tuned.

The auditory cortex, like the visual and somesthetic cortices, is organized in numerous functional columns that run vertical to the surface. Neurons in a frequency column have a best-frequency response of no more than one octave. Other variables, such as intensity, location, timbre, and pitch of sounds, are apparently plotted in similar functionally defined columns in primary auditory cortex. Adjoining cortical areas play associative roles, but also probably receive additional auditory input.

Descending Fibers

As we have seen, the auditory pathway leads from the hair cells all the way up to cortex and then back down again. There are almost as many descending as ascending fibers. But what function do such descending fibers along a supposedly sensory path serve?

The answer is that through descending fibers higher centers modulate neural activities below. The descending fibers convey excitatory or inhibitory impulses from the cortex, medial geniculate body, and inferior colliculus to the deep auditory (superior olivary-trapezoid) and cochlear nuclei, even to the bipolar neurons and hair cells. These influences refine the gathering of information, the process of hearing. To borrow the language of electronics, they increase auditory acuity, filter out "static" or background noise, "squelch" unwanted signals, and sharpen contrast. For example, stimulation of the crossed olivocochlear bundle (in which axons run from the superior olivary nucleus of the brain to the organ of Corti) has such an effect: it increases the "signal-to-noise" ratio. Conversely, lesions of this bundle reduce signal-to-noise discriminations.

The efferent system shows very much the same combined in-series, in-parallel arrangement we saw on the afferent side. By such flexible, efficient design, higher centers can control afferent input selectively, at any level. Each component, including the hair cells, can be "tuned" for greater or perhaps less sensitivity. We, too, like our neural sensory subsystems, must adjust the various instruments we use to gather information — we have to tune a radio or television set, focus binoculars or a microscope, and so forth. In the auditory system, the superior olive plays the comparable role by supplying fibers (the olivocochlear bundle just mentioned) to the inner ear which exert regulatory effects on receptor cell activity.

Efferent modulation is a key principle in the CNS. In the operation of sensory subsystems, it consists of an outgoing regulation of incoming signals to improve or suppress the gathering of information. But modulation is not confined to sensory pathways. Motor pathways show it, too. Many neurons of the brain and cord, including the motor neurons firing orders to muscles, are constantly sending back impulses (via axon collaterals) to adjoining local-circuit neurons. The effect of this feedback modulation is usually to reduce further output, or perhaps to increase it in some other group of neurons, as in synergistic muscle control.

The role of the human auditory cortex is still not well understood, and clinical evidence on this matter is scant. For example, one-sided removal or destruction of the auditory cortical area in the temporal lobe, or transection of the fibers leading to it through the thalamus, apparently does not produce deafness in either ear, as unilateral destruction of the cochlear nuclei, eighth nerve, or the ear itself clearly would. Such damage would probably only diminish certain qualities of hearing (see below), especially on the opposite side, because of the partial but extensive crossover of fibers ascending the brainstem.

Functional Correlates

In general, bilateral deficits that are difficult to pin down typify central auditory lesions — whether to lateral lemniscus, inferior colliculus, or some other structure along the path. The ability to localize sounds in space, however (particularly brief ones), may be considerably reduced by a cortical lesion. Even though interaural analysis of sound takes place subcortically (in superior olive and inferior colliculus), the auditory cortex plays a still higher and more critical role in acoustic sensory feature extraction and comparison. As long as the brainstem remains undamaged, auditory reflexes (such as head-turning, tensing of the ear drum, sudden inspiration, etc.) will probably not be lost, but may be affected in some obvious manner, depending on how much the interplay of auditory cortex and subcortical structures has been affected.

It appears that the auditory cortex is concerned in part with decoding the complex acoustic stimuli used in communication: sounds of words, intonations, and the like. Moreover, auditory cortex seems necessary if the brain is to make decisions about the significance of sounds, and when they should have access to the motor system. In man, where auditory function seems more dependent on cortical influences than in animals studied thus far, cortical auditory areas are essential for short-term memory storage and immediate recall, for identification (not detection) of novel stimuli, and for recording the temporal order of acoustic events. Although bilateral destruction of the primary auditory cortex or the auditory radiations in man is rare, with bilateral middle cerebral artery infarcts it can happen, and there is evidence that nearly total "true cortical deafness" ensues. This would probably not occur in a monkey or a cat. In fact, cats apparently have five cortical areas devoted to auditory sensations, and bilateral cortical lesions would have to be extensive to destroy them all (Fig. 3-5).

Surrounding the primary auditory cortex are additional auditory areas together with cortical association territories. The latter regions do not display a tonotopic organization, and are activated by a variety of sensory modalities. The association areas are involved in integrating many sensory stimuli, and are thus important to the understanding of one's environment and formulating speech. Strange disorders of this symbolic function may result from lesions to these regions in the hemisphere that is dominant for speech (usually the left). These interesting conditions are largely outside the scope of this book. One of them is "pure word deafness." The affected person can hear perfectly, but cannot understand spoken speech. The sounds are understood to be words, but in their lack of meaning are like the words of a foreign language. Curiously, the person's own speech, reading, and writing are normal. Other association disorders are discussed in Chapter 13.

In general, lesions of the various nuclei and tracts of the auditory pathway do not produce specific localizing symptoms. Exceptions, however, occur with thalamic lesions in or near the medial geniculate. Such damage may be associated with distortions of auditory sensations and with the experience of disagreeable qualities in sounds that are normally not bothersome. Such changes in both discriminative and affective qualities of sensation are characteristic of thalamic lesions, as we shall see in Chapter 8.

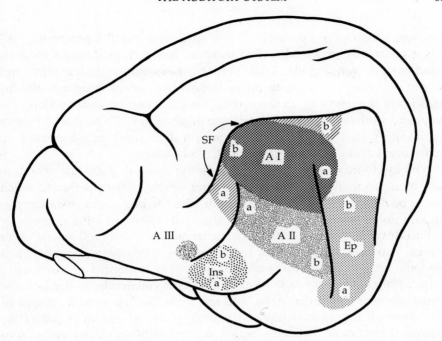

FIG. 3–5. *Cortical auditory areas.* Areas of feline cerebral cortex activated by auditory stimuli under various conditions. At least five areas receive input by way of the classical lemniscal pathway, i.e., from inferior colliculus via its brachium to medial geniculate body. Impulses reach these cortical subdivisions through various subdivisions of the medial geniculate. In addition, extralemniscal pathways through the reticular formation (not shown) have been found. In fact, a sleeping cat can be aroused by auditory stimuli after both lateral lemnisci are cut. This nonlemniscal path appears not to synapse in the geniculate, but in the older posterior and intralaminar thalamic nuclei, i.e., the nonspecific part of the thalamus.

A I = primary auditory area, A II = secondary auditory area beneath A I, Ins = insular area, Ep = posterior ectosylvian area, SF = suprasylvian fringe area. A III = small area activated by sound, but tonotopy (if present) not established. In each of these five areas, a = apex and b = base of the cochlea, or low and high frequencies, respectively. Note reversed tonotopy in A I and A II. (After C. N. Woolsey, Organization of cortical auditory system. In *Sensory Communication*, W. A. Rosenblith, ed. The M.I.T. Press, Cambridge, Mass., 1961)

General Concepts

The auditory pathway is extremely complex, probably far more than we realize. Nevertheless, it illustrates many important organizing principles of the nervous system: transduction of stimulus energy, sequential analysis of features, progressive synthesis of response, and parallel processing. All this is constantly reviewed and adjusted by feedback modulation through bundles of descending fibers that permit the system to regulate input and output. Everywhere we note the orderliness of neural design: in the intricacies of the pathway, in the cortical design of certain stations along the way, and in the ever-present tonotopic organization. To alert and protect us, auditory analysis is carried out with a divergence of information to many brain areas that helps to unify CNS function.

Why are there so many neurons along the auditory pathway — and, in fact, along so many brain pathways? One simple answer is that so much has to be done with raw sensory stimuli. The cerebral cortex, for example, doesn't deal with reports from individual hair cells, but with analyses by multitudes of midbrain and thalamic neurons. Such analyses, among other things, correlate the reports of many sensory subsystems. Another, less obvious, answer is that there must be a generous number of distributive neurons along the way to send axons, or axon collaterals, to the reticular formation of the medulla, pons, and midbrain. Such neuronal "dispatchers" drop off urgent bulletins to the brain's core at certain stages of the analytical operation. This core region is constantly regulating spinal sensory and motor excitability, adjusting forebrain activity, and mediating important auditory reflexes — such as the stapedial and tensor tympani reflexes that protect the organ of Corti against excessive stimulation.

Therefore, it should not surprise us to find that auditory impulses spread so widely and quickly through the brain. We are watching a team effort, in which each neuron in a vast organization of interdependent cells does its job. This effort is characterized by convergence of messages upon clusters of cells and then integration of this information by the cells in those clusters, over and over, as well as upward and downward, in the many auditory pathways.

Glossary

Auditory cortex: the primary auditory receiving area of the cerebral cortex on the anterior and posterior transverse temporal gyri; Brodmann's areas 41 and 42.

Basilar membrane: a delicate membrane extending the length of the cochlear duct, supporting the spiral organ of Corti; decreases in width, stiffness, and frequency response from the base (near the oval window) to the apex (at the helicotrema) of the cochlea.

Bony (osseous) labyrinth: the complex group of chambers (cochlea, vestibule, and cavities for the three semicircular canals) within the petrous part of the temporal bone.

Cochlea: a spiraling bony chamber of graduated diameter, curled 2½ times on itself so as to resemble a snail shell, and partitioned into three small tunnel-like passageways: the scala vestibuli, scale tympani, and the cochlear duct (the last containing the receptor system for hearing).

Cochlear nerve: the auditory division of the vestibulocochlear nerve (cranial nerve VIII).

Cochlear nuclei: clusters of secondary sensory neurons in the medulla oblongata; receive input from the primary auditory neurons innervating the cochlea.

Endolymph: the thin, watery fluid in the membranous labyrinth.

Eustachian tube: a tubular evagination of the pharynx connecting the air-filled middle ear cavity with the oral cavity; serves to equalize pressure between the inner ear and external environment.

External auditory meatus: the ear canal, derived from a tubular invagination of the embryonic ectoderm during the formation of the external ear.

Hair cells: the ubiquitous and generally similar receptor cells of the cochlear duct and vestibular organ; hairs comprise numerous stereocilia and one kinocilium per cell.

Inferior colliculus: a large mound of neurons in the roof of the midbrain; involved in the feature analysis of sounds and localization of sounds in binaural space.

Kinocilium: the single true cilium (probably nonmotile, however) of the hair cells, which elsewhere on their free surfaces bear stereocilia.

Lateral lemniscus: a conspicuous fiber tract ascending lateral to the brainstem reticular formation; crossed and uncrossed fibers from the superior olivary trapezoid nuclear complex ascend in it.

Medial geniculate body: a grossly visible nucleus of the thalamus and component of the auditory pathway; its fibers project topographically to the auditory cortex.

Membranous labyrinth: a delicate, thin-walled system of cavities and tubes within, and conforming to, the bony labyrinth.

Olivocochlear bundle: a distinct fascicle of fibers originating in the superior olive, traveling outward in the cochlear nerve, and terminating in the spiral organ of Corti; exerts efferent modulation of auditory input.

Ossicles: three tiny articulated bones of the middle ear; the malleus, incus, and stapes (hammer, anvil, and stirrup).

Perilymph: the thin, watery fluid in the bony labyrinth.

Pontine tegmentum: the pontine region of the brainstem core of gray matter; see tegmentum (Chap. 2).

Reissner's membrane: the membranous roof of the cochlear duct; overlies the complex of tectorial membrane, organ of Corti, basilar membrane, and adjoining shelves of bone and connective tissue.

Scala tympani: the lower tunnel, as divided by the bony spiral lamina, of the cochlea; begins at the helicotrema and ends at the round window.

Scala vestibuli: the upper tunnel, as divided by the bony spiral lamina, of the cochlea; begins at the oval window and ends at the helicotrema.

Spiral ganglion: a long, helically arranged ganglion within the cochlea; contains the cell bodies of the bipolar primary auditory neurons.

Spiral organ of Corti: a complex arrangement of epithelial cells (including the auditory hair cells) in the cochlear partition; the organ of hearing.

Stereocilia: long, nonmotile microvillous processes, resembling hairs, bristling from the free surfaces of auditory receptor cells (hair cells); deflection of the nonmotile kinocilium toward them stimulates the cells.

Superior olivary nuclei: a large auditory nuclear complex in the pontine tegmentum; input comes from the cochlear nuclei bilaterally, output goes upward over the lateral lemniscus.

Tectorial membrane: a membrane in the cochlear duct directly above the organ of Corti; with the basilar and Reissner's membranes, responsible for producing the shearing or displacement effect which deflects the stereocilia of the hair cells.

Trapezoid nuclei: a small auditory nuclear complex in the pontine tegmentum near the superior olivary nuclei; input comes from the cochlear nuclei of both sides; output passes to the superior olive.

Tympanic membrane (eardrum):   a thin, deflectable membrane between the external and middle ear; its vibrations, set up by sound (air) waves, move the ear ossicles and set up vibrations of the perilymph in the scala vestibuli and scala tympani.

Vestibulocochlear nerve: cranial nerve VIII; consists of vestibular and cochlear divisions, which serve the vestibular organ and cochlear duct, respectively.

The Vestibular
System

4

The vestibular system deals with sensory impulses that result from movements and positions of the head. Such input enables the nervous system to keep the eyes on target, the visually most effective regions of the retinae centered (foveation), and the body on an even keel. This is accomplished largely automatically, at a subconscious level, but the vestibular system also mediates a sensation that we seldom think about, our sense of stability of the space around us and of the ground beneath. Barring earthquakes, we take this sense of stable space and solid ground for granted. Thus the sensation of stability is part of a spectrum of bodily sensations — of vibration, motion, contact, and sound; of shapes and movements of things around us; of our own posture and locomotion.

The Inner Ear and Vestibular Receptors

As described in Chapter 3, all the receptors in the inner ear are flask-shaped or columnar hair cells, some for hearing and some for balance. Such cells bear 50–110 hairs or stereocilia (long, specialized microvillous processes) and a single even longer kinocilium which is probably non-motile. In the acoustic organ, hair cells transduce vibrations in a column of fluid (endolymph) that bathes the organ of Corti in the cochlear duct. In the equilibratory organ, virtually identical cells in ridgelike patches (the cristae ampullares) respond to currents of fluid within slender, curved tubules (the semicircular canals) which arch in all three planes of space (Fig. 4-1; see also Fig. 3-1). At a crista, a cupula ("cap") of viscous, gelatinous mate-

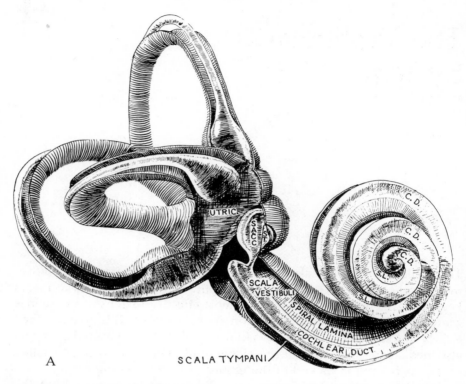

FIG. 4–1. *Stepwise dissection of right bony and membranous labyrinths.* Viewed from lateral aspect. (A) The bony labyrinth as it would appear if all but a bit of bone had been chiseled away from the right perilymphatic cavity, and that remaining bone had been partially cut away to show the enclosed membranous labyrinth.

rial (glycoprotein) lies just above the apices of the hair cells, so as to bend the hairs during fluid movement. In addition, in specialized discoid patches or spots (the maculae) within two small, membranous bags (the utricle and saccule), similar hair cells translate the inertial or gravitational pull on tiny, sandlike particles embedded with the hairs in an overlying gelatinous mass that is free to shift this way and that.

How Movements are Detected

Movements of fluid in the canals or displacements of the "stone-loaded" jelly in the utricle and saccule result from movements or changes in posi-

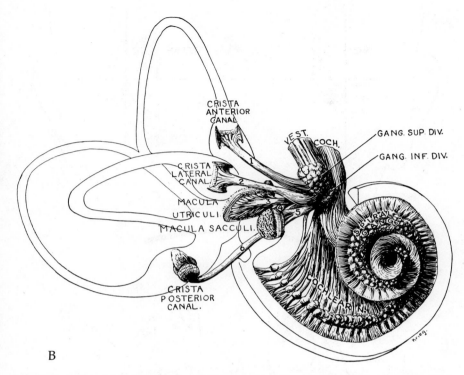

CRISTA ANTERIOR CANAL

CRISTA LATERAL CANAL

MACULA UTRICULI

MACULA SACCULI

CRISTA POSTERIOR CANAL.

VEST.

COCH.

GANG. SUP. DIV.

GANG. INF. DIV.

B

(B) The membranous labyrinth rendered transparent to show the positions of its receptor surfaces: the cristae (crests) ampullares and the maculae (spots) of the utricle and saccule. Note the relationship of these sensitive regions of hair cells to the various numbered branches of the vestibular and cochlear nerves. (From W. J. S. Krieg, *Functional Neuroanatomy*. 3rd ed. Brain Books, Evanston, Ill., 1966)

tion of the head (Fig. 4-2). The necessary details of the anatomy and the key events are as follow:

(A) The three canals in each ear are arranged in three orthogonal planes of space, like the three sides of a corner of a cube. The two lateral canals (one from each side) are in the same plane, while the anterior canal on one side is roughly parallel to the posterior canal on the other. The lateral canals are tipped up 30° anteriorly; their plane becomes horizontal when a person looks down 30° from the horizon. The anterior and posterior canals in one ear form approximately a right angle with one another, with the posterior about 55° off the midsagittal plane (accounts vary slightly).

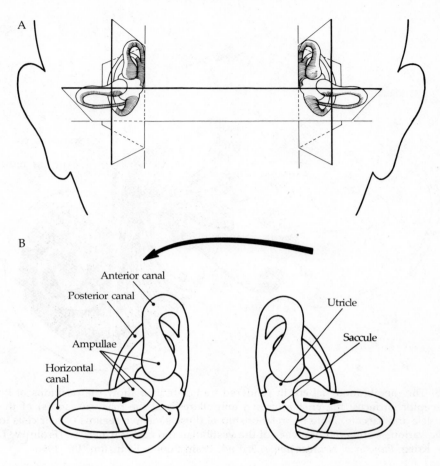

FIG. 4–2. *Vestibular receptors*. Orientation of semicircular canals in space.
(A) Orientation of semicircular canals in space, as shown in frontal view.
(B) Higher power view.

(B) Each semicircular canal has a bulbous enlargement, an ampulla
      ("jug") at one end: the anterolateral end of the anterior canal, an-
      teromedial end of the lateral canal, and posteroinferior end of the
      posterior canal. Each ampulla contains a ridgelike patch (crista ampul-
      laris) of receptors (hair cells). The effective stimulus is rotational
      movement of the head. Beginning such a movement to the right, as
      shown by the large arrow, creates a leftward current of endolymph in
      the lateral canals (small arrows). This brings about a slow leftward

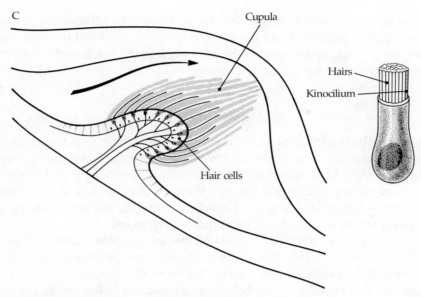

(C) Closeup of ampulla, crista, and hair cells. See Text.

movement of the eyes with subsequent rapid movement to the right. Stopping such a movement brings about reversed flow, and reversed eye movements. Because an observer cannot run in circles about someone who is spinning on a swivel chair, it is the postrotatory effects on eye movement that the neurologist examines. What happens after the individual comes to a stop is the exact opposite of what occurs when rotation begins.

(C) The current of fluid deflects the cupula over the hair cells, bends the hairs (stereocilia), and generates a receptor potential. As shown, a current which bends the hairs toward the kinocilium (motile cilium; shaded process) increases the firing rate of the unit, and vice versa. Unit response frequency changes only when rotation starts or stops.

The most effective stimuli for the hair cells of the cristae ampullares of the semicircular canals are rotational movements of the head, or angular accelerations (through an angle). The most effective stimuli for the hair cells of the maculae of the utricle and saccule, on the other hand, are probably (see comments below) straight-line movements of the head (up-down, front-to-back, etc.), or linear accelerations. It is important to realize that stopping these rotational or straight-line movements, i.e., deceleration, is an equally effective stimulus. Furthermore, the utricular and saccular maculae appear to signal the static position of the head in space on a continuing basis. In any event, the messages to the brain begin with minute voltage changes in hair cell membranes.

The Unified Function of the Membranous Labyrinth

The parcellation of functions for the various chambers that make up the vestibular part of the membranous labyrinth outlined above is greatly oversimplified. Any kind of movement or position of the head must obviously have some effect on the fluid that fills these various cavities. It is probably the combination of signaling of what is happening (or not happening) in all the chambers at any given moment that is important.

For example, the ampullary crests of the semicircular canals may serve partly to detect straight-line movements, although to lesser degree than they respond to angular acceleration, the most effective stimulus for their excitation. Conversely, the macular sensory patches of the utricle and saccule are probably affected to some degree by rotation, even though linear movements and positions are their most effective stimuli. It is hard to see why angular acceleration would not set the endolymph in motion in these baglike cavities, as it so easily does in the canals.

The saccule is still a place of mystery: its role in static equilibrium has never been as clear as that of the overlying utricle. Some investigators think that in man, at least, the saccule serves as a vibration detector — a function resembling that of the nearby cochlea (to which it is joined by a tiny duct, as mentioned earlier). Although an earthquake would probably stir them up, neither the utricle nor the saccule seem to be as efficient static sensors in man as they are in other animals.

The Close Relationship of Auditory, Vestibular, and Somatic Sensations

As we said earlier, the inner ear is a complex of structures derived from a patch of embryonic surface ectoderm. This membranous region invaginates, pinches off, and sinks beneath the surface to form a small, buried sac of specialized "skin." The close developmental relationship of ear and skin is reflected in the organization of their respective sensory subsystems. There is an interesting similarity, in some respects a continuity, in the modalities of hearing, equilibration, and cutaneous sensation. Sound produces pressure waves, which set up perturbations in a column of incompressible fluid and ultimately in hair cells of the organ of Corti. Cutaneous stimuli, such as touch, exert their mechanical effects on the epidermis and dermis, or perhaps more deeply. We could say that touch, pressure, movement, vibration, and sound all lie along a spectrum of the mechanical influences of our environment.

Central Circuitry

A paramount role of the vestibular system is to provide for rapid, reflex eye movements: to maintain proper eye position, to keep the eyes on target, and to center the image on the regions of highest visual acuity, the retinal foveae. An equally important role is to orient the head and body in space: to provide a stable ocular platform. The system accomplishes these tasks through coordinated ocular, cervical, and truncal muscle contractions which regulate eye and head movements, head position, and posture. The system also works to reinforce the appropriate tonic activity of axial and appendicular muscles, so that we may keep our balance and not fall.

All sensory subsystems must work together in the above tasks. Visual, tactile, and other sensory inputs take part in the action and feed into the circuitry, so that all the senses are integrated in the moment-by-moment task of maintaining posture and adjusting body position. The visual input is particularly important. A fixed, steady image promotes visual activity and feature analysis, whereas a wavy, bouncing image precludes efficient sensory processing. With the help of the cerebellum, the vestibular system integrates its input from all the hair cells which, in their turn, are transducing movements of fluid in the membranous labyrinth. Then the system issues commands to the oculomotor, trochlear, abducens, spinal accessory, and spinal motor neurons to bring about the correct eye, head, and trunk movements.

Central Projections of the Vestibular Nerve

Bipolar neurons of the vestibular nerve (one division of cranial nerve VIII, the cochlear nerve being the other) monitor signals from the hair cells of the vestibular receptors and carry them to four vestibular nuclei (superior, lateral, medial, and inferior; Fig. 4-3). Some fibers go directly to the cerebellum; others synapse in the vestibular nuclei, which then give rise to cerebellar projections. As mentioned in Chapter 2 and spelled out in Chapter 9, the cerebellum is critically involved in the regulation of movement and

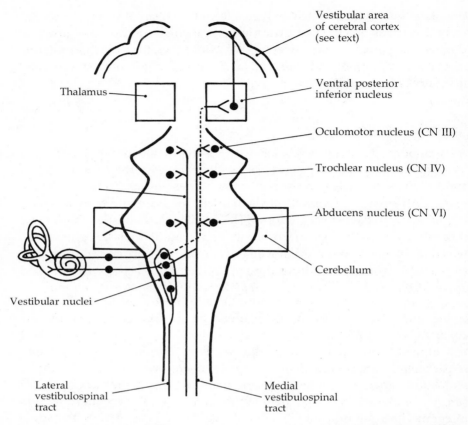

FIG. 4–3. *Principal connections of the vestibular system.* Pathways to the thalamus (ventral posterior inferior nucleus) and cerebral cortex (a region near the face area of the primary sensory homunculus) are not well known anatomically, but the subjective feelings of dizziness and vertigo are assumed to depend in part on such ascending connections.

posture. Thus, the midline cerebellum (vermis and flocculonodular lobe) receives a constant update on rotational and linear accelerations of the head, as well as on its static positions. The results are the refinements of all those ocular, cervical, and truncal movements and positions called for by vestibular input.

Output of the Vestibular Nuclei

Neurons of the vestibular nuclei project to areas involved in ocular and axial motor control. Thus, they project to the spinal cord via two tracts, the lateral and medial vestibulospinal tracts (see Fig. 4-3), and through the mediation of spinal interneurons affect the activity of the alpha and gamma motor neurons of the cord (see Chap. 10). Similarly, they project to the brainstem via the medial longitudinal fasciculus, and thereby affect the activity of motor neurons controlling the eye muscles. They also send fibers to the cerebellum (flocculonodular lobe) and reticular formation. There are additional ascending connections that probably are important to our conscious sense of stability in the space around us (the normal but unnoticed reciprocal to dizziness and vertigo). These fibers proceed via poorly known brainstem pathways to the thalamus (ventral posterior inferior nucleus) and then to the cerebral cortex — to the head region of the homunculus on the postcentral gyrus and a region near the auditory area.

In the vestibular system, as in the auditory system, descending efferent fibers play an important regulatory role. Outgoing fibers from the vestibular nuclei terminate directly on the hair cells of the vestibular organs, thereby providing for efferent modulation of sensory input (see below).

Reflex Actions of the Vestibular System

The vestibular system provides information on spatial orientation that is important for the control of volitional movement. In addition, it triggers reflexes that tend to stabilize the eyes, head, and body in space. Two important reflexes are the vestibulospinal reflex and vestibulo-ocular reflex or VOR.

In the vestibulospinal reflex, muscles act to counter or oppose an unwanted movement. For example, if you suddenly start falling to your right, the extensor muscles of your right leg will contract more strongly, while those on the left will relax. Your neck muscles will also contract to keep your head in its normal position. The vertibulo-ocular reflex, on the other hand, has a different but closely related function. As your head turns to one side, this reflex drives your eyes in the opposite direction, in order to maintain a stable retinal image and keep it on the fovea.

During rotation of the head, slow eye movements in one direction (opposite to that of the movement) are followed by rapid ones in the other direction, both generated by vestibular input. This combination of involuntary, alternating slow and rapid movements of the eyeballs is called nystagmus. The slow ones keep the eyes trained on target as long as possible, while the rapid movements serve to foveate new targets. As we have said, a stable visual world is essential to visual analysis, and the vestibulo-ocular reflex helps to provide this stability.

The vestibular system also participates in a set of righting reflexes. For example, a kitten always lands right side up when it falls, due to vestibular reflexes. The first compensatory movement involves a movement of its head toward its normal position. Other righting movements follow in sequence. Vestibular reflexes thus work in concert with various reflexes of the motor system (stretch and segmental reflexes) and with visual input to maintain body attitude, to preserve when desirable our postural *status quo*.

Basic Design Concepts of the CNS

Neural circuitry follows many principles that have found wide use in engineering and computer design, and the vestibular system provides suitable illustrations of these familiar principles.

Feedback Control

The vestibulospinal reflex illustrates the concept of a feedback control system (Fig. 4-4). In such systems, the controller of the process to be controlled is built directly into the path of the circuit, and the output is returned to the input. The vestibulospinal reflex is such a system; signals related to the sequence of corrective postural events triggered by displace-

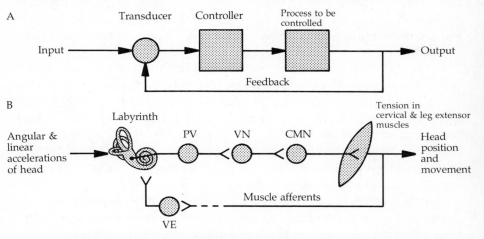

FIG. 4–4. *Reflex arc as a feedback control system.* (A) Block diagram for a feedback control system.
(B) General neuronal connections for the vestibulospinal reflex. PV, primary vestibular neuron; VN, cell of vestibular nucleus; CMN, cervical motor neuron, VE, efferent cell of vestibular system. (After M. Ito, The control mechanisms of cerebellar motor systems. In *The Neurosciences. Third Study Program.* F. O. Schmitt and F. G. Worden, eds. The M.I.T. Press, Cambridge, Mass. pp. 293–303)

ment of the head or falling to one side are fed back on the vestibular system which detected the disturbance in the first place. These signals nullify the neural activity generated by such a disturbance, and thus feedback promotes stability. Feedback control is a basic form of control in the nervous system. It is used in whole systems, as well as in parts of systems. It is used even at the single-cell level. A neuron with a recurrent axon collateral may inhibit, either directly or through a local interneuron, activity in adjacent neurons — in some instances, it may even (usually indirectly) suppress its own activity.

Feedforward Control

Some systems, in contrast, operate on a feedforward control system. Such systems, in which the controller is built into a side-arm of the circuit, are even more sensitive to external disturbances and changes than feedback systems. The vestibulo-ocular reflex is an example; it can be viewed as a three-neuron arc (Fig. 4-5), in which the cerebellum provides a side-arm of the loop. In this circuit, the cerebellum can enhance the magnitude of the response, so that even slight, barely detectable vestibular input can have a

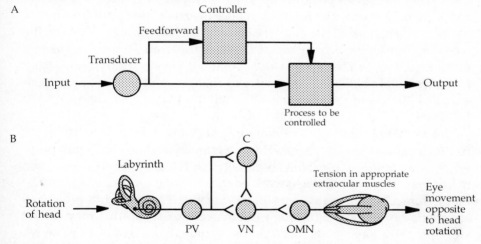

FIG. 4–5. *Reflex arc as a feedforward control system.* (A) Block diagram for a feedforward control system.
(B) General connections for the vestibulo-ocular reflex. VN, cell of vestibular nucleus; PV, primary vestibular neuron; OMN, oculomotor neuron; C, cerebellar Purkinje cell. (After M. Ito, The control mechanisms of cerebellar motor systems. In *The Neurosciences. Third Study Program.* F. O. Schmitt and F. G. Worden, eds. The M.I.T. Press, Cambridge, Mass., pp. 293–303)

strong effect on eye movement. If the resulting cerebellar output is stronger, the response is stronger. There is thus an opportunity for output enhancement when a circuit has such a side-arm.

Feedforward control systems have another feature: with each occurrence there can be a central "memory" in some neural repository of the consequences of the particular pattern of neural activity associated with the event. In fact, there is evidence that in the vestibulo-ocular reflex the "gain" imposed by the cerebellum can be reset, depending on the appropriateness of the response. For example, people or animals kept with telescopic lenses over their eyes are served poorly by the normal VOR. Initially, however, they use visual feedback to couple eye movements to head rotation. In time, the cerebellum comes into play, adjusting the gain to compensate for the effect of the lenses.

In certain instances, feedback and feedforward control systems work together. The microcircuitry of the spinal cord and cerebral cortex offers many examples.

General Concepts

The vestibular system provides the essential input for control of reflex eye and head movements and for maintenance of certain aspects of posture. Its receptors, like those of the auditory system, are hair cells. In this case, the receptors transduce movements of fluids as the head rotates, moves in a given direction, or changes position. As in all sensory subsystems, these receptors seem to be more responsive to changes (accelerations and decelerations), than in the steady state, although this particular system is geared to both.

The vestibular pathways provide excellent examples of feedback and feedforward systems of control. These servomechanisms must work properly if other neural subsystems, especially the visual system (Chap. 5) and motor system (Chap. 9), are to work properly. When these crucially important gyromechanisms of the vestibular system are subjected to prolonged stimulation or damaged (through trauma or disease) so that they cannot work properly, the results — dizziness, vertigo, nausea, motion sickness, past-pointing (to one side of a target), and falling — are all too clear and troublesome.

Glossary

Ampulla: a bulbous enlargement at one end of each semicircular canal, containing a ridgelike elevation (crista) in its wall.

Bony (osseous) labyrinth: the complex group of chambers (cochlea, vestibule, and cavities for the three semicircular canals) within the petrous part of the temporal bone.

Crista ampullaris: a ridgelike elevation in the ampulla of a semicircular canal with hair cells on its surface.

Cupula: a mass of viscous gelatinous material (glycoprotein) capping the hair cells of a crista ampullaris, a moveable wedge of "jelly" hinged on and running the full width of the crista; its deflection by fluid moving within the semicircular canals bends the processes of these cells.

Endolymph: the thin, watery fluid in the membranous labyrinth.

Flocculonodular lobe: a phylogenetically old lobe of the cerebellum, comprising the hemispheric flocculus and vermian nodulus; interconnected with the vestibular nuclei and adjacent reticular formation.

Hair cells: specialized receptor cells of the inner ear; some (in the cochlea) serve the sense of audition, and others in the utricle, saccule, and semicircular canals detect movement.

Kinocilium: the single true cilium (probably nonmotile, however) of the hair cells, which elsewhere bear stereocilia on their free surfaces.

Macula: a small, disc-shaped patch of hair cells; one is found within both the utricle and saccule.

Medial longitudinal fasciculus (MLF): a small but important tract interconnecting the somatic motor nuclei (oculomotor, trochlear, abducens, and hypoglossal) of the brainstem; conveys vestibular input to ocular motor neurons and to spinal motor neurons mediating trunk movements.

Membranous labyrinth: a delicate, thin-walled system of cavities and tubes within, and conforming to, the bony labyrinth.

Perilymph: the thin, watery fluid in the bony labyrinth.

Saccule: the lower membranous chamber within the vestibule, containing a patch of hair cells (macula sacculi) that may serve in sensing deep vibration.

Semicircular canals: three bony, slender tubules (anterior, lateral, and posterior) of the inner ear, oriented at right angles to each other, springing from the upper part of the utricle; detect angular (rotational) accelerations of the head.

Stereocilia: long, nonmotile microvillous processes, resembling hairs, bristling from the free surfaces of vestibular receptor cells (hair cells); deflection of them toward the nonmotile kinocilium stimulates the cells.

Utricle: the upper membranous chamber within the vestibule, containing a patch of hair cells (macula utriculi) that detect straight-line (linear) accelerations of the head.

Ventral posterior inferior nucleus (VPi):   a thalamic nucleus receiving ascending vestibular projections and sending fibers to the vestibular cortex.

Vestibular cortex: the primary vestibular area of the cerebral cortex; located in a temporoparietal region near the primary auditory receiving area.

Vestibular nerve: the equilibratory division of the vestibulocochlear nerve (cranial nerve VIII).

Vestibular nuclei: four elaborately subdivided brainstem nuclei; receive input directly from primary vestibular neurons, as well as from the cerebellum and send fibers into the vestibulospinal tracts.

Vestibular organ: the organ of equilibration; the utricle, saccule, and three semicircular canals.

Vestibule: that part of the bony labyrinth of the inner ear that encloses the utricle and saccule of the membranous labyrinth.

Vestibulospinal tracts: two tracts, medial and lateral, that convey vestibular impulses downward to spinal motor neurons; the medial tract, a prolongation of the MLF, innervates axial motor neurons down to the midthoracic cord, while the lateral tract extends the length of the cord and mediates appendicular muscle extensor tone.

The Visual System

5

The visual system deals with sensations of great importance to effective neural function. Vision exerts strong, often prepotent influences on the activity of our nervous system, as when we stand erect, run, or drive a car. It makes indispensable contributions to our posture, locomotion, and skilled movement. With one's eyes closed, standing and walking soon become difficult, and except by luck a task such as threading a needle is virtually impossible. And our sense of sight is of priceless value in other ways that we need not belabor here.

Stimulus Transduction

Like a camera, the eye captures fixed or fleeting light images for us (Fig. 5-1). It is an almost completely light-tight, spherical compartment with a three-layered wall. At the front, there is a lens system that focuses rays of light on the retina, the sensitive layer at the back of the eye. The pupil is the adjustable lens aperture; this optic diaphragm controls the amount of light entering the eye, to facilitate vision in dim light by widening and, conversely, to prevent damage to the retina (such as burning of its elements by the sun) by narrowing. When constricted, the small aperture eliminates refractive errors introduced by the peripheral part of the lens and acts to give greater depth of field (as in accommodation to nearby objects).

The retina is like a screen, a film plane where constantly changing images are focused and recorded. If you peeled off the outer opaque layers of the eye (sclera and uvea) as the ancient anatomists did, and looked at the back of the eyeball, you would see on the translucent retina a tiny, inverted image of the visual field.

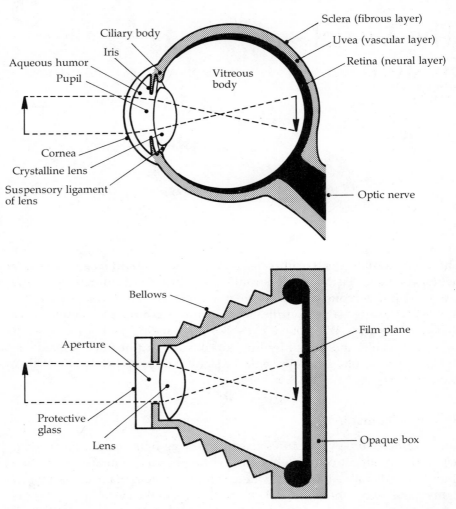

FIG. 5–1. *The eye as a biocamera.* The pupil (aperture) is recessed behind the transparent cornea, which is both protective and refractive in function. Its diameter is regulated by contraction and relaxation of smooth muscle in the iris, effectively changing the "f-stop" with great speed. The lens (like that of a camera) is made up of several elements: the cornea/aqueous humor and crystalline lens provide the major refractive surfaces. Contraction of muscles in the ciliary body, and consequent narrowing of the ciliary ring, reduces the outward pull of the suspensory ligament of the lens, thus allowing the lens to assume greater biconvexity by virtue of its intrinsic viscoelastic properties. The more rounded curvature of the lens enables the eye to focus on near objects; a similar result is obtained in the camera by increasing the bellows-draw. The vitreous body has no refractive power, but plays important supportive and metabolic functions. At the focal or "film" plane of the

But the retina must not be regarded merely as a camera film or photosensitive emulsion, nor the whole eye as a camera. The retina not only receives focused images; as a part of the brain, it starts to interpret them. While such visual interpretation continues progressively in other parts of the brain (thalamus, cerebral cortex, and superior colliculus), the process of feature analysis begins through the activity of large neuronal populations right in the retina, which (by moving the eyes) can be turned to facilitate such analysis.

Retinal Structure

Light falls on the retina, and out the optic nerve comes a torrent of neural activity: a coded pattern or train of action potentials, an electrical abstraction of the image. The retina is unsurpassed in orderliness and complexity of neural organization. It is a multilayered arrangement of specialized cell types (Fig. 5-2). Curiously, the receptor cells (rods and cones) are at the very back of the eye. If one mentally reverses the process of development — the formation of the two-layered optic cup and the involuted neural tube from which it evaginates (see an embryology book) — the original position of these receptor cells is within the sheet of ectoderm that forms the surface of the embryo, a place where photosensitive elements are thought to have arisen in our invertebrate ancestors. To reach this surface once it has been buried during neural tube closure and optic vesicle outgrowth, light must pass through the other elements of the retina (ganglion cells and bipolar cells) before activating the rods and cones.

In man, each eye has approximately 6 million cones and about 120 million rods. The density of receptors is highest in the posterior region of the retina and decreases toward the anterior edge (ora serrata). Cones prevail at the center of the retina, almost exactly in line with the optical axis of the eye, while rods dominate the periphery. In the central retina a tiny depressed region (the fovea) within a yellowish spot (the macula) represents the focal point of the eye and the area of highest visual acuity. The fovea contains only cones, and their density is extraordinary — 150,000 per square millimeter! (A television screen has only about 250,000 independent phosphorescent elements, spread over perhaps a 24-inch screen.)

Rods and cones have complementary properties. Cones have a higher

---

ocular "camera" lies the neural retina, which transduces the visual image, subjects its features to neuronal analysis, and transmits information centrally via the optic nerve. The sclera is comparable to the light-tight box of the camera.

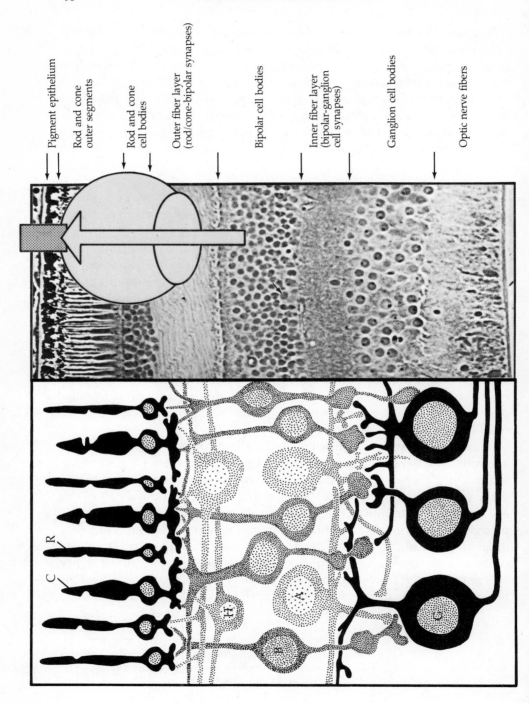

Pigment epithelium

Rod and cone outer segments

Rod and cone cell bodies

Outer fiber layer (rod/cone-bipolar synapses)

Bipolar cell bodies

Inner fiber layer (bipolar-ganglion cell synapses)

Ganglion cell bodies

Optic nerve fibers

threshold, and are stimulated by light of relatively high intensity. They handle sharp vision and color vision in good light. Rods are very sensitive to light, but their resolution is limited and they are insensitive to color; they are receptors for twilight and night vision.

Rods and cones are connected synaptically to long fusiform elements — bipolar cells. These small neurons in turn synapse with larger ones, the retinal ganglion cells, whose axons pass into the optic nerve head (papilla). Thus, retinal circuitry is primarily vertical: receptor cells to bipolar cells to ganglion cells. Integration starts right in the retina, where the approximately 126 million receptor cells converge onto 800,000 to a million ganglion cells.

The retina also has a horizontal organization, in which horizontal cells and amacrine (axonless) cells play additional integrative and sharpening roles that are important for contrast functions (Fig. 5-2). Most laminated structures in the CNS have both vertical and horizontal organizations; certainly the cerebral and cerebellar cortices do. Indeed, the retina is a diencephalic cortex, no less complicated in its intrinsic articulations of neurons than other cortical neuronal assemblies.

Although anatomically similar, the ganglion cells are not all alike. Three major functional types are known: W, X, and Y. The W cells have the slowest conducting axons, and their function remains enigmatic. (In early development, some of them may be direction-selective.) The X cells are "private lines" from the fovea to the lateral geniculate body of the thalamus; they are necessary for high visual acuity. The Y cells seem to be involved with foveation of new visual targets; their axons project to both the lateral geniculate and the optic tectum (superior colliculus). Y cells

---

FIG. 5–2. *Principal layers and cell types of the human retina.* The right-hand panel shows the major layers of cell bodies and fibers of the neural retina as they appear in the light microscope. The left panel shows diagrammatically how the major cellular elements articulate synaptically. The pigment epithelium is the outer light-absorbing and light-reflecting wall of the indented optic cup (see an embryology text). The inner wall of this cup becomes the neural retina, an outward peering and moveable eye of the brain. For orientation with respect to the globe and lens of the eye, see inset at upper right.

Abbreviations for cells: A = amacrine cell (local integrative cell without an axon), B = bipolar cell, C = cone (color photoreceptor cell), G = retinal ganglion cell (with axon passing along anterior surface of retina toward optic nerve), H = horizontal cell (like the amacrine cell, performs intraretinal integrative functions), R = rod ("black-and-white" photoreceptor cell). Arrangement and variety of retinal neurons and receptors greatly oversimplified.

appear and develop later in neurogenesis than the other two types, and are markedly affected by visual deprivation.

These three classes of retinal ganglion cells illustrate an important principle: parallel processing. Whatever their exact contributions to vision are, these groups of neurons obviously represent functionally distinct pathways running in parallel from the retina to other CNS regions. Although their cell bodies are confined to one layer, this lamination does not preclude individual neuronal variation. Each ganglion cell oversees a part of the retinal surface (defined as its receptive field; see below), has an assignment of things to look for (respond to), and must report these events centrally over its particular channel (W, X, or Y).

Receptive Fields

In many sensory networks, such as the retina, the task of reassembling complex stimulus patterns begins at the receptor. Individual rods and cones respond to the wavelength and intensity of light. But these responses are scarcely an image. Such single bits of information must all be put together to create a neural representation of the visual world for the brain to interpret.

What does the retina do with photic stimuli? We saw that there are far fewer ganglion cells than photoreceptor cells, so some convergence of responses must take place. Moreover, we noted that the retina contains horizontal circuitry, as well as vertical linkages, and that different types of ganglion cells respond only to certain stimuli. The response depends on the type of stimulus (form of objects, color, direction of movement, etc.) that falls on their particular area of the retina and the intensity of that stimulus. The term used by neurophysiologists to describe the region of the retina over which a particular stimulus can influence the firing of a single cell is "receptive field." This concept must not be confused with the clinical terms "retinal field" and "visual field," which refer to the retinal surface of one eye and the visual world viewed by the two eyes, respectively (Fig. 5-3).

Retinal receptive fields are fairly simple, at least the common ones are. The most frequently encountered fields are circular, with an excitatory or inhibitory center and a functionally opposed area surrounding it. Thus, when a circular group of photoreceptor cells behind a given ganglion cell is illuminated at its center, the ganglion cell (which is usually active anyway) may increase its rate of firing (an "ON-center" cell). Then, as the spot of light moves to the periphery of this cluster, the ganglion cell reduces its

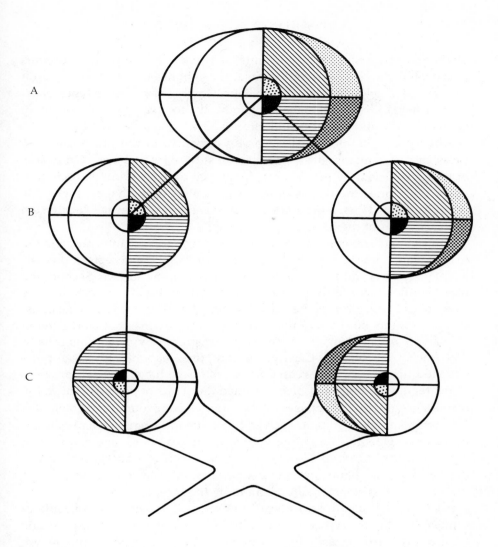

FIG. 5–3. *Visual and retinal fields*. In clinical usage, the term "visual field" usually connotes the binocular field of view of both eyes (A). It is divided into four quadrants with a central area of highest visual acuity demarcated. The binocular visual field consists of two monocular visual fields, the areas seen by the two eyes independently (B). Each of these fields has a monocular crescent laterally that cannot be seen by the other eye because of the presence of the nose. The retinal fields are exact horizontal opposites and vertical inversions of the monocular visual fields (C). Clinicians always describe vision, or the lack of it, in terms of the visual field. To a neurologist, it is what the patient can or cannot see that counts.

discharge frequency ("OFF-surround"). Eventually, when the stimulus falls outside the circular receptive field, the light has no effect whatever on that ganglion cell's normal spontaneous activity. Many other types of receptive fields exist; with some ganglion cells, for example, the center response is OFF and the surround effect is ON.

A receptive field encompasses a very tiny area of the retina (in many cases, less than a pinpoint), so the retinal surface (retinal field) is a mosaic of receptive fields. By means of its frequency coded responses, each ganglion cell informs the brain's other visual centers of the happenings in its receptive field. Thus, a group of retinal cells renders a partially abstracted representation of the image.

Some generalizations can be made about the process of integration in the mammalian retina. First, the neural output from the receptors onward maintains order, and so preserves a spatial map of the surface. Second, the receptive fields are fairly simple, thus providing building blocks for the assembly of more comprehensible images at higher levels — thalamus, cortex, or midbrain. For example, the image of a fly may not be registered by a frog's retinal ganglion cells, but is recognized by certain neurons in that frog's optic tectum. Clearly, the receptive fields of such tectal cells, gathered up from simpler retinal receptive fields, have, through progressive integration of bits and pieces, gained the status of pictures. Third, the unambivalent retinal responses (ON-center, OFF-surround) screen out diffuse or meaningless stimuli, such as those coming from an evenly illuminated area. Flooding the retina with light, for example, has no effect in eliciting center/surround responses, but only increases background activity. On the other hand, providing a pattern will lead to enhancement of that pattern of contrasting illumination by the receptive cells.

Anatomically, as we said above, the retina illustrates the principle of cellular lamination. Why are certain brain cells so neatly ordered? At one level of explanation, lamination is probably the most efficient framework for the development of orderly circuitry: incoming fibers can end in one layer, outgoing axons collect in another, and in still other layers local circuits may prevail. In another sense, lamination offers a suitable plan of organization for progressive analysis, much like a factory assembly line where at each station the end-product is more nearly realized.

The most important answer, however, at least with respect to the human brain, seems to be that lamination is tied to redundancy. In layered arrangements of nerve cells, many parallel circuits perform similar functions, and these circuits can cross-react and progressively integrate sensory or other modes of information.

Whatever its advantages to the nervous system, lamination is a boon to the experimenter. The layered plan makes structures easier to investigate. The various neuronal components (cell bodies, dendrites, specific terminal fields, etc.) are segregated in the various layers, for selective impalement by microelectrodes or regional study under the electron microscope. The presence of sharply defined layers is one of the reasons why the hippocampus and cerebellar cortex have attracted such attention, and why such progress has been made toward understanding their neatly ordered "wiring diagrams."

Central Circuitry

As shown in Figure 5-4, the axons of retinal ganglion cells project to the lateral geniculate body (nucleus), the cells of which in turn project to the primary visual cortex (area 17). This area of cortex sends impulses to other visual cortical areas (18 and 19) for higher visual analysis, as well as to more distant areas of cortex for the integration of vision with other sensory modalities and for the elaboration of complex responses such as speech and writing. It also sends axons back down to the geniculate, presumably for modulating thalamocortical input.

An enormous amount of knowledge has been derived from unit-recording electrophysiological studies (responses of single cells impaled by a microelectrode) on the ways in which simple visual stimuli of various sorts (bars, circles, etc.) are handled at various levels of the system. One principle that has emerged from such studies is that information processing takes place progressively along the visual pathway. Each station (retina, thalamus and/or tectum, cortex) performs specific analytic functions, and at higher levels of organization the responses of groups of cells become more and more general. We do not as yet, however, understand the ultimate transaction—that of visual perception itself.

We can characterize the visual pathway to a large extent as long, private, and precise. It is also partly crossed. We shall examine each of these features and compare the visual and auditory pathways for interesting similarities and differences.

Crossed Connections

As a result of the crossover at the optic chiasm, the visual cortex of each occipital lobe is able to analyze the opposite half of the visual field. The optic nerves enter the cranial vault, exchange fully half their total two

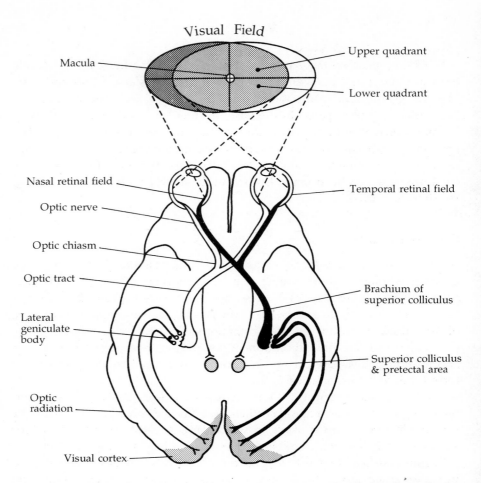

FIG. 5–4. *The monocular visual field as seen by the visual brain.* Axons of retinal ganglion cells collect as an optic nerve, partially cross in the optic chiasm, and continue in the optic tract to the lateral geniculate body, where many of them terminate. Some retinal fibers run through the brachium of the superior colliculus to the superior colliculus and pretectal area. Visual orientation responses, eye movements, and pupillary reflexes depend on these connections. Visual discrimination depends on the geniculate connections, which lead by way of the optic radiation to the visual cortex.

Because of the partial crossing of fibers in the chiasm, information pertaining to events occurring on (for example) the left side of the visual field, and activating the right side of both retinas (shaded nasal and temporal retinal fields of the left and right eyes, respectively), is transmitted to the right cerebral hemisphere. Due to the inverting effect of the lens, the upper quadrants of the visual field are projected through the lower (inferior) parts of the entire visual projection, ultimately to the lower bank of the calcarine fissure. Each half of the tiny but enormously important retinal macula is "blown up" to a huge region of the appropriate occipital pole.

million fibers in the optic chiasm and continue as optic tracts around the cerebral peduncles to the lateral geniculate bodies. (The chiasm, or chiasma, resembles the Greek letter *chi* or *X*, hence the name). By thus combining the corresponding sides of the two retinas, the pathway enables each hemisphere to survey the opposite side of the visual field. Another example of such partial crossing is the outflow of the motor cortex, as we shall describe in Chapter 9.

These crossed visual connections have obvious significance. Combining the congruent halves of what both eyes see on each side of the brain is highly important in integrating visual stimuli: such decussations, as occur at other points along the neuraxis, afford routes that unify CNS activity and thus integrate the body.

In keeping with this principle, fibers from the nasal half of each retina (which looks outward past one's temple) cross, while those from the temporal half (which looks inward toward the nose) stay on the same side. In this way, each side of the brain has a binocular view of the opposite half of the visual field.

Length of Pathway

The visual pathway is clearly one of the longest communications routes in the brain. By sweeping all the way from retina to occiput, it determines one of the two major axes of the brain — the horizontal axis, from front to back. The entire pathway may thus be surveyed in one horizontal plane, as depicted in Figure 5-5. The corticospinal pathway is the other chief axis; it runs vertically through the CNS, from top to bottom. That these two pathways are both so long is of clinical significance and diagnostic value: brain lesions of any appreciable size are almost bound to encroach on one or the other, if not both, and thus result in evident symptoms. To evaluate such disturbances in function and to determine the place of damage, physicians must learn these pathways well. Fortunately, both the visual and corticospinal pathways are laid out in a more or less orderly manner; their retinotopy and somatotopy facilitate location of the pathologic insult (Fig. 5-6).

Privacy of Pathway

Another feature of the visual pathway is its privacy. Except for recently discovered inputs to the hypothalamus that are important to neuroendocrine control mechanisms, few fibers depart from the optic nerve tract or optic radiation. At one point, however, a contingent of axons leaves for the

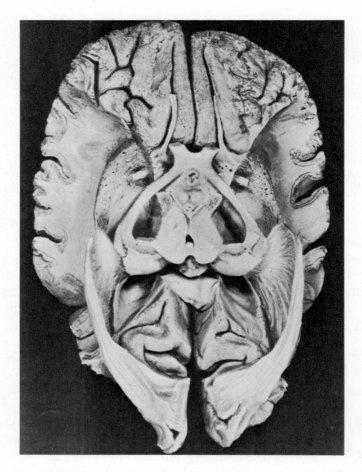

FIG. 5–5. *The visual pathway.* In this beautiful dissection by the late Joseph Klingler, almost the entire visual pathway may be seen at a glance; only the eyes and proximal parts of the optic nerves have been cut away. The optic tracts lead backward from the chiasm toward the lateral geniculate bodies at the extreme lateral margins of the thalamus. From the lateral geniculates, the compact geniculocalcarine tracts abruptly expand into the optic radiations that curve backward toward the occipital poles (see Fig. 5-4 for labels of structures shown). Note Meyer's loop, the part of the radiation that curves anteriorly and inferiorly, then posteriorly through the anterior region of the temporal lobe. The medial geniculate body of the auditory system lies immediately medial to the lateral geniculate, and the pulvinar is the large mass of gray matter at the rear of the thalamus, directly behind both geniculates. Also shown are the olfactory tract and trigone, anterior commissure, infundibulum, mammillary bodies, oculomotor nerves, and a transverse view of the midbrain surmounted by the pineal gland and splenium of the corpus callosum. Can you identify all these important structures? (From E. Ludwig and J. Klingler, *Atlas Cerebri Humani*. Little, Brown and Company, Boston, 1956, plate 61)

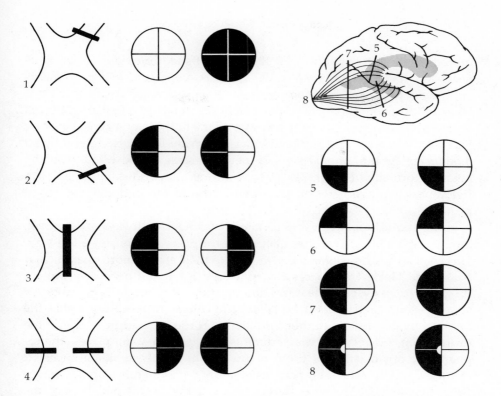

FIG. 5–6. *Anatomical basis of commonly encountered visual field defects.* (1) Right monocular blindness due to transection of right optic nerve. (2) Left homonymous hemianopsia due to section of right optic tract (a lesion destroying the left lateral geniculate body would have a similar result). (3) Bitemporal heteronymous hemianopsia due to encroachment on fibers crossing in the optic chiasm (e.g., by pituitary tumor). (4) Binasal heteronymous hemianopsia from pressure on the edges of the optic chiasm, and hence on the uncrossed fibers (e.g., due to the presence of a carotid aneurysm; rare, and included only for instructional purposes). (5) Left lower homonymous quadrantanopsia due to interruption of fibers in the upper part of the right optic radiation. Because the radiation is much more spread out than the optic tract, such partial homonymous "field cuts" are commonly encountered with cerebral lesions. (6) Left upper homonymous quadrantanopsia due to interruption of fibers in the lower part of the right visual radiation. Defects 5 and 6 illustrate the axiom that "Upper parts of the visual pathway look down, and lower parts look up." (7) Left homonymous hemianopsia due to complete interruption of the right optic radiation as the fibers converge on the occipital pole. As shown, this defect is exactly like number 2, but in practice macular vision is usually spared (see number 8). (8) Left homonymous hemianopsia with macular sparing, owing to incomplete destruction of the extensive territory of occipital polar cortex devoted to analysis of macular vision. (After Maurice W. Van Allen, *Pictorial Manual of Neurologic Tests.* Year Book Medical Publishers, Inc., Chicago, 1969)

pretectal area and superior colliculus. This offshoot provides connections necessary for pupillary and ocular reflexes, conjugate eye movements (both eyes together), and complex behavioral patterns. Thus some optic fibers (Y ganglion cell axons and possibly collaterals of other ganglion cell axons) peel away from the pathway just rostral to the lateral geniculate (see Fig. 5-4). But otherwise the pathway is a private line, lacking any direct monitoring by multimodal sensory neurons such as those found in the reticular formation (Chap. 11). In fact, during a brain dissection, one can freely pass a probe between the optic tract and the underlying cerebral peduncle.

In the auditory pathway and certain somesthetic pathways, by contrast, innumerable fibers leave the main routes at many points along the way. These sensory subsystems seem to handle their affairs more openly, as it were. The "leaks" are necessary, not only for reflex purposes, but for progressive analyses of features (localization of sounds, recognition of stimulus source, etc.) that the cochlear and cutaneous receptors, unlike the retina's brain cells, cannot provide. These departures from the mainstream, however, perhaps diminish, at least in some places, the to-pographic organization of these pathways. In largely avoiding such en-tanglement with other components, the optic nerve enjoys an advantage over the other craniospinal nerves — by being an integral part of the forebrain to begin with.

Precision and Topography of Pathway

The visual pathway is beautifully ordered. "Precision" could be its epi-graph. The retina has "point-to-point" connections to the lateral geniculate nucleus and visual cortex (Fig. 5-7).

We can see this exquisite order if we mentally look back down the path-way from the cortex. Lower parts of the visual cortex (inferior bank of the calcarine sulcus) survey the upper half of the visual field, and hence "look up." Upper parts (superior bank) "look down." Because of the partial decussation at the chiasm, the entire right field of vision is projected as a map of two combined retinal halves (one from each eye) upon the left hemisphere, and vice-versa. Note in Figure 5-7 that the map of the retina twists and turns somewhat as it passes inward through the optic pathway. For example, it is the lateral (not the lower) part of the geniculate that surveys the upper half of the visual field, and the medial (not the upper) part of this nucleus that "looks down."

Moreover, retinal regions important to visual acuity occupy an increas-

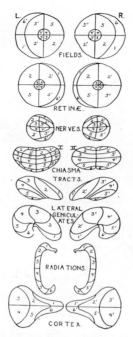

FIG. 5–7. *The retinotopy of visual projections.* Due to the partial crossing at the optic chiasm, fibers from the nasal halves of the retina (temporal parts of the visual field) cross and project to specific regions of the contralateral geniculate, whereas those from the temporal halves (nasal parts of the visual field) remain uncrossed as they proceed to those same regions (follow the numbers on the illustration). The lateral geniculate, in turn, projects in a similar orderly manner through the optic radiation to the cerebral cortex. (From W. J. S. Krieg, *Functional Neuroanatomy*, 3rd ed. Brain Books, Evanston, Ill., 1966, p. 202)

ing proportion of the pathway. The amount of cortex devoted to macular vision represents almost the entire occipital pole, even though the macula itself is a mere spot upon the retina (Fig. 5-8). In contrast, the cortex devoted to peripheral vision (including the monocular crescents) is restricted to the banks of the calcarine fissure, even though peripheral vision is mediated by most of the photosensitive surface of the retina, right out to its edge (ora serrata).

This neural magnification of the macula illustrates an extremely important principle of brain organization: the amount of feature-analyzing region of the brain devoted to a receptive surface of the body is proportional to the sensory importance of that surface, not to its area. In central neural analyzers, like the lateral geniculate nucleus or visual cortex, it is the sensory

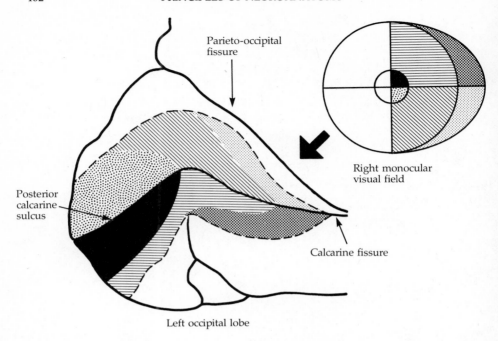

Parieto-occipital
fissure

Right monocular
visual field

Posterior
calcarine
sulcus

Calcarine fissure

Left occipital lobe

FIG. 5–8. *Cortical retinotopy.* Right monocular visual field (that is seen by the right eye) as mapped on the visual cortex in the left occipital lobe of the human cerebrum. Note extensive territory allotted the macula, retinal area of keenest vision. Peripheral regions of retina are represented to far less extent along the upper and lower banks of the calcarine fissure. Also note inversion of quadrants and anteriorly represented monocular crescent. (Redrawn from G. Holmes, 1951 in *The Self and Its Brain*, by K. R. Popper and J. C. Eccles. Springer International, 1977)

value (not the size) of a body part that counts. Thus, surprisingly large lesions of the occipital lobes may not abolish effective vision as long as central vision is spared — which it often is, a phenomenon called "macular sparing" (see Fig. 5-6 legend).

This centrally preserved retinotopy is more pronounced than the tonotopy of the auditory path. Anatomically, the difference is quite apparent, especially if one compares the respective geniculate bodies of the visual and auditory subsystems under a microscope. The lateral geniculate body has a more distinct arrangement of neurons than the medial geniculate, and is really a kind of thalamic cortex. It has six definite cell layers, with respect to which there are evident constraints on incoming retinal fibers. Fibers from X ganglion cells on the same side are directed to certain layers (2, 3, and 5) and to those only, while fibers from X cells of the opposite eye go to certain other layers (1, 4, and 6). Furthermore, compounding the complexity, the axons of W and Y retinal ganglion cells each seem to have quite different laminar distributions, based on recent studies in experimental animals. In contrast to the almost wandering appearance of afferents in some brain regions (such as the brainstem reticular formation), incoming fibers show an obviously formal distribution in the highly ordered edifice of the lateral geniculate.

Columnar Organization of Visual Cortex

Like the lateral geniculate, the visual cortex is itself laminated. It consists of six layers of specialized neurons, designated (from the surface down) by Roman numerals, I to VI. These layers are distinguished by the organization and types of neurons they contain, as well as by the presence of other neuronal elements. For example, the dendrites of the cells in one layer may extend upward, beyond the confines of their own layer and into one or more overlying layers. In a cortex, each layer of neurons obviously receives a different mix of inputs and, less obviously but nonetheless true, each layer projects to a different combination of targets.

Geniculate fibers connect only to small cortical pyramidal and stellate cells in layer IV. From that port of entry to the cortex, the connections are arranged in a vertical mode, as they seem to be in all areas of the cerebral cortex. This unit of cortical organization is called a "functional column." The various pyramidal and stellate cells are intimately interconnected within the confines of such a column.

Two important types of columns are ocular dominance columns (in which a particular region of one retina is studied) and orientation columns (in which a particular stimulus orientation is analyzed). These columns are shown in Figure 5-9. When plotted on a map of visual cortex, such columns have a striped or swirled appearance in surface view. It is generally believed that ocular dominance and orientation columns overlap and mix in some way to form a basic module of visual analysis called a hypercolumn: a small, vertical cylinder of gray matter (about one square millimeter) that receives input from a point on the retina and has all the essential neural machinery to reassemble ocular dominance and orientation features of the image.

There is more, however, than cortical columns to this interdigitating order. Each neuron of the visual system is most sensitive to a particular kind or configuration of visual stimulus: onset or cessation of illumination, concentric rings of different colors, a straight bar of special length and

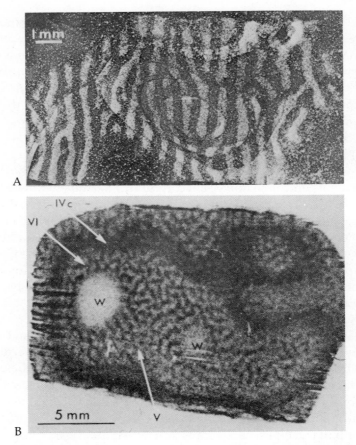

FIG. 5–9. *Ocular dominance and orientation columns.* (A) Ocular dominance columns, in which a particular region of the retina of one eye is represented, are shown by autoradiographic techniques that demonstrate the passage of radioactive protein synthesized from amino acid precursors injected into the contralateral eye. If sufficient amounts are injected, some label is transported transynaptically into lateral geniculate neurons and on up to the cortex, as shown in this horizontal slice, tangential to layer IV.
(B) Orientation columns, in which a particular stimulus orientation is analyzed, are demonstrated by the 2-deoxyglucose technique. This glucose analogue accumulates in the metabolically active neurons. In this case, the neurons had been subjected to the effects of prolonged presentation of a stimulus of a given orientation. The letters and Roman numerals indicate the structures through which this horizontal slice passes, i.e., IVc, V, and VI are the deeper cortical layers and W is the underlying white matter. (A, from D. H. Hubel, T. N. Wiesel, and S. LeVay, *Philos. Trans. R. Soc. Lond.*, Ser. B. *278*: 377-409, 1977; B, from D. H. Hubel, T. N. Wiesel, and M. P. Stryker, *Nature (London) 269*: 328-330, 1977)

width tipped at a certain angle and moving in a given direction, etc. At retinal and geniculate levels of analysis, receptive fields are small, circular spots. The distinguishing feature of cortical neurons is their orientation selectivity. A bar or edge of light must be at a particular angle to get a good response. In fact, certain cortical cells in layer IV respond to simple shapes of objects visualized, as long as these objects are oriented in a particular way. This orientation preference is retained in neurons of other layers in that column.

Thus, the visual cortex illustrates the key principle of neural teamwork — essentially modular organization. In many systems in the brain, cells participating in a given task are grouped together in vertical or horizontal columns, or some other form, such as a cell cluster. The components of some modules may be widely separated, thus constituting a "distributed system" that may include cerebral and spinal team members. In a sense, we are beginning to see some weakening of the neuron doctrine here: a single neuron is not so much a basic functional unit as the group is.

In the visual system, the prerequisites for cell response become more and more complex as information flashes from retina to geniculate to cortex. And in secondary and higher-order visual cortex (see Chap. 13), the feature extraction becomes even more comprehensive. Somewhere a great distance from area 17, there may be, as some have speculated, a cell that will respond to the sight of a particular object — a hairbrush, perhaps a hand, even (as has been suggested) one's grandmother!

Eye Movements

Our eyes, and hence our retinal brain stalks, are always moving about, taking in the world. We follow objects, scan scenes, and study things at will through coordinated eye movements.

In fact, we must keep our eyes moving to permit continued image analysis; an immobile pair of eyes leads quickly (for reasons we don't have time to go into) to fatigue of sensory processing. The complete circuitry underlying eye movement is not yet known in detail. It is clear, however, that there are complex well-defined circuits, involving both the cerebral cortex and the brainstem, which are distinct from those participating in normal pattern recognition.

Some of the connections involved in eye movements are illustrated in Figure 5-10. As previously mentioned, the axon of a Y ganglion cell branches, and one branch goes to the superior colliculus where it terminates in its proper place on a retinotopic map. Some of the fibers leaving

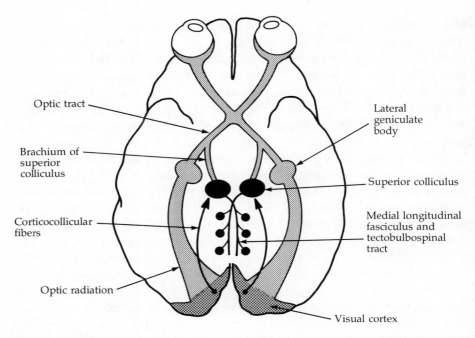

FIG. 5–10. *Connections involved in eye movements.* Certain retinal ganglion neurons (Y cells) send their axons through the brachium (arm) of the superior colliculus into that tectal structure, a complex many-layered cortex in the roof of the midbrain. Axons of collicular cells pass into the medial longitudinal fasciculus and also into the contralateral tectobulbospinal tract to brainstem and spinal motor nuclei mediating eye and head movements, as well as postural adjustments (connections highly oversimplified in figure). Corticocollicular fibers provide additional control over these movements and over reflex adjustments to visual input.

the colliculus lead (through the medial longitudinal fasciculus and the underlying tectobulbospinal tract) to those brainstem and spinal nuclei (oculomotor, trochlear, abducens, spinal accessory, cervical motor cell clusters, etc.) concerned with eye movements, head orientation, and postural adjustments. The superior colliculus also receives inputs from the visual cortex. Thus the colliculus receives direct visual information, as well as highly abstracted and well-processed information from the cortex. Moreover, it reports up and back to the visual cortex, through a thalamic "tectal recipient zone" that includes the lateral posterior (LP) nucleus.

   Some movements of the eyes are reflexly controlled by movements of the head, so as to maintain foveation, to "keep the eyes on target." As the head turns sideways, the vestibular ocular reflex (VOR) brings about movement of the eyes in the opposite direction so that gaze remains fixed, at least for a moment (see also Chap. 4). Eye position then is reset "straight-ahead" by a rapid eye movement, a saccade. This is the fastest movement in the body.

Pupillary Responses to Light

The instant and normally invariant response of the pupil to light is a marvelous safety and regulatory feature of the visual system, and as such is one of the body's vital signs. It is of cardinal importance to the protection and proper function of the sensitive retina, as well as of great diagnostic value to the clinician. When a beam of bright light shines directly into the eye, the pupil constricts, due to contraction of circumferentially arranged smooth muscle fibers in the iris. The response occurs in both eyes, even though only one eye may have been illuminated.

Such bilateral pupillary responses are reflexes — completely automatic (involuntary and unconscious) as well as swift. They are mediated by midbrain structures, specifically by neurons in the pretectal area in front of the superior colliculus, and do not involve the participation of thalamus and cortex, at least not directly. Recent studies, however, demonstrate numerous connections from the pretectal area to the pulvinar of the thalamus, hence mesencephalic information concerned with pretectal mediation of eye movement does appear to reach cortex. These bilateral ocular reflexes depend on the integrity of an essentially four-neuron arc (Fig. 5-11): retinal ganglion cell (type Y?), pretectal cell, pupillomotor cell in the Edinger-Westphal nucleus of the oculomotor nuclear complex, and postganglionic parasympathetic neuron in the ciliary ganglion.

The pupillary response to light is consensual (takes place in the nonilluminated eye) as well as direct (occurs in the illuminated eye) for three reasons: (1) some retinal fibers involved cross in the optic chiasm, (2) the two halves of the pretectal area richly interconnect through the posterior commissure (as shown in the figure), and (3) the pretectal efferent fibers are distributed to both pupillomotor clusters of neurons, the nuclei of Edinger-Westphal in the oculomotor complex (again, as indicated in figure).

Dilation of the pupil in the absence of light or for other reasons (such as fear or anger) is effected by a different reflex arc involving descending sympathetic fibers in the brainstem that synapse with sympathetic preganglionic neurons in the lower cervical and upper thoracic levels of the cord. Axons of these cells pass into the sympathetic chain to postganglionic sympathetic neurons, the efferent processes of which in turn travel along

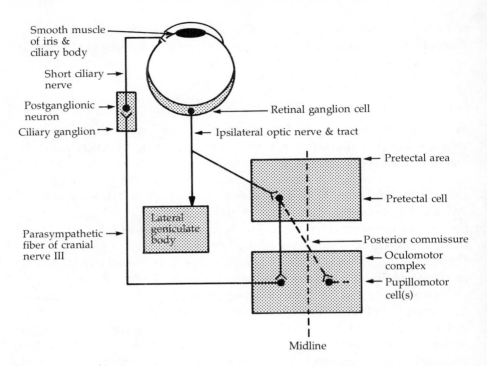

Smooth muscle of iris & ciliary body

Short ciliary nerve

Postganglionic neuron

Ciliary ganglion

Retinal ganglion cell

Ipsilateral optic nerve & tract

Pretectal area

Pretectal cell

Lateral geniculate body

Parasympathetic fiber of cranial nerve III

Posterior commissure

Oculomotor complex

Pupillomotor cell(s)

Midline

FIG. 5–11. *Pupillary responses to light and accommodation.* (1) The first neuron in the light reflex is a retinal ganglion cell (Y type?); its axon passes through the optic nerve and tract to the pretectal area (rostral to the superior colliculus) on the same or opposite side, depending on whether the fiber crosses in the optic chiasm. (2) The second neuron is a pretectal cell which sends its axon into the underlying oculomotor nuclear complex, again on the same or opposite side depending on whether the fiber crosses in the posterior commissure. (3) The third neuron is a pupillomotor cell, a tiny visceral motor neuron found in certain parts of the oculomotor complex; collectively such cells comprise the accessory oculomotor nucleus, or nucleus of Edinger-Westphal. The slender, lightly myelinated axon of this preganglionic parasympathetic neuron travels to the rear of the eyeball through cranial nerve III and synapses upon a postganglionic nerve cell body in the ciliary ganglion. (4) This fourth neuron innervates, by way of a short ciliary nerve, the iridial constrictor and ciliary musculature.

The pupillary response to accommodation involves three of the same levels of neurons, specifically levels (1), (3), and (4). It is, however, a longer and more complex route, with added connections lying between levels (1) and (3). The axons of retinal ganglion cells pass to the lateral geniculate, and from there impulses proceed to visual cortex and thence back down to superior colliculus (not to the pretectal area). From the colliculus, fibers go to the Edinger-Westphal nucleus, and from there on the circuit is the same.

branches of the internal carotid artery to the radially arranged dilator muscles of the iris.

Pupillary Responses in Accommodation to Near Objects

Closely related to, yet distinctly different from, the pupillary light reflexes are the adjustments in the size of the pupil and curvature of the lens necessary to bring a nearby object into focus. These adjustments comprise the accommodation reflex. Although this arc involves some of the same neurons (retinal ganglion cells, neurons of the Edinger-Westphal nuclei, and ciliary ganglion cells) as the pupillary reflex to light, it is a longer, more complex route, involving first the thalamus (lateral geniculate nucleus), next the visual cortex, and then the superior colliculus, instead of the pretectal area. And although it is a largely involuntary and unconscious response, a person can exercise some control over it in selecting the object for visual study.

Over this long route the pupillary aperture can be narrowed, through action of the circular constrictor muscles in the iris, thus eliminating peripheral lens aberrations and enhancing depth of field. Simultaneously, the biconvex, viscoelastic lens rounds up to increase its curvature and refractive power. How is this greater convexity accomplished? Through contraction of the ciliary muscle, which pulls forward, and consequently closes, the ring of suspensory fibers that reach from the ciliary processes to the margin of the lens, thus allowing the latter to assume a more rounded shape. Both of these adjustments — "stopping down" the aperture and focusing the lens — are necessary to focus nearby objects on the retina, just as similar adjustments in f-stop and lens extension are made when a camera is used for close-up shots.

Adaptability and Plasticity

An Interdependent Hierarchy

So much visual analysis takes place in the occipital cortex that a person is virtually blind after its destruction or removal. With smaller lesions of visual cortex, clearly definable blind spots (scotomata) result. Such deficits would be noted by a neurologist, but the person affected is often unaware of them. Such a curious lack of self-recognition of serious sensory loss illustrates the interdependent hierarchy of associated functions in the

CNS. Seeing is one thing, recognizing what we see (or don't see, as with injury to the visual cortex) is another.

The lack of awareness of serious sensory loss, however, is also due to a remarkable compensatory capacity of our nervous system. The brain seems to be able to "fill in" patches of missing sight, even if "holes" or scotomata in the visual field are demonstrable by clinical testing. Such restorative capacities may derive from resynthesizing neural patterns from incomplete information, pressing little-used pathways into full service, and/or reorganizing damaged pathways through axon sprouting to replace lost connections or modify residual connections.

Pupillary and ocular reflexes are little affected by lesions of visual cortex. Other responses, however, such as orientation of the eyes and head to sources of illumination, may be altered to varying extents. These functions are associated with the less recently evolved optic tectum — the superior colliculus and pretectal area of the mesencephalon. A contemporary interpretation is that the optic tectum and visual neocortex discharge two different tasks: the tectum is concerned with the chiefly automatic localization and tracking of visual targets, while the cortex analyzes and interprets features, ultimately in man at the conscious level. Through newly discovered connections in the posterior thalamus (pulvinar and LP), tectal activity reaches cortex, and thus the two major analyzers of the visual subsystem — optic tectum and visual cortex — work in a unified manner.

In nonmammalian vertebrates, the tectum apparently must perform both functions, because these animals have almost no cortex as we know it, with most of the forebrain made up of basal ganglia. But they often have an enormous tectum, as is most evident in birds of prey. In mammals, a division of labor seems to have taken place, although, as we have mentioned, close communication between tectum and cortex is established through the intervening thalamic tectal recipient zone.

Such evolutionary changes, though hard to trace, are an extraordinary expression of biologic adaptability in the nervous system. They put "old" structures to "new" uses, and while the original connections of these structures are discernible, the greater number of acquired connections attests that little of the original function for these parts remains.

Developmental Plasticity

From a few cells in the embryo, intricate and precise circuitry rapidly takes shape in each new person: newly germinated neurons glide into position along glial guiderails, differentiate in myriad spidery configurations, and make connections, sometimes at a great distance, point-to-point. . . . Many factors combine to build our visual brain. Some come from the archives of the genes, others from forces created by the developing brain itself, and still others from the environment, which models and refines the youthful substance of the growing brain.

However much is genetically determined, the mature visual system is clearly also a product of its early experience, and the visual cortex is the most plastic part. Abnormal visual experience during certain periods early in life can have profound and permanent effects on neurons in the visual cortex. Whatever these abnormal experiences, experiments indicate that the effects are exerted on two basic parameters: ocular dominance columns and orientation columns. For example, depriving one eye of light disturbs the development of orientation columns in the cat's visual cortex. Or, if environmental stimuli are restricted to stripes of one orientation, fewer cortical cells will respond to other orientations, thus changing the composition of orientation columns. This modifiability seems limited to a period of a few weeks early in life, the so-called "critical period." Similar critical periods during development probably exist to some degree for all neural subsystems.

In the developing visual system, much of the circuitry is laid down before birth, with its normal development depending on early experience for enforcement. Ocular dominance columns, for example, are not present from the start, but segregate from a mixture of thalamocortical fibers. Balanced binocular experience is necessary for their normal maturation. Deprivation of one eye puts it at a competitive disadvantage, and its columns fail to develop their normal width, as we just said. It has been proposed that this early plasticity may be necessary to bring cortical circuitry up to the level of precision needed for accurate binocular interactions, as for example in depth perception. In this way, experience seems to provide the ultimate fine tuning.

There are currently two conflicting schools of thought about plasticity in the visual system. One school postulates an innate catalog of patterned circuits from which visual experience selects appropriate connections and erases inappropriate ones. Normal experience brings out the full built-in potential of the system, whereas abnormal and/or deprived experience does not. The other school says that experience, of whatever kind, is the key thing, with the intrinsic circuits poorly defined. For this group, visual experience pressures and forces cells to make connections most representative of that experience, drawing out a plan where little plan previously existed. Only time will tell which school is right, but the first enjoys more favor.

In addition to its adaptability in the course of a lifetime and in the evolution of biologic structure over generations, neuronal circuitry is plastic in another sense: it is self-repairing after injury. Such repair can occur through axon sprouting over short (not long) distances to effect local restitution of some connections, and by reoccupation of vacated synaptic sites. The capacity for such self-repair seems to vary with the part of the nervous system involved, and in some instances the re-established connections are ones that do not exist in the normal brain and are therefore maladaptive in function.

General Concepts

The visual system illustrates many key principles of brain organization: crossed transactions that act to unify the body and integrate environmental stimuli; long-distance, secure, and orderly lines over which to transmit detailed reports of sensory events; delegated assignments and specialized neurons to discharge them; distorted projections to magnify important sensory surfaces (the macular region of the retina); interdependent but hierarchical levels of feature analysis; developmental plasticity and flexibility, to meet challenges from moment to moment and to adapt continually and frugally in the continuing process of evolution.

Glossary

Amacrine cells: small, axonless neurons of the retina located within and anterior to the bipolar cell layer; more generally, any axonless neuron (e.g., retinal, olfactory, etc.).

Bipolar cells: one of the three major classes of retinal neurons; interposed between the rods and cones (receptor elements) and the retinal ganglion cells.

Calcarine fissure: a prominent fissure in the occipital lobe; along its upper and lower banks lies the primary visual cortex.

Ciliary ganglion: a parasympathetic ganglion just posterior to the globe of the eye, involved in the control of pupillary diameter; innervates iridial constrictor and ciliary smooth musculature.

Cones: receptor cells of the retina that respond to colors in good light; in man and primates, concentrated in the fovea centralis.

Edinger-Westphal nucleus: the accessory oculomotor nucleus of the mesencephalic brainstem; its preganglionic parasympathetic neurons act, via postganglionic neurons in the ciliary ganglion, to constrict the pupil and increase lens convexity.

Fovea centralis: a depressed area or pit near the center of the retina, within a yellowish cone-rich patch, the macula lutea.

Ganglion cells: the output cells of the retina, projecting to the thalamic lateral geniculate body and mesencephalic tectum; there are at least three types (W, X, and Y).

Lateral geniculate body: a grossly visible, prominently laminated nucleus of the thalamus; receives input from the retinal ganglion cells and projects to visual cortex.

Layer IV: the layer of visual cortex which receives input from the lateral geniculate body; displays a dense population of small, dustlike neurons (stellate cells; see Chap. 13).

Lens: a transparent, flexible member of the dioptric media of the eye; serves to adjust focus by changing shape, becoming more curved for near objects and flatter for far ones.

Macula lutea: a yellow, pigmented (rich in carotene) region at the bottom of the fovea, where the retinal ganglion cells and bipolar neurons are offset to uncover a patch of pure cones; the region of maximal visual acuity and resolution.

Ocular dominance columns: tiny cylindrical modules (about 30 μm diameter) of neurons in the visual cortex in which a particular region of the retina in one eye is represented.

Optic chiasm: the place of crossing (decussation) of half of the fibers of each optic nerve at the base of the diencephalon; combines information from homonymous parts of both retinas for transmission to each side of the brain.

Optic nerve: the massive bundle (over a million fibers) of retinal ganglion cell axons leading from the eye to the optic chiasm.

Optic radiation: a broad fan of fibers projecting topographically between the lateral geniculate and visual cortex.

Optic tract: that part of the visual pathway between the optic chiasm and lateral geniculate body; differs from optic nerve only in that it contains axons of ganglion cells in homonymous parts of the two retinas.

Orientation columns: similar to ocular dominance columns (see above), except that in these functional modules of visual cortex the orientation of a particular stimulus, like a tilted line, is analyzed.

Pretectal area: a region between the superior colliculus and the thalamus; important to visual motor responses, e.g., pupillary constriction, accommodation, etc.

Primary visual cortex: the occipital cortex on the upper and lower banks of the calcarine fissure; Brodmann's area 17 (see Chap. 13).

Pupil: a round aperture in the center of the iris; under autonomic control (cervical sympathetic and oculomotor nerves), it opens and closes like a diaphragm to control the amount of light entering the eye.

Retina: the innermost layer of the three-layered eye; includes the neural retina, composed primarily of four major cell types (rods, cones, bipolar neurons, ganglion cells) organized in discrete sublayers.

Rods: photoreceptor cells of the retina which respond best in dim light intensity, but not to colors.

Sclera: the outermost, tough connective-tissue coat of the eye; in the cornea, at the anterior pole of the eye, its arrays of collagen fibers and degree of hydration are specialized to provide transparency.

Superior colliculus: a tectal area receiving retinal input and connecting to brainstem and spinal motor nuclei, as well as back to visual cortex via thalamus; important center for control of eye movement.

Uvea: the choroid coat, or intermediate, vascular layer of the eye, vital to the nourishment of the highly active retina.

The Somesthetic System

6

Acoustic, visual, and olfactory stimuli come to their appropriate "distance" receptors after passage through space. In contrast, body sensations arise from changes in the mechanical or thermal energy states impinging on or originating in the body itself. This incessant rain of stimuli falling on the body and ceaseless welling up of events inside it pose immense tasks of detection, analysis, and synthesis for the nervous system. The peripheral nervous system is responsible for the detection, through a wide variety of specialized, ingenious, and virtually ubiquitous receptors. The central nervous system carries out the analysis and synthesis of detected stimuli into patterns of meaningful happenings, and keeps adequate records for subsequent retrieval and comparative study. Other sensory systems have similar functions, but the somesthetic system must monitor a tremendous range of stimuli coming in all over the body from all directions. Clearly, "touch" — the word used in the age-old list of "five" senses — is an inadequate label for the system's contribution to sensory perception.

Attributes of Somatic Sensation

A bodily sensation, like any other sensation, has several dimensions or attributes. One is quality, the ensuing subjective experience that enables us to call it touch, warmth, or cold and so forth. Another is intensity; without some finite strength a stimulus will not exceed a subjective threshold and no sensation will occur, while with rising stimulus intensity the sensation increases until in some cases its quality changes to painful. A third parameter is location; a sensation is referred to some part of the body or region of

115

the external environment. The affect of a sensation — whether pleasant or unpleasant — is a fourth and important attribute that involves somewhat different neural mechanisms than those used to analyze the other three. Evidence in support of this statement comes from the clinical evaluation of individuals with certain neurologic disorders, in which affective feelings normally associated with a given stimulus may become much more intense and disagreeable (dysesthesia), or perhaps changed in character (paresthesia), while appreciation of other attributes normally associated with that stimulus is diminished or possibly unchanged.

Cutaneous, Deep, and Visceral Sensations

Light touch (like that of cotton wool) is a familiar intensity and quality of external, or cutaneous, sensation. Pain, warmth, and cold are others. The changes in ambient energy levels — the stimuli — producing these sensations affect the skin, especially the outer dermis as well as the epidermis. Certain sensations, however, arise more deeply: pressure, vibration, sense of position or movement of body parts, judgments of weight, shape, and form of objects, deep pain. All these, and more, are mediated by the somesthetic system.

Internal sensations, from the viscera, also lie in the domain of the somesthetic system. These deep sensations are obviously important to that visceral effector agency traditionally, but unrealistically, treated separately as the "autonomic" nervous system. Visceral sensations are frequently hard to verbalize (a "burning feeling") and are difficult to locate precisely ("somewhere about here"). They are usually unpleasant, and whether describable or not are difficult to ignore: the need to urinate, the pangs of hunger, the discomfort of visceral distention, cramps, nausea. . . . No news is generally good news where our viscera are concerned!

Although recognized scientifically as well as in everyday life, these many bodily sensations have not received as much anatomical and physiological study as vision and hearing. Cutaneous sensation, in fact, has been called a "poor cousin" in this respect. One category of somatic sensory input, however, has been investigated extensively; for want of a more appropriate term, it may be called "muscle sense."

Muscle Afferent System

In the strict interpretation, muscle sense is not a true sensation — a consciously experienced quality of bodily sensation complete with attributes of intensity, locale-reference, and affect. Instead, it is a key part of a chiefly unconscious motor servomechanism. The input comes from stretch receptors in skeletal muscles (muscle spindles) and from tension-sensing devices in the tendons (Golgi tendon organs). It is very important in reflex and higher levels of motor control; it affords moment-by-moment reports on the status of the skeletomuscular "riggings" of the body.

Recent studies indicate that some of this information eventually reaches the thalamus and then the cerebral cortex, as occurs with visual, acoustic, or other modalities of sensation. Such forebrain connections are probably important to our sensations of muscular effort and strain. Most of the incessant signals from muscles and tendons, however, flow into reflex channels within the spinal cord or along various clearly defined routes to the cerebellum. These pathways provide a massive and highly ordered feedback system that regulates the activity of motor neurons and of related command neurons at higher levels of the neuraxis.

Receptors

How does the nervous system detect and report the innumerable changes in the wide spectrum of energy around and within the body? By transduction of these stimuli into nerve impulses, a familiar concept by now. Specialized receptors — miniature transducers — convert the flux, or sometimes steady state, of a vast range of mechanical and thermal forms of energy into electrical potentials that in turn trigger action potentials. Although the structure and mode of operation of these receptors vary widely, all such efficient sensory devices serve the fundamental purpose of gathering information.

Components of Receptors

A receptor always includes the peripheral or distal ending of a primary sensory neuron and frequently also incorporates modified epithelial cells that participate in the receptor function. These associated "sense" cells are not true neurons or excitable elements in themselves; they cannot propagate action potentials. Instead, they modulate, amplify, or otherwise help to generate the trains of nerve impulses in the sensory processes ramifying amongst them. The auditory and vestibular hair cells are examples. They interact with, and pass their electrical perturbations to, the endings of the first-order neurons: the bipolar cells of the spiral and vestibular ganglia.

Encapsulated, Expanded-tip, and Free Nerve Endings

Some somesthetic receptors (Fig. 6-1) include a group of such modified non-nervous cells spatially organized so as to encapsulate the peripheral axon terminal (Meissner's and Pacinian corpuscles are examples). Others show terminal specializations of the axon itself — endings with expanded tips (Merkel's discs and Ruffini's endings). Still others appear quite simple: tiny, tapering, unmyelinated axonal branches or endings found throughout both layers of the dermis and also in the epidermis, where they penetrate the basal lamina and extend almost to the cornified layer. These "free nerve endings" are the most widely distributed receptors in the body. The richest variety of encapsulated endings, in contrast, is found mainly in deep regions: the inner dermis, fasciae, and mesenteries.

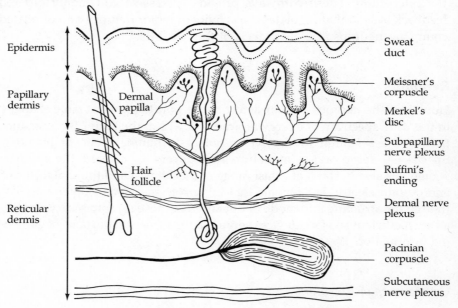

FIG. 6–1. *Examples of somesthetic receptors.* Section of hairy (left) and glabrous (nonhairy, right) skin cut transversely across papillary ridges. Meissner's corpuscles occupy uppermost layers of the skin in the papillary dermis. Merkel's discs also lie primarily there, while Pacinian corpuscles lie in the deep dermis or subcutaneous tissue. Ruffini's corpuscles are less well defined, and may appear at any place in dermis. Hair follicles have receptors which are free nerve endings. (Modified from M. E. Jabaley, in *Medical Physiology*, Vol. One, V. B. Mountcastle, ed. Mosby, St. Louis, p. 299, 1974)

Modality Specificity

In the past, the fashion was to match the various encapsulated endings, endings with expanded tips, and free endings with specific primary qualities of sensation, such as deep pressure, light touch, heat, cold, and pain, etc. We now know, however, that all these qualities may derive from regions of skin containing only fine, unmyelinated nerve fibers and free nerve endings. While the mechanism of differential (or at least preferential) sensitivity of different nerve fibers to mechanical, thermal, or noxious stimuli is not understood, it seems to be a property of the axon terminal itself.

It has long been believed that the distinctive corpuscles or lamellated structures which encapsulate certain nerve endings are associated with mechanoreceptive afferents. Such an encapsulation, however, does not seem to determine mode specificity, but rather to modify the discharge of the sensory nerve fiber inside: the firing rate will vary with different degrees of deformation of the fluid-filled, turgid, and almost incompressible surrounding mass of cells. This seems to set the selective and dynamic sensitivity of the ending — its lowered threshold of response to certain temporal stimulus parameters and its speed of accommodation (slowly-adapting, fast-adapting).

Speed of adaptation is important to signaling the displacement and time parameters of physical stimuli. The distinctly lamellated Pacinian corpuscle is an example. It responds best to accelerating mechanical displacement with respect to time (ramp stimuli), not to uniform velocity displacements. In man, Pacinian corpuscles are known to subserve high-frequency vibration sense in the skin.

Thus, the specific sensitivity of a sensory nerve fiber to a particular form of stimulus is considered an intrinsic property of the fiber, not of its capsular adornment. In turn, the specific quality of sensation experienced in a body region under a given set of conditions is thought to be built up from the activity of groups of modality labeled sensory fibers differing in their dynamic sensitivities and central connections. Our sensations emerge from central elaboration, at various hierarchical levels from spinal cord to cerebral cortex, of patterned activity in many overlapping, mode-specific mosaics of nerve endings in the skin and hypodermis. Each peripheral mosaic signals its own preferred type of stimulus. In such signaling, several means of encoding are postulated: a simple "on-off" signal for transient events, a periodic burst of spikes for stimulus frequency, a rate or frequency code for stimulus intensity, and other codes for movement, direction, speed, and configuration of stimulus, etc.

Distribution of Receptors

Whatever their form and however they encode activity for transmission centrally, receptors are sprinkled in greater or lesser density throughout the body, not merely in the skin. In fact, they are found almost everywhere except in the nervous system itself. And even though the CNS is insensitive, numerous receptors are found in the meninges and along the intracranial blood vessels. Furthermore, in certain parts of the CNS (notably the hypothalamus and adjoining regions), specialized neurons and attending structures act as sensors of the internal milieu of the body, monitoring blood sugar, fluid and electrolyte content, circulating hormones, body temperature, and so forth. Conventionally, such central sensing devices are not classified as receptors, but they serve no less the purpose of gathering information. We also know that receptors of another description exist throughout the CNS, keeping track of and responding to amounts of chemical substances in the neuraxis itself: catecholamines, amino acids, peptides, opiate or morphinelike compounds, and so forth. We will discuss such intraneural receptors, which are really specialized regions on and beneath the postsynaptic membranes of nerve cells, in relation to pain transmission below and also in Chapter 14.

Classification of Receptors

Because of their structural variety, differential distribution, and mode specificity, receptors are classified in three main ways. Structurally, there are the free, expanded-tip, and encapsulated endings just described. Topographically, exteroceptors serve the body surface, interoceptors the viscera, and proprioceptors the muscles, tendons, and joints. ("Proprio-" means "its own," in this case the body's own; such receptors are thus those activated primarily by movement or action of the organism itself.) Functionally, receptors are given prefixes to indicate the form of energy to which they preferentially (at the lowest stimulus intensity) respond, i.e., to show "what turns them on." Thus, there are mechanoreceptors, thermoreceptors, photoreceptors, chemoreceptors — even, as we saw in the vestibular system, gravireceptors (or graviceptors, for short). And we must not forget nociceptors: this collective term embraces all receptors which respond, either preferentially or at sufficient stimulus intensity, to painful stimuli (mechanical and thermal) and concomitant products of cell injury and tissue destruction.

Role and Mode of Action of Receptors

Receptors, as we said, detect and monitor the energy constantly flowing and ebbing around and through the body. They respond chiefly, but not exclusively, to changes in this flow. Exceptions include certain mechanoreceptive afferents that continue to signal maintained deformation of the skin.

The initial results of stimulus transduction are local electrical events called generator potentials. Such stimulus-evoked potentials occur in the distal terminal ramifications of the primary sensory axon. (If specialized "sense" cells are present, receptor potentials in these non-neural elements precede, and largely resemble, the generator potentials.) When strong enough, such localized, graded differences in voltage across the axon membrane induce an action potential in a nearby trigger zone of the sensory nerve fiber. At this point, the amplitude of the incoming signal, as reflected in the amplitude of the generator potential, is converted ("abstracted") to frequency modulation — to an axonal firing pattern, a coded train of nerve impulses.

Such "spikes" transcend the local, graded electrical events. These propagated, "all-or-none" signals speed along the nerve to the CNS, where they stimulate further activity that ultimately leads to bodily sensations.

Sensory Coding

Somesthetic information is coded for both time and place. As we shall see, primary sensory fibers project in a topographically precise manner to the CNS. Thus, signals from a particular fiber inform the spinal cord or brain of happenings at a particular place in the body. The geographical space of the body surface and mass is mapped in neural space, just as the retina and organ of Corti are. The quality or mode specificity of somatic sensation is also achieved by place coding in peripheral and central mosaics, as indicated earlier.

Temporal coding is widely and effectively used to abstract events for a brain and spinal cord that cannot experience them directly. We said above that stimulus frequency and intensity are so encoded. Temporal coding can be extremely precise; in joint receptors, for example, a given change in axonal firing frequency may signal with mathematical exactitude a minute change in the angle of the joint. A simple frequency code, however, is only one of the many types of codes which relay news from the receptors to the CNS. One reason (among others) for the wide range of temporal codes is that some receptors are sensitive to more than one type of stimulus, even though they respond selectively to one by a lowered threshold for that type.

Primary Somesthetic Neurons

The nerve cell bodies of the first-order somesthetic neurons lie in the dorsal root ganglia of peripheral nerves or in comparable ganglia along certain cranial nerves (V, VII, IX, and X). The peripheral territories of innervation by these primary somesthetic neurons strikingly illustrate the embryonic segmental nature of the body in the pattern of so-called dermatomes (Fig. 6-2).

Dorsal root ganglion cells have a special morphology: they are pseudounipolar (Fig. 6-3). Because its cell body is offset from the centrally coursing axon, a pseudounipolar cell seems to be a more efficient sensory neuron than the primitive bipolar cell it derives from during embryonic development. In a bipolar neuron, the cell body (which receives no synapses from other neurons, and is hence purely trophic in function) lies along the course of the axon, where it must be traversed by the action potential and wrapped loosely in myelin. We saw such cells in the auditory and vestibular systems.

FIG. 6–2. *Segmental innervation of the skin.* The axons of primary somesthetic neurons (dorsal root ganglion cells) in each dorsal spinal nerve root have a specific territory of peripheral cutaneous innervation: a *dermatome*. While adjacent dermatomes overlap to some extent, the overall pattern of this segmental innervation of the skin of the head and body is as shown in the illustration. Roman numerals I–III refer to the three divisions of the trigeminal nerve: ophthalmic, maxillary, and mandibular. No territory for C1 is shown because the first spinal nerve usually has no dorsal root. The remaining dermatomes from C2 through S2 follow in a logical sequence; in the extremities, the numbers lead down the preaxial side of the arm or leg and progress back up the postaxial side. S3, S4, and S5 are not visible; they surround the perineum in a concentric "bullseye" manner with S5 (and the first coccygeal segment) in the center. Injury to one of the dorsal roots, such as that caused by compression from a herniated intervertebral disc, will produce an area of cutaneous sensory disturbance (paresthesia or, if complete denervation occurs, anesthesia) in the corresponding dermatome (e.g., L5 or S1, or both, as commonly encountered with low lumbar herniations). (Modified from W. Haymaker and B. Woodhall, *Peripheral Nerve Injuries*. Saunders, Philadelphia, 1953)

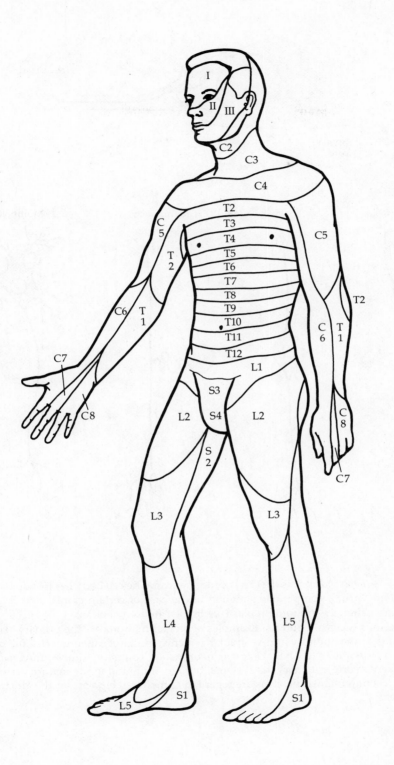

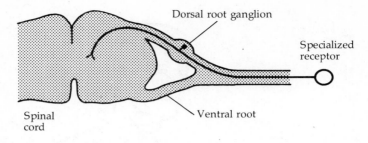

Dorsal root ganglion

Specialized receptor

Spinal cord

Ventral root

A

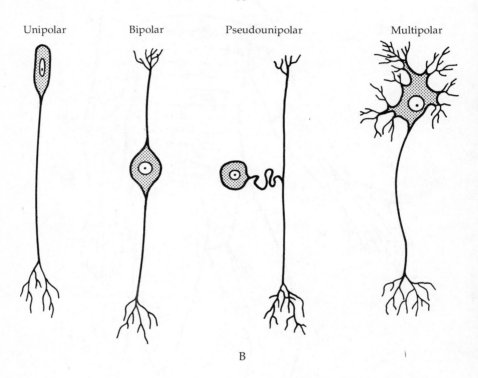

Unipolar   Bipolar   Pseudounipolar   Multipolar

B

FIG. 6–3. *Types of Neurons.* (A) First-order neuron. The cell body lies in a dorsal root ganglion, or in a comparable ganglion in the case of certain cranial nerves. Such cells are generally pseudounipolar (see bipolar neurons below).
(B) Various types of neurons. Examples of bipolar neurons are the primary sensory neurons of the auditory and vestibular systems; multipolar neurons are the dominant type within the CNS. Unipolar neurons are common, almost universal elements in invertebrate nervous systems, but are not found in the mature vertebrate CNS. Pseudounipolar neurons are regarded as modified bipolars, as the illustration suggests.

Secondary Somesthetic Neurons

The entering fiber of each primary sensory neuron has an ascending and descending branch, and both branches emit numerous collaterals like the tines of a garden rake. These features are extremely important to the divergence (upward and downward spread) of information arriving in the CNS. The second-order somesthetic neurons that the branched central process of a dorsal root ganglion cell synapses with lie entirely in the CNS, in layers in the spinal gray matter or in clusters (like the cochlear nuclei of the auditory system) in the brainstem. They keep track of events in different body regions, perhaps concentrating on one sensory modality, but also blending and coding afferent information as mentioned earlier. These cells transmit their integrated responses to other somesthetic neurons at higher levels (midbrain and thalamus), and those in turn to still higher ones (sensory and association regions of cerebral cortex). As we pointed out in Chapter 1, all these central neurons have the multipolar design that facilitates integration.

Central Organization of Somesthetic Pathways

Somesthetic pathways are organized in a general plan (Fig. 6-4). The primary sensory neuron lies outside the CNS, in a ganglion located along the dorsal root of a peripheral nerve or in a similar cell cluster of a cranial nerve. The peripherally directed process (axon) of the primary neuron ends (with or without short dendritic arborization or encapsulation) in or as the receptor, as the case may be. The centrally directed process synapses with a secondary sensory nerve cell in the spinal cord, medulla oblongata, or pons. Axons of these second-order neurons chiefly, although not invariably, cross the midline (decussate) to the opposite side of the neuraxis and terminate at some higher level. Some run all the way up to the somesthetic nuclei of the thalamus, but most have destinations closer to the level of origin — in the spinal gray matter or within the reticular core of the brainstem. Certain thalamic neurons serve as third-order sensory neurons, and their axons project to a primary somesthetic area of the cerebral cortex where fourth-order neurons begin analyses that will involve many additional levels of cortical and subcortical neurons (see Chap. 13).

Duality of Somesthetic System

As we have said, the ascending fibers may terminate in spinal gray or reticular core, or at least give off collaterals that synapse there or in other

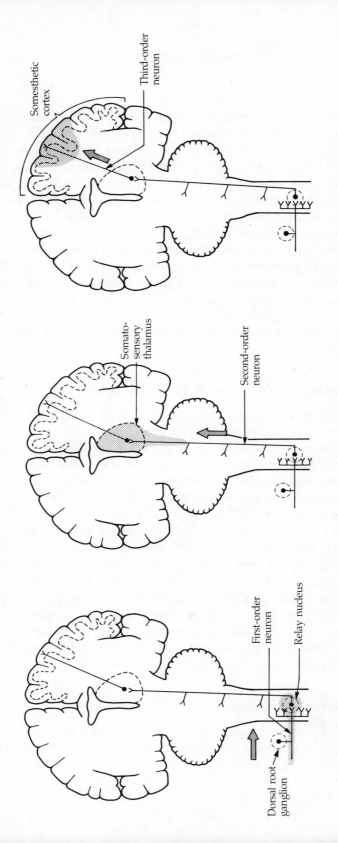

FIG. 6–4. *General plan of organization of somesthetic pathways.* A first-order neuron has its cell body in the dorsal root ganglion. It collects sensory information from a receptor in the skin, or in the viscera, joints, muscles, etc. Its fiber enters the CNS to synapse on a second-order neuron in the spinal cord (as shown), or in the medulla aud pons. The second-order fiber generally crosses the midline in its ascent to higher centers (such as the brainstem reticular formation) and the thalamus. In this illustration, a thalamic third-order neuron is shown projecting to the somesthetic cortex.

such places (tectum). Thus, there can be more than three orders of neurons between periphery and cortex, with parallel processing in offshoot pathways comprising variable numbers of intercalated neurons. Moreover, there are uncrossed as well as crossed upward projections — even "double-crossed" routings in some cases. Despite these complexities, we can resolve matters by recognizing an important duality of the somatic afferent system: bodily sensations are transmitted up the neuraxis over two differently organized types of pathways, lemniscal and reticular, which have correspondingly different functional characteristics (Fig. 6-5).

The lemniscal pathways begin with the ascending central branches of large caliber, well myelinated primary fibers that enter the spinal cord over the medial division of each dorsal root filament (a fingerlike strand that with other similar strands makes up a nerve root). At least one in four (perhaps more) of these thick, rapidly conducting axonal branches reaches all the way up the posterior white columns of the cord (fasciculus gracilis and fasciculus cuneatus) to the corresponding posterior column nuclei (gracilis and cuneatus) of the medulla oblongata and (to an extent undetermined in man) to the lateral cervical nucleus of the upper cervical cord. Axons from these three nuclei decussate and pass upward through the medial lemniscus, a ribbon of closely packed large fibers, to the somatosensory thalamus, from which projection fibers run to the somesthetic cortex. The upward passage of the second-order axons by such direct and distinct routes as the medial lemniscus is the reason certain somatic afferent pathways are called lemniscal. By the same criteria, the major auditory and visual inputs to thalamus and cortex are lemniscal systems, even though the optic nerve/tract is not a lemniscus in the strict sense.

The reticular pathways arise indirectly from a massive offshoot of afferent fibers at the level of dorsal root entry. Some of these fibers are collaterals of large myelinated fibers, while others are smaller myelinated fibers and unmyelinated fibers. Many of these smaller fibers and all the unmyelinated ones enter the cord through the lateral division of a dorsal root filament, synapsing at or near the level of entry with various interneurons of the spinal gray matter. In part, these immediate connections upon entry subserve local and intersegmental spinal reflexes. But an important and diversified group of ascending projections rises up from these spinal interneurons, and these pathways, as they run toward the thalamus, make numerous connections with intervening structures — especially with the brainstem reticular formation. Because of such core connections, made by collaterals of the ascending fibers or by fibers that leave the mainstream, these pathways may be classified as reticular.

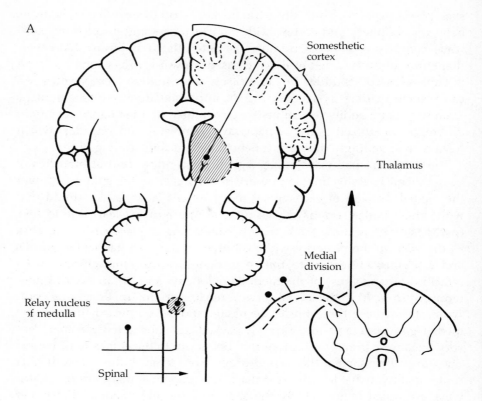

FIG. 6–5. *Duality of the somesthetic system*. (A) A lemniscal pathway. The primary afferent fiber enters over the medial division of a dorsal root filament and synapses on a second-order neuron in a relay nucleus of the medulla oblongata. The second-order fiber crosses the midline and synapses in the contralateral somatosensory thalamus with a third-order cell, which in turn sends fibers to the somesthetic cortex.

(B) A reticular pathway. The primary afferent fiber enters over the lateral division of a dorsal root filament and synapses on a second-order neuron in the spinal cord. The second-order axon crosses the midline and gives off numerous collaterals to higher regions of the cord and to the brainstem reticular formation. In fact, the fiber may terminate long before it reaches the thalamus, and other neurons will pass the information upward. In the example illustrated, the second-order axon eventually synapses on a third-order neuron in the thalamus, as in the lemniscal system. The difference, however, is that much information has been disseminated en route. The third-order neuron projects to somesthetic cortex as before.

B

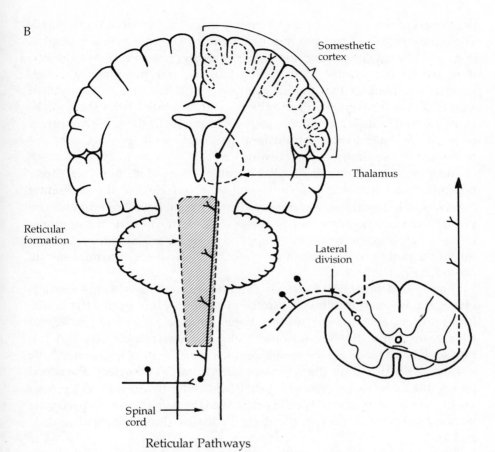

Reticular Pathways

Conceptually, this classification is useful; it expresses the indirect and widespread upward percolation of spinal sensory signals through the reticular core as compared to their rapid transit over the expresslike lemniscal pathways. It is not, however, reflected in the usual terminology. A less descriptive name for the spinoreticulodiencephalic pathways enjoys greater popularity: the anterolateral system. This term is purely anatomical; it signifies the concentration of several reticular-type tracts differing in functional organization (see below) in the anterolateral region of the spinal white matter.

Lemniscal Pathways

The lemniscal pathways are the posterior column/medial lemniscus pathway and the lateral cervical system (spinocervical tract). The latter is well developed in the cat, but its importance in man has not been determined. These long pathways conduct impulses rapidly over their medium-sized to large myelinated fibers. From the viewpoint of a communications engineer, they are reliable routes, in that they transmit information in a direct, somatotopic manner that favors analysis of the source and strength of stimuli at the destination. Practically no signals "leak" from these pathways into the reticular formation; instead, impulses flash up the brainstem over private lines to the contralateral lemniscal receiving region of the thalamus: the ventrobasal complex, or VB.

The posterior column/medial lemniscal pathway (Fig. 6-6) is a three-neuron chain. Initially, it is composed of about 25% of the ascending branches of large caliber, heavily myelinated spinal dorsal root fibers. The primary sensory neurons that give rise to these fibers respond to movement of hairs, touch, or pressure applied to the skin; some report movement of a joint or stimulation of deep receptors. Noxious or painful stimuli are generally ineffective.

The upward branches travel via the posterior columns to the medulla oblongata, where they terminate in the posterior column nuclei: the gracile (thin) nucleus and cuneate (wedge-shaped) nucleus. Axons of gracile and cuneate neurons, the second-order cells, decussate, obliquely but immediately, and travel up the medial lemniscus to the principal somesthetic nucleus of the thalamus: the ventral posterolateral (VPl) nucleus, the lateral part of the ventrobasal complex (VB). Third-order neurons in VPl project via the internal capsule and corona radiata to the somesthetic cortex on the postcentral (parietal) bank of the Rolandic fissure (Brodmann's areas 3, 1, and 2).

The spinocervical pathway (Fig. 6-7) is a less well understood route by which primarily mechanoreceptive information from the level of the spinal cord reaches the brain. In contrast to the foregoing pathway, it is a four-neuron chain, with the "extra" junction located at the point where the primary sensory fibers enter the spinal cord. Second-order fibers proceed, via the posterior columns like the first-order fibers in the medial lemniscus pathway, from neurons in the posterior spinal gray matter to the lateral cervical nucleus, which adjoins the posterior horn of the first and second cervical segments. Third-order fibers from this nucleus join the contralateral medial lemniscus and terminate within a thin layer of cells surrounding VB, from which fourth-order axons reach the somatosensory cortex.

Spinocervical tract neurons, like those of the posterior column/medial lemniscal pathway, are excited by movements of hairs, touch, or pressure to the skin. Unlike the other pathway, however, proprioceptive stimuli are ineffective, and these cells are also influenced by pain and temperature.

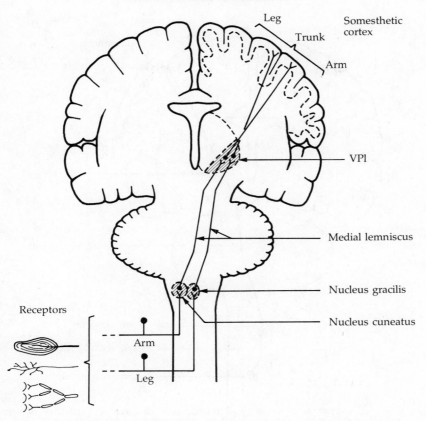

FIG. 6–6. *The posterior column/medial lemniscal pathway.* Axons of primary sensory neurons from different parts of the body (here the arm and leg) synapse in the posterior column nuclei (nucleus gracilis and nucleus cuneatus). Such axons come primarily from Pacinian corpuscles (which are specialized to pick up vibration), Meissner's corpuscles (for two-point or fine tactile discrimination), and Merkel's discs (also thought to subserve precise localization of mechanical stimuli), as well as from joint receptors. Axons of second-order sensory neurons cross the midline and terminate in the contralateral ventral posterolateral nucleus (VPl), which in turn projects to particular somatotopic regions of the primary somesthetic cortex.

Nevertheless, both routes are rapid and direct, and offer few axon collaterals over which impulses could filter into the brainstem core.

Reticular Pathways

Despite their speed and directness, the lemniscal pathways have serious limitations. They are essential to analysis of sensory features by the cortex, but offer few side routes to places along the way to cortex and no provi-

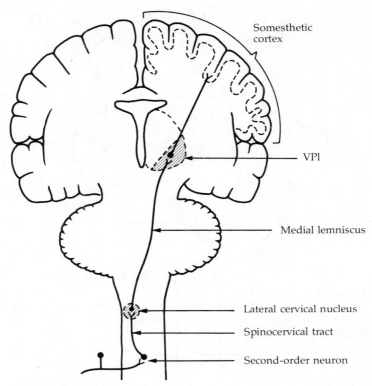

FIG. 6–7. *The spinocervical pathway.* This recently discovered pathway is a four-neuron chain, in contrast to the three-neuron sequence of the posterior column medial/lemniscal pathway. The extra neuron is a second-order cell somewhere in the posterior horn of the spinal cord at the level of entry of the primary fiber. The second-order axon passes to the lateral cervical nucleus (LCN) by way of the spinocervical tract. The LCN corresponds in position in the circuit to the nucleus gracilis and nucleus cuneatus of the posterior column pathway, but in this instance contains third-order neurons. The third-order axons cross to join the medial lemniscus and run to the contralateral ventral posterolateral nucleus (VPl), from which a fourth-order cell projects to somesthetic cortex.

sions for local traffic of impulses. Yet an immediate, extensive spread of sensory information over short local connections is crucial for reflexes (which must be carried out almost instantaneously) and for generalized brain functions, such as arousal and alertness, that allow effective use of the lemniscal systems.

Here the reticular mode of disseminating information comes in. These routes have less somatotopy and show cross-modality convergence, but they exert stronger, longer, and more generalized influences on the CNS. The best known reticular pathways are the lateral and anterior spinothalamic tracts, said to mediate painful and tactile sensations, respectively (Fig. 6-8). This distinction, however, has little anatomical or physiological basis; thus, they are now subsumed under the heading of anterolateral system.

This system consists of a diffuse group of small-caliber, lightly myelinated, slowly conducting axons. The assorted receptors report touch, pain,

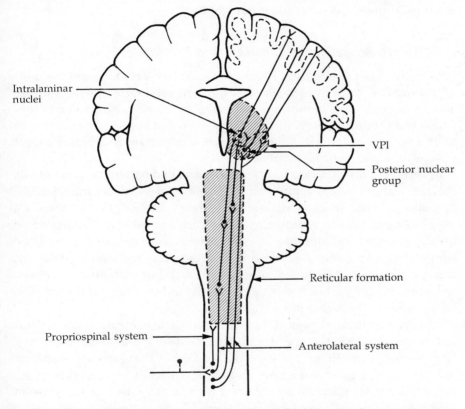

FIG. 6–8. *The spinothalamic tracts.* A group of poorly demarcated nociceptive and tactile pathways ascend in the anterolateral white column of the spinal cord, and are thus referred to as the anterolateral system. In some of these pathways, impulses filter upward through the reticular formation, primarily to the intralaminar nuclei of the thalamus. In other instances, impulses are carried upward more directly, arriving in both intralaminar and posterior groups of nuclei. A small number of anterolateral system fibers run directly to the thalamus: chiefly to the ventral posterolateral nucleus (VPl), but also to the posterior nuclear group.

or temperature. Primary afferents enter through the dorsal roots at all spinal levels and synapse with second-order neurons in various regions of the spinal gray. These fibers are largely but not completely crossed, the decussations taking place in the anterior white commissure of the cord. As the fibers ascend the neuraxis, multiple connections are made by profusely branching axons: at higher cord levels (where such fibers enter the propriospinal system), within the reticular formation of the medulla, pons, and midbrain and in several nuclei of the thalamus, including VB as well as the intralaminar and posterior groups of nuclei.

Evolutionary Perspective on Lemniscal and Reticular Pathways

We can think of the lemniscal routes as neural freeways to speed the traffic of information to the phylogenetically recent cerebral cortex and to preserve an orderly flow of messages, all traveling in their correct somatotopic lanes, from different parts of the body. Such fast routes are essential for critical sensory judgments, but perhaps less important to affective aspects of sensation and general awareness.

In their less direct, branched, and polysynaptic pattern of connectivity, the reticular pathways typify archaic features of brain organization that probably evolved in early marine vertebrates. Interruption of them can alter our feelings as to whether sensations are agreeable or disagreeable or impair alertness and attention — even abolish consciousness. Anesthetics suppress transmission over these pathways, while the lemniscal systems continue to conduct impulses, much as normal, but without awareness of sensation on the part of the person. (One could envision all that freeway traffic flowing through a sleeping city.)

Apparently, these slower, diffuse routes are still evolving: some reticular pathways approach the speed and directness of the lemnisci thought to have sprung from them. For example, certain of the spinothalamic tracts are more direct, fast-conducting, and topographically organized than others. Although they should be regarded with healthy skepticism, the terms "neospinothalamic," "paleospinothalamic," and "archispinothalamic" signify these differences. Moreover, many spinothalamic fibers infiltrate the lemniscal nuclei of the thalamus, and thus seem to have acquired additional connections and functional interactions with the newer pathways. Thus the old fabric of the nervous system is not only retained, but woven into the new, thereby unifying our neural mechanisms of bodily inquiry and self-awareness.

The Trigeminal System

We seldom stop to think, perhaps, how important facial sensations, such as a splash of cold water, a rub with a towel, a fresh breeze, a kiss, one's own smile, are to our daily sensory experience. The fibers conveying cutaneous and deeper sensations from the face comprise a distinct, almost separate network: the trigeminal system (Fig. 6-9). As might be expected,

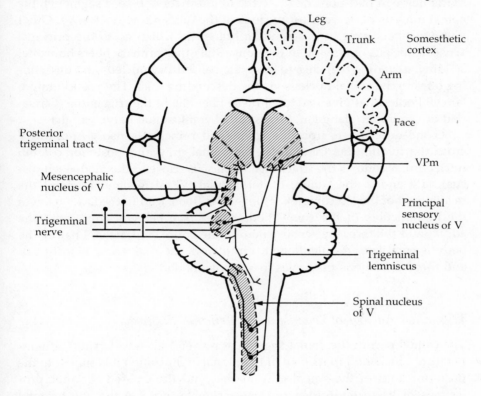

FIG. 6–9. *The trigeminal system.* First-order neurons with cell bodies in the trigeminal ganglion synapse in the spinal nucleus and principal sensory nucleus of nerve V. Second-order fibers from these two sensory trigeminal nuclei cross the midline to the trigeminal lemniscus and course upward to synapse in the thalamus (ventral posteromedial nucleus, VPm), cells of which in turn send third-order axons to the facial area of the primary somesthetic cortex. Some fibers from the principal sensory nucleus ascend to VPm ipsilaterally, via the posterior trigeminal tract.

The mesencephalic nucleus of nerve V is a curiosity, in that it contains primary sensory neurons, normally found only in ganglia. The central processes of these pseudounipolar cells run caudally (see text).

its make-up is dual, with two modes of connections similar to the lemniscal and reticular (anterolateral) systems.

Primary trigeminal nerve fibers have sharply defined cutaneous fields on the face, oral cavity, and nasal passages. Centrally, many of these fibers have only descending branches; these synapse in a long cylindrically shaped nucleus of second-order neurons extending from the level of entry of the nerve in mid-pons down to the first few cervical cord segments, the spinal nucleus of nerve V (or nucleus of the descending tract of V). Other entering fibers have only ascending branches, which go to the principal sensory nucleus of nerve V in the pons. Still other primary fibers bifurcate, sending ascending branches to the principal sensory nucleus and descending ones to the spinal nucleus via the descending tract. The pseudounipolar cell bodies that give rise to all these fibers lie in the trigeminal (Gasserian or semilunar) ganglion, largest of all craniospinal nerve ganglia.

Second-order fibers from the spinal and principal sensory nuclei of V cross the midline (as those from the spinal gray and posterior column nuclei do), ascend as the trigeminal lemniscus (close to the medial lemniscus), and end in the ventral posteromedial (VPm) thalamic nucleus, the medial part of the VB complex. Third-order fibers lead to the face region of the homunculus in the somesthetic cortex (see below). Thus, with the addition of the face, the sensory map of the entire contralateral half of the body is complete. As mentioned, input from the oral cavity is included, and these sensations play roles in swallowing and speech.

Trigeminal Analogs of Lemniscal and Reticular Pathways

The caudal part of the spinal trigeminal nucleus subserves pain and temperature sensibility. In its plan of functional organization it is similar to the posterior horn of the spinal gray matter, and the crossed thalamic projections of its second-order neurons resemble those of the anterolateral system — they pass to the intralaminar and posterior groups of thalamic nuclei, as well as to the VB complex.

The principal sensory nucleus of the trigeminal nerve, together with the oral region of the spinal nucleus, subserves discriminative cutaneous sensation in a manner like that of the gracile and cuneate nuclei. Second-order projections are comparable to the lemniscal system, passing principally to the contralateral ventral posteromedial nucleus (with a small contingent of fibers to the ipsilateral VPm).

A Unique Feature of Trigeminal Neuroanatomy

Deep pressure sensation from the teeth and gums, together with stretch input from the muscles of mastication, are conveyed to the slender, fusiform mesencephalic nucleus of V — a unique nucleus, because it represents a cluster of primary neurons (complete with characteristic pseudounipolar configuration) inside the CNS, an intramesencephalic ganglion, as it were. Why these cell bodies were not sequestered in a peripheral cluster in or near the trigeminal ganglion is a mystery. Elsewhere, primary neuron precursors (neural crest cells) migrate during embryogenesis to form such sensory ganglia — in the case of other primary trigeminal neurons, to form the trigeminal ganglion just mentioned. Whatever the reason for its central location, the arrangement permits the proximal process of the pseudounipolar cells to establish a number of direct connections of strategic importance to feeding: to the motor trigeminal (masticator) nucleus, the salivatory nuclei, ambiguus (swallowing) nucleus, dorsal motor vagal (general visceromotor) nucleus, and so forth.

Efferent Modulation

An important similarity shows up in the lemniscal and reticular systems. Both types of pathways illustrate efferent modulation of afferent signals, the same kind of regulation of incoming information we described in the auditory system. In the somatosensory system, signals from higher centers act to improve the process of somesthesis by filtering out background stimuli, sharpening contrast, enhancing acuity, and other means. For example, cells in the gracile and cuneate nuclei are facilitated in their activity by excitatory fibers from the cerebral cortex that accompany the cerebral motor pathway (pyramidal tract) down to the brainstem.

Similar cortical efferents go to the trigeminal nuclei and somatosensory nuclei of the posterior horn of the spinal cord — even to secondary gustatory/visceral sensory neurons, such as those in the nucleus of the solitary tract. Few regions of the neuraxis, in fact, lie beyond the reach or influence of the cerebral cortex (Fig. 6-10); motor neurons are by no means its only cortical targets.

Thus, the functional effects of impulses delivered over cortical efferent fibers is not always "motor," i.e., selective facilitation of certain motor neurons. Influences may be exerted upon the receptive fields of sensory neurons, perhaps to narrow (through facilitation of neuronal activity) the

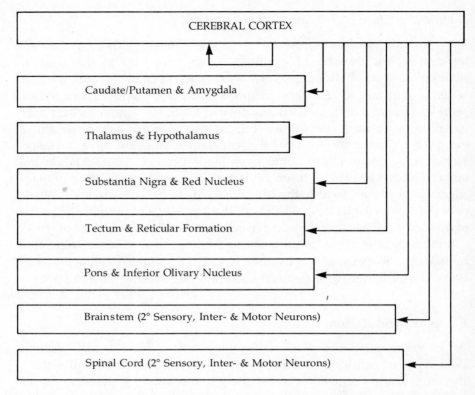

FIG. 6–10. *Organization of cortical efferents.* The cerebral cortex is notable for its direct lines to all major structures and levels of the neuraxis, including association and commissural connections to other cortical areas. Thus, cortical fibers modulate activity in all regions of the CNS, including the activities of sensory and motor neurons — somatic and visceral.

area of skin that a particular tactile cell is monitoring. For example, a cell in nucleus gracilis, prompted by the cortex, might "zoom in" its receptive field from a large area of tactile receptors on the skin to a small spot where we fear a spider may be crawling. From such efferent modulation of sensory cell activity comes attention to focal stimuli and enhanced discrimination, as well as heightened alertness.

Pain Pathways – A Special Kind of Efferent Modulation

The affective aspects of pain are associated especially with the deep spinoreticular pathways, the "archispinothalamic" and "paleospino-

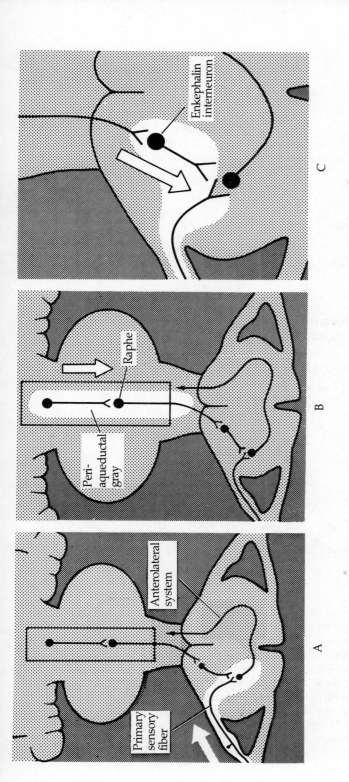

FIG. 6–11. *Pain pathways and modulation of pain.* (A) Pain signals monitored by receptors travel to the spinal cord (laminae I–III) via primary sensory fibers. Some of these axons appear to use substance P as their transmitter. The pain signals travel on up the CNS, primarily via the anterolateral system.

(B) Pain signals can be modulated. Neurons in the periventricular hypothalamus and periaqueductal gray activate serotoninergic raphe neurons. These raphe neurons send fibers to enkephalinergic interneurons in the posterior horn of the spinal cord which terminate presynaptically on primary afferents.

(C) Enkephalin terminals inhibit synaptic transmission at the primary afferents, and thus prevent incoming signals from acting upon spinal neurons.

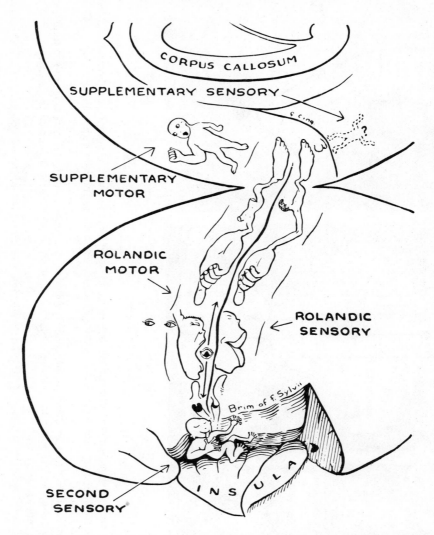

FIG. 6–12. *The sensory homunculus in primary somesthetic cortex (S I)*. Except for the face, the primary sensory representation or homunculus of the opposite half of the body is chiefly upside down. The many receptive surfaces of the body are mapped on the somesthetic cortex in proportion to their importance in sensory analysis, not their physical size. Thus certain parts, such as the genitals, feet, legs, torso, and upper arm, have rather limited territories on the medial and upper surfaces of the somatosensory cortical strip. In contrast, the major sensory exploratory surfaces of hand, fingers, face, and lips are greatly magnified. These distortions in the representation of certain body parts reflect the degree to which our cerebral cortex extracts and analyzes features of somesthetic events.

Below the face region lie a variety of alimentary analyzing regions; underneath

thalamic" tracts that comprise the innermost sensory systems leading up the neuraxis. Recent evidence has uncovered powerful and relatively specific brainstem controls over spinal pain-transmission neurons: inhibitory tracts descending from midline regions of the midbrain, pons, and medulla.

Apparently, there is an endogenous brainstem analgesia system. It can be activated by systemically administered morphine, stimulation at certain places in experimental animals, or, under physiological conditions, by the liberation of endogenous opiates (endorphins and enkephalins; see Chap. 14). The system involves a region surrounding the cerebral aqueduct of the midbrain (periaqueductal gray) and nearby midline areas of the forebrain (preopticohypothalamic area), which are rich in opiate receptors. Also included are several other areas near or in the brainstem raphe, a "seam" or medial strip of the medullopontine (bulbar) reticular formation that gives rise to well-defined bulbospinal inhibitory fiber systems. One of these exerts its effects through the action of serotonin, but the neurotransmitters for the other two are not known. Figure 6-11 shows the basic circuitry believed to be involved in pain control.

While details remain matters for future research, it is now clear that efferent modulation of input holds true for pain, as well as other stimuli. It apparently regulates more than just the discriminative qualities of painful information filtering up the neuraxis, the information that facilitates analysis of the damage to the body and identification of the traumatic agent. Efferent modulation — whether activated from outside the body by "pain-killing" drugs, acupuncture, or some other means; or from within through some mental activity that possibly promotes endorphin-release — may reduce or abolish the unpleasant, compelling feelings that are the affective aspects of pain. Thus, when faced with painful stimuli that are intolerable, the CNS may be able to take measures to shut them off at or near their source.

Thalamic and Cortical Topography of Somesthesis

Eventually, through the lemniscal and reticular routes up the spinal cord and brainstem, information concerning body sensations reaches the VB nuclear complex in the thalamus. From VB, fibers pass in somatotopic

---

them (in the parietal operculum) is the secondary somesthetic area (S II). The sequence of body parts in S II is largely the reverse of that in S I, but their territories are much less clear and representation of the body is bilateral. (From W. Penfield and H. Jasper, *Epilepsy and the Functional Anatomy of the Human Brain*. Little, Brown & Co., Boston, 1954)

array through the fanlike superior thalamic radiation to the primary somesthetic cortex (S I) in the parietal lobe, just behind the central sulcus (Fig.
6-12; see also Fig. 9-1). S I adjoins the motor cortex, with which it works so
closely that it is in fact inseparable. A functionally appropriate (if anatomically grotesque) picture of the opposite side of the human body is represented in the primary somesthetic cortex. This extremely distorted,
largely upside-down image of half a body is in fact the way a cerebral
hemisphere "sees" its side of the somesthetic world.

Another sensory homunculus, the secondary somesthetic cortex (S II),
lies beneath the first (Fig. 6-13; refer also to Fig. 6-12). It is largely hidden
by the Sylvian fissure that runs between the frontoparietal region and the
underlying temporal lobe. Its arrangement of body parts is reversed, i.e.,
right-side up. The representation of certain parts (face, mouth, and throat)
has not yet been confirmed in man, apparently because these cortical fields
lie so close to their primary counterparts, while other body parts are represented in a less distinct way in man. It is as if the first figurine had been
mirrored in a muddy pool. Moreover, bilateral mapping of the body is
present, and input to this secondary somesthetic cortex comes only from
superficial and not from deep receptors.

Multiple Representation – Another Principle

Multiple representation occurs in many functional subsystems of the CNS.
Visual signals, for example, are processed both in the midbrain tectum and
in the visual cortex; the two regions seem to work on different tasks —
orientation and identification, respectively. Division of labor occurs also
along the auditory pathway, where feature analysis and organization of
response patterns are begun immediately and carried out simultaneously
by diverse cell groups.

We have already seen that multiple representation, or parallel processing, is an important organizing principle of the nervous system. As an
outgrowth of neuronal specificity and individuality, entire networks of
neurons are given specific jobs to perform, so that we have fast and slow
tracts, private and public lines of communication, numerous homunculi,
etc. Moreover, secondary and tertiary auditory, visual, and somesthetic
cortical areas are recognized, though their functional contributions are not
entirely clear. They are served by recently discovered auditory, visual, and
somatosensory routes to cortex that parallel the classical lemniscal pathways.

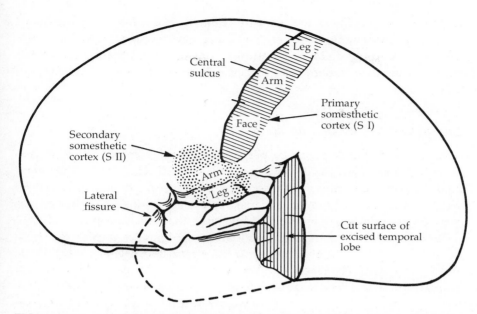

FIG. 6–13. *General relationship of primary and secondary somesthetic cortex.* The broad cortical strip S I (see Fig. 6-12) lies just behind the central sulcus; face, arm, and leg territories are indicated. S I is actually larger than shown, and includes some frontal cortex anterior to the central sulcus where the motor homunculus (M I) is located (see Chap. 9). The various corresponding body regions of S I and M I are intimately interconnected by short association bundles (U fibers) looping beneath the central sulcus.

The sequence of body parts in S II, which lies just beneath S I, is just the reverse of the S I pattern, as indicated by the placement of labels for the arm and leg. The face region in S II tends to blend with that in S I, but in general the area is difficult to explore due to the proximity to the insula and the risk of damaging branches of the middle cerebral artery. Representation of the body is bilateral in S II, and there are other differences relating to the types of somesthetic submodalities analyzed here.

Columnar Organization of Somesthetic Cortex

Somesthetic cortex, like visual cortex, is organized in columns, located at right angles to the cortical surface. All neurons in a given column tend to respond to stimulation of the same region of the body surface. Such columnar organization depends on the somatotopic organization of thalamic afferents entering the cortex. It provides for integration of place or modality labeled information throughout the cortical column, and for cross-integration of cognate information in adjacent columns. Some columns are devoted to body surface, others to deeper structures and still others to sensations as specific as temperature changes of the tongue. Neurons of secondary somesthetic cortex are particularly responsive to touch or pressure; some are polymodal, responding to several kinds of peripheral input. But whatever their specific role, cortical columns provide the units of function.

Clinical Correlates: Blending the Senses

Not only is the body mapped, perhaps over and over for different purposes, in the ventrobasal thalamus and somesthetic cortex. The many kinds of body sensation must also be blended: touch, pressure, vibration, sense of position and movement, heat, cold, and pain. Pain is charted less precisely than most submodalities, but more than adequately.

That the cortex is extremely important to this synthesis is shown from the clinical study of individuals with injuries to the primary somesthetic area. They can feel objects handled with their eyes closed, but cannot evaluate their textures, shapes, weights, or temperature; in short, they cannot recognize them. Nor can they correctly and precisely localize sensations, appreciate locations and attitudes of body parts, or sense their movements as easily as before. And comparison of stimuli with those previously experienced is difficult.

Even more striking losses, of awareness of half of the body, may result (see Chap. 13). Obviously, such individuals have lost an ability to analyze and alloy many concurrent bits of information. Still, they may do a fair job if given time, illustrating again the brain's ability to compensate for losses. Those discriminative functions that remain intact after S I injury remind us that the cerebral cortex is not the only brain structure that blends sensations. Other areas, especially the thalamus, play important roles. The cortex completes pictures already sketched elsewhere. Let us take a closer look at this progressive system.

The Hierarchical Organization of Somesthetic Feature Analysis

Somesthetic neurons, like visual and auditory neurons, are organized in an interdependent hierarchy. An apparent difference, however, is that somesthetic neurons must keep track of so many kinds of stimuli from so many places. While the variety of visual and auditory stimuli and the number of receptors for them is considerable, the surface area of the body far exceeds that of the retina or cochlear partition.

At the lowest levels of the somesthetic system, in the secondary sensory nuclei, the coded signals probably represent incoming data which may not deserve the term "raw" but are nonetheless just so many reports of deviations from the status quo. At higher levels, perhaps in spinal gray or reticular core, rough sketches are made: the presence, perhaps, of some nearby object in a certain sector of extrapersonal space — just beyond the left shoulder for example. At mesencephalic levels, bigger pictures are formed (see Chap. 11). Specialized neurons respond only to certain features in combination: the simultaneous presence, perhaps, of several colder spots and well-defined regions of pressure on the palm of the hand. At the highest neuronal echelons, in the ventrobasal complex and S I, a clear image appears. It is through such progressive analysis that we recognize a dime in a pocket or purse, the weights and textures of objects hefted and handled, our finger positions on the neck of a violin. At each level, the features selected by somesthetic neurons represent increasingly complex combinations. Selection consists of a distinctive change in neuronal response; like tiny slot machines, neurons "pay off" when the right combination comes up!

As we have said, such high-level combinations of signals are more important in determining the nature of a sensation than the neural lines over which the signals arrive, although clearly there are limits (somesthesis does not come in over the optic nerve). Moreover, combinations of signals determine the affective quality of a sensation. The experience of pain as severe and calling for protective responses necessitates a synthesis of information, much as appraisal of a fire as a serious blaze would.

For the sensory miracles of texture discrimination and judgment of weight (or the mysteries of tickle and itch), these simplistic explanations are inadequate. Such complex, subjective evaluations are surely the work of a multitude of neurons dealing with a tremendous amount of past and present data. Such decisions cannot be made by a few nerve cells. They require searching analysis of many matters and progressive integration of the findings on the part of the brain.

General Concepts

The somesthetic system illustrates many important principles of CNS organization: somatotopy, parallel processing, modular organization (cortical columns), progressive feature extraction and analysis, magnified images, crossed connections, and efferent modulation of input. Somesthetic receptors respond best to changes in stimulus activity, deviations from the steady state ("novelty"). Somesthetic neurons employ fibers of various caliber and path of entry, as well as dual central channels to provide for fast, accurate long-distance signaling and local reflex functions. The central synthesis of diverse submodalities, however, seems more important than these labeled lines and channels in determining the nature and quality of sensations. Certainly such synthesis underlies pattern recognition.

Pattern recognition lies at the heart of neural function. Neurons detect, interpret, and act upon patterns of environmental stimuli and inward occurring events. With few exceptions, as in the retina or hypothalamus, the brain does not face the external surroundings or internal milieu of the body directly. It recognizes only electrical and chemical signals and their coded patterns.

Glossary

Anterolateral system: a somesthetic pathway for pain, temperature, and crude tactile sensibility, ascending through the anterolateral region of the spinal cord and reticular formation to the diencephalon and comprising the lateral and ventral spinothalamic tracts; an example of a reticular pathway (see below).

Anterolateral white column: the ventrolateral sector of the lateral funiculus of the spinal cord; a region of spinal white matter occupied in part by the lateral and ventral spinothalamic tracts.

Corona radiata: see Chap. 2.

Cuneate (wedge-shaped) nucleus: the more lateral of two nuclei of the medulla oblongata receiving ascending fibers of the posterior columns of spinal white matter; the medullary "relay" in the posterior column/medial lemniscus pathway up to somatosensory thalamus and cortex, mediating sensation from the upper extremities and upper half of the trunk.

Dorsal root ganglion cells: primary somesthetic neurons; cell bodies of these pseudounipolar neurons lie in the sensory ganglia, with distal and proximal branches of the axon directed toward the periphery and the spinal cord, respectively.

Gracile (thin) nucleus: the more medial of the two posterior column nuclei of the medulla oblongata (see *Cuneate nucleus*); mediates sensation from the lower extremities and lower half of the trunk.

Internal capsule: see Chap. 2.

Intralaminar nuclei: small, indistinct clusters of neurons in the internal medullary lamina of the thalamus; receive spinothalamic and reticulothalamic fibers and are thus important components of the diffuse thalamocortical activating system.

Lateral cervical nucleus: a group of nerve cell bodies adjoining the posterior gray horn of the first and second cervical spinal cord segments; the third echelon of a sequence of four levels of neurons projecting tactile impulses up to somesthetic cortex.

Lemniscal pathway: an ascending somatosensory pathway composed of large-diameter, fast-conducting myelinated fibers projecting upward through a minimum of interposed neural centers (one or two) to thalamus and cerebral cortex; more direct and secure as to information transfer than a reticular pathway.

Medial lemniscus: a ribbonlike tract of closely packed, large-diameter, fast-conducting somesthetic fibers; courses upward through the brainstem from the gracile and cuneate nuclei of the medulla oblongata to the contralateral ventroposterolateral nucleus of the thalamus.

Meissner's corpuscle: a specialized sensory receptor located in the papillary dermis and encapsulating the axon terminal of a primary somatosensory neuron; believed important to precise localization of mechanical stimuli, and may serve vibration sense as well.

Mesencephalic nucleus of nerve V: a cluster of somatosensory nerve cell bodies in the upper pons and midbrain, located lateral to the fourth ventricle and cerebral aqueduct and mediating afferent impulses conveyed by the trigeminal nerve from the ipsilateral jaw muscles; its pseudounipolar cells are the only primary sensory neurons within the CNS, hence the nucleus is equivalent to a dorsal root ganglion.

Pacinian corpuscle: a large, specialized sensory receptor, resembling an onion in its shape and lamellated structure, located in the reticular dermis or hypodermis and encapsulating the axon terminal of a primary somatosensory neuron; believed important to vibration sensibility.

Periaqueductal gray: a cylindrical region of gray matter, interlaced with extremely fine, poorly myelinated fibers, surrounding the cerebral aqueduct of the midbrain; contains diffuse conduction pathways for pain and provides part of the neural substrate for affective responses to painful stimuli.

Posterior column/medial lemniscus pathway: a fast-conducting, direct, three-neuron pathway up to somesthetic cortex, involving primary sensory neurons at all spinal cord levels, cells of the gracile and cuneate nuclei of the medulla oblongata, and cells of the ventral posterolateral nucleus of the thalamus; important to rapid, high-resolution reporting of tactile and position sensations.

Posterior columns: the collected bundles of nerve fibers comprising the posterior funiculus of the spinal white matter; the gracile and cuneate fasciculi, many axons of which travel all the way up the cord to synapse in the gracile and cuneate nuclei, respectively.

Primary somesthetic cortex (S I):   an extensive, somatotopically organized region of parietal cerebral cortex just posterior to the central sulcus; site of the so-called sensory "homunculus" of the opposite side of the body.

Principal sensory nucleus of nerve V: a nucleus at the level of entry of the trigeminal nerve in mid-pons, containing cell bodies of second-order neurons serving discriminative tactile sensibility from the ipsilateral half of the face.

Raphe (seam) nuclei: small clusters of serotonergic nerve cell bodies within a prominent midline strip of myelinated fibers in the medullopontine reticular formation; important in mediating modulatory influences of the upper brainstem on the reception of painful stimuli in the spinal cord.

Reticular pathway: an ascending somatosensory pathway composed of medium-diameter and small, moderately fast to slowly conducting myelinated fibers which project upward through numerous intermediate centers (in the spinal cord and brainstem reticular formation) to thalamus and cerebral cortex; less direct and secure as to information transfer than a lemniscal pathway.

Rolandic fissure: see *Central sulcus* (Chap. 2).

Ruffini's ending: a specialized sensory receptor located throughout the dermis and near joints, possibly representing an expanded tip of the axon terminal of a primary somatosensory neuron; believed important to joint sensation.

Secondary somesthetic cortex (S II):   located in the insular margin of the parietal lobe, beneath S I; features a less distinct somatotopic representation of both sides of the body, opposite in sequence of body parts to that in the primary somesthetic area.

Spinal nucleus of nerve V: a long, cylindrical nucleus, extending caudally from the point of entry of the trigeminal nerve into the cervical spinal cord; contains cell bodies of second-order neurons serving pain and temperature sensations from the ipsilateral half of the face.

Spinocervical pathway: a four-neuron, fast-conducting, tactile/pressure pathway from spinal cord up to somesthetic cortex; involves primary sensory neurons in the spinal ganglia, second-order cells in the spinal gray, third-order neurons in the lateral cervical nucleus, and fourth-order cells in the ventrobasal thalamus.

Trigeminal lemniscus: second-order ascending fibers from the principal and spinal nuclei of nerve V to the contralateral ventroposteromedial nucleus of the thalamus; trigeminal analog to the medial lemniscus.

Trigeminal sensory fibers: primary somatosensory fibers from the face traveling centrally over the ophthalmic, maxillary, and mandibular divisions of the fifth cranial nerve; cell bodies of these axons lie in the trigeminal (Gasserian, semilunar) ganglion.

Ventral posterolateral nucleus (VPl): the more lateral of the two nuclei in the ventrobasal complex of the thalamus; somatotopically organized, it mediates somatic sensations from the body and projects to the body region of the homunculus in primary somesthetic cortex.

Ventral posteromedial nucleus (VPm): the more medial of the two nuclei in the ventrobasal complex of the thalamus; somatotopically organized, it mediates somatic sensations from the face and projects to the face region of the homunculus in primary somesthetic cortex.

Ventrobasal complex: the somesthetic nuclear complex of the thalamus, made up of the ventroposterolateral and ventroposteromedial nuclei.

The Olfactory System and Taste

7

Smells and tastes are processed by the olfactory and gustatory systems, respectively. Less is known of them than of other sensory systems.

Olfaction

The Olfactory Brain

The olfactory system, sometimes called the rhinencephalon (nosebrain), includes the olfactory bulb and those tracts, nuclei, and cortical areas that serve the sense of smell. The rhinencephalon lies in the telencephalon, or endbrain, close above the nasal cavity. Phylogenetically, it is the oldest part of the forebrain, and thus has been of great importance to its plan. This nosebrain corresponds to the primitive endbrain of earlier vertebrates: a rostrally located sensory analyzer drawn up to meet the need for detecting, studying, and responding to odors. In man, it is buried beneath other forebrain regions that are far larger and more imposing. How did this happen? With the passage of millions of years and adaptative modification of the vertebrate neuraxis, visual, somesthetic, and other sensory tracts entered the forebrain by way of the thalamus and spurred the development of extensive cortical analyzer/effector fields. Such new inputs and outputs greatly complicated the original structural and functional layout of the forebrain. In man, many parts of the forebrain have no direct connections with olfactory structures and little, if anything, to do with olfaction.

The Importance of the Sense of Smell

It might seem that the sense of smell is a luxury and that we could fare quite well without it. Civilization has blunted whatever meager ancestral gifts of smell we may have had, and our olfactory acuity is poor. Still, we have retained and enhanced our power of olfactory association: a scent can lead one to recall something unexpectedly and in vivid detail, frequently with strong and inexplicable overtones of emotion. Furthermore, there are probably powerful subconscious effects of smell. For example, a sudden instinctive like or dislike on our part for someone at first meeting may derive from an attractive or disturbing odor or pheromone that does not reach consciousness (see below). Finally, olfaction is obviously important to us in maintaining personal hygiene and a clean or safe environment.

In animals, if less obviously in "civilized" humans, the sense of smell plays three vital everyday roles in the preservation of self and species: a nutritive role, involving the location of acceptable food, taking hold of it, and reflex-stimulated secretion of digestive enzymes; a protective role, important in detecting enemies or other threats to survival; and a reproductive role, goading toward mating and copulation, with concomitant excitation and preparation of the genital organs. Olfaction has other well-documented functions in animals that relate to territorial behavior, social ordering, and sensory gratification. All the above considerations attest to the wealth of interconnections between the olfactory system and other parts of the brain, and give us pause before we dismiss olfaction as a luxury for chiefly gastronomic pleasure.

The Layout of the Olfactory System

In overview, the olfactory system is laid out as follows. The olfactory receptors within the nasal cavities are the peripheral tips of true neurons ("olfactory rods" or bipolar ganglion cells) serving as distance receptors themselves, without any interposed sense cells. The central processes of these exposed surface neurons connect with the nearby overlying olfactory bulbs of the cerebral hemispheres. From there, the olfactory tracts of the two sides run posteriorly and mostly laterally to paired regions of primary olfactory cortex on the medial surface of each temporal lobe and to the underlying amygdaloid nuclei (see Fig. 7-1). We shall examine these structures briefly in turn.

Olfactory Receptors

The olfactory receptive membrane consists of several yellow-brown patches of specialized pseudostratified columnar epithelium in the upper regions of the nasal cavities. The olfactory cells, small bipolar receptor neurons, lie among supporting or sustentacular cells that have hexagonal surface profiles and a microvillous border, (Fig. 7-2). The coarse peripheral

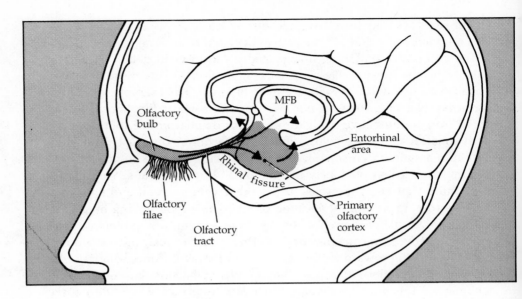

FIG. 7–1. *Medial view of olfactory brain (rhinencephalon).* Delicate central processes of some 25 million olfactory receptor cells collect and pass as small fascicles through the cribriform plate of the ethmoid bone into the overlying olfactory bulb. Collectively, these fascicles comprise the olfactory nerve, or cranial nerve I. The output of this primitive, yet intricately wired, region of the cerebral hemisphere passes posteriorly and chiefly laterally to the primary olfactory cortex on the medial surface of the temporal lobe and to the underlying amygdaloid nucleus.

FIG. 7–2. *The olfactory epithelium and receptor cells.* (A) The olfactory membrane is a specialized pseudostratified columnar epithelium in which bipolar receptor elements (olfactory cells) lie among supporting cells with hexagonal surface profiles. The peripheral process of an olfactory cell bears short hairlike bristles (modified cilia) on its swollen tip, resembling a tiny spiked club or mace. These macelike endings protrude from alternate angles of the supporting cell hexagons into the solvents (water and mucus) for odoriferous substances that coat the free surface.

The delicate central processes of rod cells pass through the basal lamina of the epithelium and then combine in fascicles (fila olfactoria; see Fig. 7-1) en route to the olfactory bulb. These receptor cells, which actually confront the environment directly, are strikingly similar to elements of simple nervous systems and represent the most primitive true neurons in our brain. (From W. J. S. Krieg, *Functional Neuroanatomy*, 3rd Ed. Brain Books, Evanston, Ill., 1966)

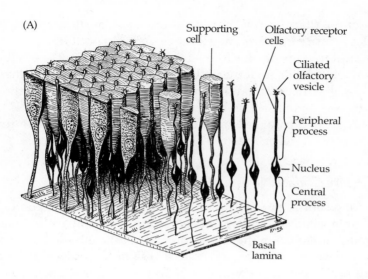

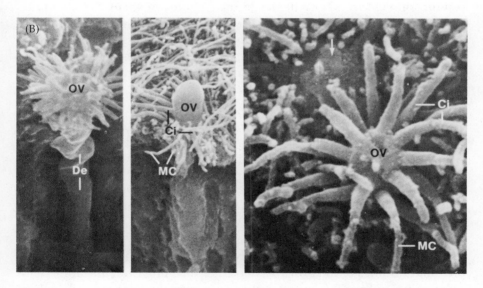

(B) Scanning electron micrographs showing a portion of the lateral surface of the olfactory epithelium. It can be seen that the olfactory cell's peripheral process or dendrite (De) ends in a bulbous expansion (the olfactory vesicle, OV) from which approximately one to two dozen cilia (Ci, MC) protrude. In some species, e.g. dogs, up to one hundred cilia may extend from the olfactory cell. (From R. G. Kessel and R. H. Kardon, *Tissues and Organs: A Text-Atlas of Scanning Electron Microscopy*, W. H. Freeman, San Francisco, 1979)

process of an olfactory cell, bearing many short bristles (modified cilia), protrudes from every other angle of the supporting cell hexagons into the watery mucous film on the free surface. This secretion is produced by special tubular glands underneath the olfactory mucous membrane, and is probably augmented or modified by the secretions of the supporting cells. The water and mucus act as solvents for odoriferous substances. Small, irregularly located basal cells in the epithelium are of uncertain function; they may serve to regenerate the olfactory and supporting cells.

The Olfactory Cranial Nerve and Clinical Correlates

The delicate central processes of these receptor cells form poorly myelinated ("unmyelinated") fibers or fila olfactoria, which pass as small fascicles through foramina in the cribriform plate of the ethmoid bone into the inferior surface of the olfactory bulb. These axons collectively form the olfactory nerve (cranial nerve I or CN I). Its tiny fibers have the slowest conduction velocity of any nerve. In man, there are about 25 million filaments from each side of the nose.

Unlike the rich assortment of sensory and motor fibers in a mixed spinal or cranial nerve, olfactory nerve fibers are all alike — central extensions of primitive neurons (found nowhere else in the human nervous system) serving as chemoreceptors.

The Olfactory Bulb

This flattened, ovoid body could be thought of as the "nucleus" of termination of CN I. But it is really a highly specialized, primordial region of the cerebral cortex positioned and designed for direct entry of sensory impulses from the nose. In macrosmats (keen-scented animals), the bulb has a complex, strikingly laminar organization. The layers, however, are difficult to make out in microsmatic man (Fig. 7-3).

Within the bulb, primary olfactory fibers synapse (in glomeruli) with brushlike endings of the principal dendrites dangling from the large, triangular mitral cells. (The mitral cell is so-named because its cell body is shaped like a bishop's mitre; a mitral cell resembles an inverted pyramidal cell of the cerebral cortex, the tip of the pyramid giving rise to an axon rather than an apical dendrite.) Additional mitral cell dendrites run horizontally. These accessory dendrites enter into reciprocally communicating dendrodendritic synapses with small amacrine (axonless) neurons nearby, the internal granule cells. Such cells seem to provide for lateral inhibition and contrast — perhaps for discrimination of odors.

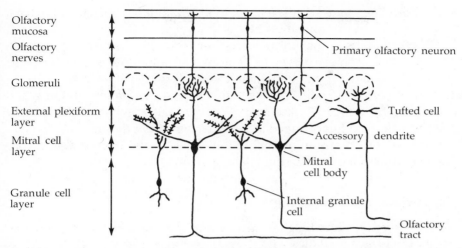

Olfactory
mucosa

Olfactory
nerves

Primary olfactory neuron

Glomeruli

External plexiform
layer

Tufted cell

Mitral cell
layer

Accessory dendrite

Mitral
cell body

Granule cell
layer

Internal granule
cell

Olfactory
tract

FIG. 7–3. *Neural elements of mammalian olfactory bulb.* Primary olfactory fibers synapse in glomeruli with brushlike arborizations of principal dendrites extending vertically from the large triangular mitral cells. Mitral cell axons depart from the bulb in the olfactory tract. Most of these fibers pass over the lateral olfactory stria to the amygdala and periamygdaloid cortex in the region of the uncus.

Accessory mitral cell dendrites extend horizontally to form two-directional dendrodendritic synapses with small amacrine cells, the interal granule cells. These unusual connections, by which mitral cell activity is quickly and directly suppressed by adjacent cells, seem to provide lateral inhibition and contrast. Not illustrated are several other types of local-circuit interneurons and other "unconventional" synapses that give the olfactory bulb an extraordinarily complex structure for what we often dismiss as "primitive" cortex.

Teeming numbers of other small interneurons are present in the olfactory bulb. Like interneurons elsewhere, these dwarf cells act in various ways to modify the output of the bulb, for example, amplifying signals, converting excitation into inhibition, and enhancing signal-to-noise ratio. And there is a rich variety of so-called "unconventional" synapses—dendrodendritic, axodendrodendritic, somatodendritic, and dendrosomatic (these compound terms signify the pre- and postsynaptic parts of the nerve cell in apposition) — as well as the familiar, "conventional" types. Thus the intrinsic circuitry of the olfactory bulb is quite complex.

The Anterior Olfactory Nucleus

The output of the bulb is carried centrally by the axons of the mitral cells and also by those of tufted cells. Olfactory information passes chiefly to a region of the temporal lobe known as the uncus (see below). Along the way, however, many fibers terminate at the anterior olfactory nucleus, which lies along the course of the tract.

Olfactory fibers do not show the evident orderly arrangement found in the optic and cochlear nerves (retinotopy and tonotopy) and somesthetic pathways (somatotopy). How, then, are smells coded? One answer seems to be: by temporal coding in the trains of axon potentials entering and emanating from the bulb. But spatial coding is also probable. One orderly feature is that modulatory feedback connections from the anterior olfactory nucleus to the amacrine internal granule cells in the ipsilateral and contralateral bulbs show a striking bilateral symmetry.

The Accessory Olfactory Bulb

An accessory olfactory bulb lies just behind the olfactory bulb. In rodents, recent tract-tracing studies with modern techniques show that its connections are quite different from the main bulb. These techniques, which are revolutionizing neuroanatomy, reveal the nerve cell bodies of origin of tract fibers by cellular uptake of the finely particulate enzyme horseradish peroxidase and the target structures of such fibers by axon transport of radioactive amino acid.

The results of such studies suggest that there may be two distinct, separate olfactory systems. The accessory system might act to perceive pheromones: externally secreted, biologically active substances which transmit information between individuals of a species. In insects and certain other animals, pheromones are considered highly important to sexual behavior and reproduction. Recently, ethologists and other scientists have wondered about their possible existence and significance in humans.

The Olfactory Tract and Striae

The prominent ribbon of the olfactory tract (not to be mistaken for the olfactory nerve) runs caudally to the anterior perforated substance, where the striate branches of the anterior and middle cerebral arteries penetrate the base of the forebrain (see Chap. 15). There, the tract divides into lateral, medial, and intermediate olfactory striae (Fig. 7-4). The striae travel along the surfaces of corresponding olfactory gyri, which are extremely thin, rudimentary bands of gray matter. In man, the intermediate stria is poorly defined.

The largest number of bulbar efferents travel via the lateral stria. Interestingly, reciprocal connections pass over this route — from higher centers

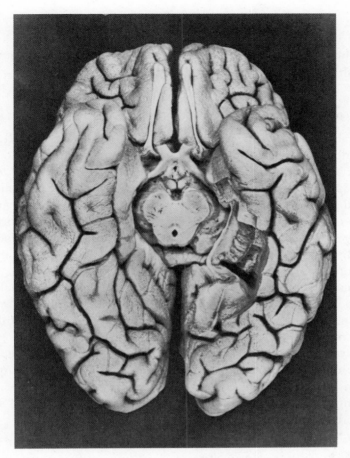

FIG. 7–4. *Basal aspect of olfactory system.* In this inferior view of the human cerebrum, the olfactory bulb, tract, and trigone (division of the tract into lateral, medial, and intermediate striae) are clearly visible. Most of the impulses arising in the bulb travel over the lateral olfactory stria, which leads by way of a hairpin turn (barely visible on the left) to the primary olfactory cortex of the uncus and the underlying amygdaloid nuclear complex.

Many nonolfactory structures may be seen in this beautiful preparation: the optic nerves, chiasm and tracts; the tuber cinereum and mammillary bodies; a cross-section of midbrain showing inferior colliculi, cerebral aqueduct, medial longitudinal fasciculi, tegmentum, and crus cerebri; the oculomotor nerves emerging from the posterior perforated substance; and numerous other parts of the brain, including part of the hippocampus as uncovered by dissection of the right hemisphere. (From E. Ludwig and J. Klingler, *Atlas Cerebri Humani*. Little, Brown and Company, Boston, 1956, plate 77)

back to the olfactory bulb. Presumably, these outgoing fibers provide the brain with means for modulating olfactory input.

The Olfactory Cortex

The lateral stria takes a hairpin turn at the threshold (limen) of the insula and distributes fibers to the uncus and underlying amygdaloid nuclear complex. These destinations on the medial face of the anterior temporal lobe are as far as mitral cell axons go. A larger region, the entorhinal area (bounded laterally by the rhinal fissure) lies just behind the primary olfactory area of the uncus. It serves as the olfactory "association" cortex, and has other polysensory associative roles related to the limbic system (see Chap. 12); it receives olfactory impulses indirectly from the primary cortex in front of it.

In macrosmats, the olfactory bulb and the uncinate/entorhinal cortical regions have a pear-shaped outline in their inferior aspect, and are hence known collectively as the pyriform lobe (or area). The term is frequently encountered.

Numerous other olfactory connections are present — to the septal area, olfactory tubercle, hypothalamus, habenular nuclei, etc. Such complex and largely indirect routes are beyond the scope of this chapter and, for the time being at least, have little clinical relevance. But the lateral stria is a major portal to the limbic system.

Functional and Clinical Correlations

As one might expect, the delicate olfactory nerve fibers are easily damaged or torn with violent movements of the head, and are so affected in 7 to 10% of all head injuries. CN I is the most commonly injured cranial nerve. The damage is usually bilateral, and 40% of the injured fibers recover (75% of these within three months). These fibers seem to die off at a slow rate during life, as do fibers in other craniospinal nerves. Such fiber loss probably accounts for our increased threshold for odors with age. In rats, it has been noted that olfactory primary axons are capable of regeneration to some extent. The satellite position of groups of these "unmyelinated" axons about a common Schwann cell (an arrangement similar to that seen in peripheral nerve regeneration) may possibly favor such regrowth.

Nevertheless, trivial head injuries (those which occur without loss of consciousness) can produce permanent anosmia in man. This does not happen often, but one in five persons so afflicted probably lost olfaction in this way. With more severe head injuries, the duration of unconsciousness and severity of trauma to the back of the head (occipital coup) correlate with increased damage to the filaments. They are torn, or compressed by edema or hematoma.

The paired olfactory bulbs, lateral olfactory striae, and primary olfactory cortical areas (uncus) provide the requisite neural substrate for olfactory perception and discrimination. Thus, as long as the olfactory nerve filaments are intact, fairly extensive and bilateral damage to the base of the frontal and temporal lobes is necessary to destroy these functions. But clinically the olfactory system is of minor importance. In certain instances, however, testing the nostrils for odors separately is useful. Asymmetrical responses can help one to diagnose fractures of the cribriform plate of the ethmoid bone; hemorrhages, meningitis, or abscesses of the frontal lobes; meningiomas of the sphenoidal ridge or olfactory groove, and hypophysial tumors extending beyond the sella turcica.

Irritative processes (such as epilepsy) in the entorhinal area and adjoining uncus can lead to olfactory and gustatory hallucinations. The odors and tastes that the patient experiences are usually disagreeable, and are accompanied by certain feeding-type oral acts (licking, lip-smacking, and tasting movements) and an abnormal, frequently fearful state of consciousness. The foregoing trilogy is known as an uncinate fit; it may precede a general seizure.

Taste

The Interdependence of Taste and Olfaction

Taste and olfaction, as common experience at the dinner table tells us, work in concert to produce the final gustatory result. Recall the bland or even indefinite "taste" of foods when you have a cold. Curiously, considering all the complexities of gustatory sensation, there are only four fundamental tastes: sour, bitter, salty, and sweet. Receptors for these basic qualities transduce stimuli in the oropharynx, primarily from the tongue, but also from additional receptors in the epiglottis. Sensory signals are carried centrally via cranial nerves VII, IX, and X to the medulla oblongata (nucleus solitarius), passed upward via largely uncharted multisynaptic pathways to the thalamus, and thence to the gustatory area of the cortex. As a result of a progressive station-by-station integration, we experience the sensation of taste. We shall attempt to describe each main station in turn, but in general very little is known about the gustatory pathway(s).

Gustatory Receptors

The surface of the tongue is covered with numerous small protuberances called papillae. Within their crevices lie the receptors, descriptively named and popularly known as taste buds. Taste buds are pale, ovoid multicellular bodies about 70–75 μm long, embedded in the epithelium of the tongue. They contain lightly staining Type I cells and dark-staining Type II cells. The Type I cells are possible sensory, and the Type II cells may be supportive, but at present one cannot assign a definite functional role to these cells. The Type I cells have a short "taste" hair (3 μm long) on the outer end which projects to the surface of the tongue through the taste pore. The opposite end of a Type III cell (a cell somewhat like the Type I) is innervated by a sensory nerve fiber, but this recent finding applies only to the rabbit at present.

Turnover and Specialized Properties of Taste Buds

Taste buds appear to die, and their cells are replaced throughout life. It is not known whether food intake influences their turnover one way or the other, but it is tempting to speculate on the effects of a steady diet of gourmet, bland, spicy, or other foods on taste receptors.

As mentioned above, the fundamental tastes are sour, bitter, salty, and sweet. Taste buds seem to be more or less specialized for each quality, and are topographically ordered: those on the lateral regions of the tongue respond preferentially to sour substances, those at the base to bitter ones, and those on the upper surface to sweet and salty elements. In some manner not yet understood, the sensory cells respond selectively to a specific chemical and structural property for each gustatory modality and transduce them to electrical impulses, which are then carried to the brain by cranial nerves.

Cranial Nerves Involved in Taste

Afferent fibers of three cranial nerves mediate gustatory sensations from the tongue, as well as general visceral sensation (Fig. 7-5). These nerves are the facial (VII), glossopharyngeal (IX), and vagal (X). The pseudounipolar cell bodies of the primary neurons which give rise to the peripheral gustatory fibers are located in certain sensory ganglia of those nerves: the geniculate ganglion of nerve VII, petrosal ganglion of nerve IX, and nodosal ganglion of nerve X. The VIIth nerve mediates taste from the

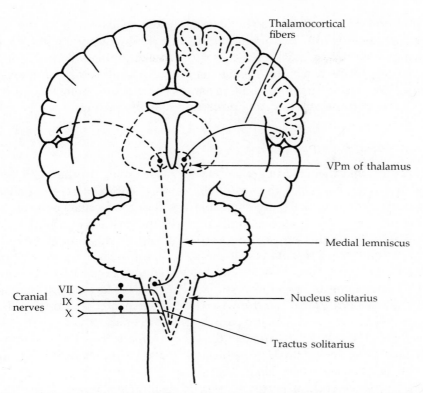

Thalamocortical
fibers

VPm of thalamus

Medial lemniscus

Cranial nerves VII IX X

Nucleus solitarius

Tractus solitarius

FIG. 7–5. *Gustatory pathway*. Afferent fibers of the facial (VIIth), glossopharyngeal (IXth), and vagal (Xth) cranial nerves mediate taste from the anterior two-thirds of the tongue, posterior one-third, and epiglottis, respectively. Central processes of ganglion cells of these three nerves extend to the medulla oblongata, join the tractus solitarius, and synapse in the oral part of its nucleus. This part is sometimes called the gustatory nucleus; it represents an enlargement of the lateral group of neurons found alongside the entire length of the solitary tract.

Axons of central gustatory neurons project rostrally, apparently via multisynaptic pathways that lie close by the medial lemniscus, to the ventroposteromedial (VPm) nucleus of the thalamus, possibly bilaterally. From there, thalamic fibers probably project to the parainsular and overlying opercular regions of the cerebral cortex.

anterior two-thirds of the tongue, the IXth nerve from the posterior one-third, and the Xth nerve from the epiglottis.

Central Gustatory Projections

Central processes of the ganglion cells described above pass into the medulla oblongata, swing caudally, join the tractus solitarius, and synapse in the oral part of the nucleus solitarius (often called the gustatory nucleus). Axons of solitarius neurons project rostrally, apparently via multisynaptic pathways that lie close to the medial lemniscus. Many of these ascending fibers reach the medial part of the ventrobasal complex, or somesthetic nuclear region, of the thalamus (ventral posteromedial nucleus or VPm). In some animals, this projection may be bilateral.

Cortical Representation of Taste

It appears that thalamic fibers conveying taste project to the parainsular and overlying opercular regions of the cerebral cortex. These regions lie adjacent to the lateral fissure — in the region of the frontal, parietal, and temporal lobes. This putative location places the gustatory cortical area in good accord with the sensory homunculus (Chap. 6), adjacent to the center for the sensory representation of the tongue and near the cortical motor centers for mastication and tongue movements. It is interesting to note how correlations of viscerosomatic activity are made possible by these strategic meeting places of otherwise clearly demarcated and often widely separated visceral and somatic pathways of the brain. Many other examples of such evident "crossroads" for viscerosomatic integration might be cited, as in the amygdaloid, preopticohypothalamic, and habenular regions of the limbic system (see Chap. 12).

The putative cortical representation of taste given above, however, is only a best guess from present electrophysiological findings, not a universally agreed upon localization. Findings which indicate that other cortical areas play a central role in the conscious sensation of taste include the uncinate fits mentioned earlier in this chapter. These seizures, which involve the uncus and adjacent temporal lobe cortex, are frequently associated with gustatory hallucinations.

General Concepts

The predominately olfactory forebrain of early vertebrates has been largely overshadowed and, in fact, usurped during neural evolution by the ingrowth of other sensory subsystems. We shall see in our study of the limbic system (Chap. 12) that the human forebrain, although still allotting territory to olfactory analysis and association, has taken on functions that call for extraordinary degrees of integration — much more complex than determining whether a smell represents food, danger, or a potential mate. Nevertheless, we still experience the power of suggestion conveyed by culinary aromas, noxious odors, or fragrant perfumes. Though some olfactory structures in man, including the bulb, seem (at least anatomically) to have been downgraded almost to vestiges, others, notably the amygdala and entorhinal cortex, have acquired new connections and functional roles.

Functionally, what we have defined as rhinencephalon is clearly necessary for the detection and differentiation of odors, which apparently are laid out in some scheme of both topographic and temporal representation — some combination of place coding and spike train coding that we do not yet understand. And clinical examination of the olfactory system has definite though limited utility, in the diagnosis of traumatic, vascular, infectious, neoplastic, and irritative lesions to structures in its immediate vicinity.

Central processing of the qualities of taste seems to follow the lines of classical sensory pathways, especially the somesthetic pathway. Taste buds pick out the four basic properties of substances in the mouth — sourness, bitterness, saltiness, and sweetness. Afferents from primary neurons in the sensory ganglia of cranial nerves VII, IX, and X respond to electrical signals from the sensory cells and send impulses centrally to a medullary nucleus (nucleus solitarius), clearly a main integrative and relay station on the way to thalamus. Just what happens next, and where, is not clear; the thalamus and cortex obviously play important roles, and the hypothalamus seems to offer a "crossroads" for taste and smell.

Glossary

Accessory olfactory bulb: a small, primitive cortical structure immediately posterior to the olfactory bulb; differs in connections and possible function.

Amacrine cells: neurons without an axon; common in the olfactory bulb.

Amygdaloid nuclear complex: a group of 8–10 nuclei immediately beneath the uncus of the temporal lobe; receives prominent olfactory input via the lateral olfactory stria.

Anterior olfactory nucleus: the most rostral of several cell groups located along the course of the olfactory tract.

Entorhinal area: the most rostral third of the parahippocampal gyrus; serves as olfactory association cortex and receives numerous nonolfactory association fibers from the remainder of the cerebral hemisphere.

Facial nerve: cranial nerve VII: mediates taste sensations from the anterior two-thirds of the tongue.

Fila olfactoria: small fascicles of proximal processes (axons) of olfactory cells, leading from the olfactory mucous membrane to the overlying olfactory bulb.

Glomeruli: complex synaptic articulations of primary olfactory axons (central processes of bipolar cells) and principal (vertical) mitral cell axons in the olfactory bulb.

Glossopharyngeal nerve: cranial nerve IX; mediates taste sensations from the posterior third of the tongue.

Gustatory cortex: a region of the parainsular and overlying frontoparietal opercular cortex which receives thalamic fibers (from VPm) conveying taste information.

Internal granule cells: small, amacrine neurons in the olfactory bulb; have dendrodendritic synapses with the accessory (horizontal) dendrites of mitral cells and apparently act to inhibit mitral cell activity so as to provide for contrast enhancement.

Mitral cells: large, triangular neurons, resembling inverted pyramidal cells of the cerebral cortex, in the olfactory bulb; principal neurons of the bulb and secondary sensory neurons of the olfactory system, projecting to uncinate cortex, amygdala, and numerous other forebrain targets.

Nucleus solitarius: a long column of secondary sensory neurons surrounding the tractus solitarius and receiving input from first-order neurons of the VIIth, IXth, and Xth nerves; subserves gustatory (special visceral) sensation in its oral part, general visceral sensation caudally.

Olfactory bulb: a knoblike extension of the olfactory tract on the undersurface of the frontal lobe; the initial forebrain analyzer of olfactory nerve signals.

Olfactory cells: slender, ciliated, bipolar neurons held together by supporting cells in a pseudostratified columnar epithelium; the modified cilia at the free surface apparently have receptor sites for primary odors, and the thin axon emerging from the base of such cells conducts impulses centrally in cranial nerve I.

Olfactory cortex: the primary olfactory analyzer area of the cerebral cortex, found mainly in the uncinate region of the temporal lobe but also along the course of the lateral and medial olfactory striae.

Olfactory epithelium: a specialized pseudostratified columnar epithelium containing ciliated olfactory sensory cells, secretory supporting cells, and basal cells of uncertain function; found in yellow-brown patches on the upper surfaces of the nasal cavities and covered by a film of mucus.

Olfactory gyri: thin, rudimentary bands of cortical gray matter located subjacent to and along the course of the olfactory tract and olfactory striae.

Olfactory nerve: cranial nerve I; its 25 million short, delicate fibers represent the central processes of olfactory cells leading to the overlying olfactory bulb.

Olfactory striae: three prominent offshoots (medial, lateral, and intermediate) of the olfactory tract; the lateral stria, leading to the olfactory cortex, is particularly important.

Olfactory tract: a distinct, flattened tract of nerve fibers leading posteriorly from the olfactory to the region of the olfactory trigone.

Papillae: protuberances on the surface of the tongue in which the taste buds are located.

Rhinencephalon: those parts of the forebrain receiving the axons of mitral and tufted cells and concerned with perception and discrimination of odors; in essence, the olfactory bulb, tract, and striae, together with the uncinate region of the temporal lobe.

Taste buds: pale, ovoid, multicellular structures embedded in the epithelium of the tongue and containing specialized sensory cells innervated by fibers of the gustatory cranial nerves (VII, IX, and X).

Tractus solitarius: a small, but distinct bundle of axons in the dorsolateral tegmentum of the pons and medulla oblongata, made up of descending primary fibers of the VIIth, IXth, and Xth cranial nerves; mediates general and special (gustatory) visceral sensation.

Tufted cells: a second category of projection neurons in the olfactory bulb, fusiform in shape and superficially located; possibly serve different functions than mitral cells.

Uncus: the superiorly and posteriorly directed "hook" at the anterior end of the parahippocampal gyrus, covering the amygdala primary olfactory area of the cerebral cortex.

Vagal nerve: cranial nerve X; mediates taste sensations from the epiglottis.

Ventral posteromedial nucleus (VPm): the most ventral and medial region of the somesthetic nucleus of the thalamus; gustatory neurons of the nucleus solitarius project to it.

The Thalamus

8

The thalamus is often called the gateway to the cerebral cortex. It is, indeed, the principal terminus of the great sensory subsystems, a forebrain structure (Fig. 8-1) ideally situated to serve as a central clearing house for all sensations. Even signals conveying the archaic sense of smell eventually come to the thalamus (as new techniques for tracing connections tell us), although, unlike other sensory inputs, olfactory impulses have already passed directly through a region of the cerebral cortex, the olfactory bulb. But the thalamus is not just a gateway or relay station. (Nor does any other part of the CNS have such a restricted, passive function.) It is one of the major sensory integrating centers of the brain — certainly the most concentrated, when its jam-packed mass of neurons is compared to the vastness of the association cortex or to the diffuseness of the reticular core of the brainstem. The thalamus receives sensory information, correlates it, and sends reports on to the cortex for further feature analysis and data reduction. But even then its role is not finished; it continues to "discuss" these matters with its overlying companion structure. In fact, the thalamus usually seems to lead this discussion.

Thalamocortical Data Processing

Three kinds of messages come to the thalamus: discriminative, affective, and integrative. Only the first two are directly related to sensation; they concern the details of sensory features and their pleasant or unpleasant aspects. All sensations fall somewhere on a scale from pleasurable to pain-

166

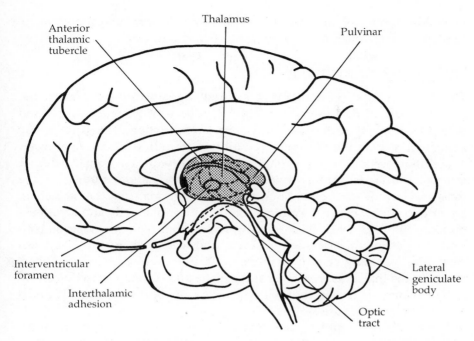

Anterior thalamic tubercle

Thalamus

Pulvinar

Interventricular foramen

Interthalamic adhesion

Lateral geniculate body

Optic tract

FIG. 8–1. *Gateway to the cerebral cortex*. The thalamus is a large mass of gray matter in the center of the forebrain. The third ventricle separates it into right and left halves, and the right half of the thalamus is visible here. The strategic central position of the thalamus allows for interconnections with the basal ganglia, amygdala, and entire cerebral cortex, as well as for inputs from the underlying hypothalamus, brainstem reticular formation, and cerebellum.

ful, even if normally dismissed as neutral. The thalamus has much to do with adjusting this affective scale.

Integrative messages come from several nonsensory parts of the brain that exploit the strategic central location and circuitry of the thalamus. Signals from the deep cerebellar nuclei, basal ganglia, and limbic system flow through nuclei in its rostral half, just as the various sensory signals (visual, auditory, and somesthetic) stream through the caudal thalamus. The anterior connections implicate the thalamus in motor control and emotion. Therefore, it serves as a key communications link for practically every major forebrain mechanism, not just the sensory ones. As clinical proof of this, lesions of the rostral thalamus may lead to tremors and movement disorders similar to those seen in cerebellar or basal ganglia disease, or to emotional problems and deficits in learning, memory, and planning resembling those which follow damage to limbic pathways.

Thalamocortical Activation

The thalamus is also important in maintaining consciousness, alertness, and attention. In these elusive but high functions, it works hand-in-hand with the cerebral cortex and the reticular formation, the core of the brainstem. Within the thalamus, the diffuse ascending reticular pathways and anterolateral system (Chap. 6) connect with an equally diffuse thalamocortical activating system. Silver impregnation studies of the thalamus in rodents show a thicket of fibers entering from the brainstem, passing to almost every thalamic nucleus, both ipsilaterally and across the midline. Similar, richly collateralizing fibers from thalamic neurons connect with other thalamic neurons and also lead forward into the basal forebrain, including certain territories of the neocortex. Still other fibers return to the thalamus from the basal ganglia and cortex. For technical and other reasons, such complex fiber systems cannot be demonstrated in man at present, but they are almost certainly present.

The functional significance of this welter of fibers leading up from the reticular formation to the thalamus and then from thalamic neurons on to the basal ganglia and cortex is that the connections provide a mechanism for regulating the general excitability of the forebrain, distributing modulatory effects on the activity of thalamic, cortical, and subcortical neurons. These connections constitute the *generalized* (nonspecific or diffuse) *thalamocortical system.* They are to be contrasted with the *specific thalamocortical system*, the various connections involved in the data processing activities mentioned above. The specific system offers a much more precise kind of "wiring" — with fibers directed to particular groups of thalamic or cortical neurons, arranged in some sort of spatial organization (such as somatotopy), and showing little tendency to give off collaterals prior to forming their terminal arborizations. These precise afferent/efferent articulations, so unlike the tangle of processes described for the generalized system, provide the kind of synaptic security necessary for feature analysis.

Thalamic Nuclei

The human thalamus is thus a highly complex structure consisting of two egg-shaped halves, joined only slightly across the third ventricle (by the interthalamic adhesion) and containing many large, small, and even minute subclusters of neurons, the thalamic nuclei (Figs. 8-2 and 8-3). While

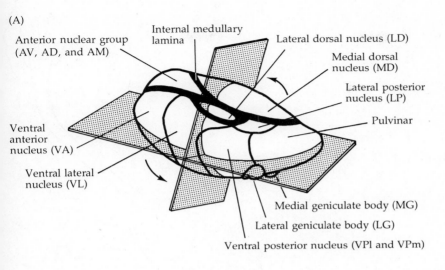

(A)

Anterior nuclear group (AV, AD, and AM)

Internal medullary lamina

Lateral dorsal nucleus (LD)

Medial dorsal nucleus (MD)

Lateral posterior nucleus (LP)

Pulvinar

Ventral anterior nucleus (VA)

Ventral lateral nucleus (VL)

Medial geniculate body (MG)

Lateral geniculate body (LG)

Ventral posterior nucleus (VPl and VPm)

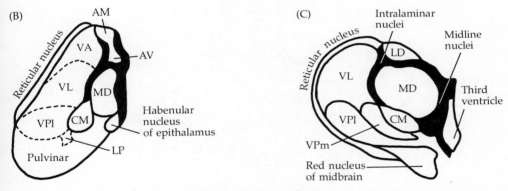

(B)

AM

Reticular nucleus

VA

AV

VL

MD

VPl

CM

Pulvinar

LP

Habenular nucleus of epithalamus

(C)

Reticular nucleus

Intralaminar nuclei

Midline nuclei

LD

VL

MD

Third ventricle

VPl

CM

VPm

Red nucleus of midbrain

FIG. 8–2. *Thalamic nuclei.* (A) Lateral view of thalamic surface showing major divisions. The thalamus is slightly rotated (arrows) so as to expose the dorsal surface. The two intersecting planes indicate the location of the horizontal and coronal sections shown in B and C. Nuclei with widespread connections are shown in dark outline.

(B) Horizontal section and (C) coronal section. Compare with (A) and Table 8–1. These sections show the three principal subdivisions of the thalamus: lateral, medial, and anterior. The ventral nuclei (VA, VL, VP1, and VPm) lie in the lateral subdivision (along with the geniculate bodies, LG and MG). The association nuclei (MD, LD, LP, and pulvinar) lie either in the medial, anterior, or lateral subdivisions or posteriorly behind the intramedullary lamina, respectively. The nuclei with widespread connections (midline, intralaminar, and posterior) lie just beneath the ventricular wall, in the intramedullary lamina itself or beneath the pulvinar; the posterior nuclear group is not shown. The reticular nucleus surrounds the lateral, anterosuperior, and anteroinferior surfaces of the thalamus like a screen; it is not found on the caudal surfaces, i.e., around the pulvinar.

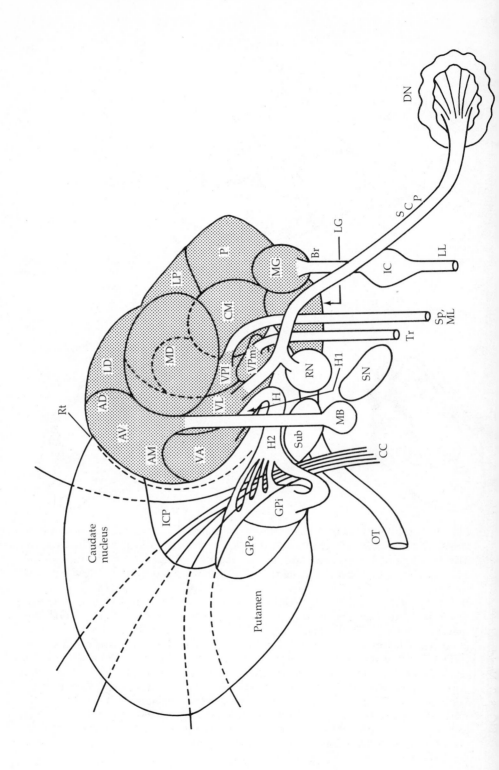

FIG. 8–3. *Nuclei and afferent fiber systems of human thalamus.* This figure represents an accurate reconstruction of the human thalamus in sagittal plane as viewed from its medial aspect (from the third ventricle).

Abbreviations (in more or less clockwise sequences):

Thalamic nuclei

AV, AM,
AD   = anterior nuclear group
MD   = medial dorsal nucleus
CM   = centromedian nucleus
Rt   = reticular nucleus
LD   = lateral dorsal nucleus
LP   = lateral posterior nucleus
P   = pulvinar
LG   = lateral geniculate nucleus
MG   = medial geniculate nucleus
VPm   = ventral posteromedial nucleus
VPL   = ventral posterolateral nucleus
VL   = ventral lateral nucleus
VA   = ventral anterior nucleus

Afferent fiber systems and associated structures

OT   = optic tract
LL   = lateral lemniscus
IC   = inferior colliculus

Br   = brachium of inferior colliculus
Tr   = trigeminothalamic fibers
Sp   = spinothalamic fibers
ML   = medial lemniscus
DN   = dentate nucleus
SCP   = superior cerebellar peduncle
GPe   = globus pallidus, external part
GPi   = globus pallidus, internal part
H, H$_1$,
H$_2$ = fields of Forel
MB   = mammillary body
MT   = mammillothalamic tract

Other important structures

Sub   = subthalamic nucleus
RN   = red nucleus
SN   = Substantia nigra
ICp   = internal capsule
CC   = crus cerebri

Note the more medial position of MD and how it covers parts of VL, VPl, CM, and LP, the outlines of which are dashed behind MD.

the anatomical and functional unity of the thalamus should not be over-looked, the task of description may be simplified by dividing these nuclei into four arbitrary categories, as follows.

Relay Nuclei

In Chapter 3 we saw that auditory fibers in the brachium of the inferior colliculus synapse in the prominent medial geniculate body (MG), a thalamic nucleus that gives rise to a short projection to the primary auditory cortex in the temporal lobe. In Chapter 5 we saw that optic tract axons of retinal ganglion cells similarly synapse in the equally prominent lateral geniculate body (LG), from which another, longer projection curves back to the primary visual cortex in the occipital lobe. And in Chapter 6 we saw that the major somesthetic tracts (medial lemniscus, spinothalamic, and trigeminothalamic) converge in the deeply situated but large ventrobasal (VB) complex of the thalamus — composed of the ventral posterolateral nucleus (VPl) and ventral posteromedial nucleus (VPm). From VB, a great fan of fibers sweeps up to the primary somatosensory cortex in the parietal lobe.

The above fiber systems mediate information relating to modalities of sensation — hearing, vision, and the various submodalities of somesthesis. The thalamic nuclei interposed along these routes obviously play a relay function; they afford diencephalic connections through which this information can flow upward to specific cortical analyzer regions. Thus, the term "relay nuclei" is correct as far as it goes, but does little to indicate the amount of integration that takes place in such thalamic cell clusters. Indeed, as we have pointed out before, there is really no such thing as a simple relay in the nervous system. Rather, input–output transformations are the rule where impulses pass along chains of neurons.

Three additional prominent afferent fiber systems to the cerebral cortex depend on such thalamic relay nuclei. An important difference, however, is that these routes do not mediate information directly related to sensation. Instead, the input comes from structures that are difficult to characterize as either "sensory" or "motor" (a problem frequently encountered when one deals with the CNS). These structures are the deep cerebellar nuclei (principally the dentate), the basal ganglia (globus pallidus), and the hypothalamus (mammillary body), and the information passing from them to the cortex is best characterized as relating to "motor control" for the first two and "limbic system activities" (drives and behavior, etc.) for the last.

As described in Chapter 9, the cerebellar input to the cerebral cortex passes from the cerebellar cortex to the deep cerebellar nuclei and from them over long ascending tracts to the rostral thalamus. The chief route is the dentatorubrothalamic tract to the ventral lateral (VL) nucleus, which in turn sends projections to motor and premotor cortex (areas 4 and 6, respectively). Also described in Chapter 9 is an input from the inner division of the globus pallidus that conveys integrated influences from the adjacent striatal components of the basal ganglia (caudate nucleus and putamen). Through a complex system of efferent fibers (the fields of Forel) that loops back tightly upon itself beneath the oral pole of the thalamus, the inner pallidum connects with the ventral anterior (VA) nucleus, which in turn projects widely upon the frontal cortex (including the motor and premotor areas). Thus, the two nonsensory relay nuclei described above, VL and VA, afford routes to frontal cortex for cerebellar and basal ganglia influences, and, by their proximity in the rostral third of the thalamus, permit internuclear interactions for subcortical integration of these messages. Hence these two nuclei are important to motor control, as stated.

The mammillary body connection through thalamus to cortex is one of the most important routes of the limbic system, covered in Chapter 12. Through the short, direct mammillothalamic tract (one of the most clearly defined tracts to be found in the brain), hypothalamic activity that has been regulated by the fornix projection from retrohippocampal structures reaches the anterior nuclear group of the thalamus. This complex of three nuclei (the relatively large anterior ventral or AV nucleus and the small anterior medial and anterior dorsal nuclei, AM and AD) receives additional direct connections from the adjacent fornix and projects this information in an orderly spatial manner to the dorsal sector of the limbic lobe, the cingulate gyrus. These thalamocortical relay nuclei are essential components of the famous "Papez circuit" for emotion: from the hippocampal region via fornix, mammillary body, thalamus, and limbic lobe back to hippocampus (see Chap. 12). As such, the anterior nuclei are thalamic components of the limbic system.

All of the above nuclei are thalamic cell clusters which receive input over clearly defined, fast conducting, and direct routes or lemniscal systems, and are therefore classified as relay or lemniscal nuclei. That these nuclei and their incoming tracts are all grossly or almost grossly visible attests to the importance of the auditory, visual, somesthetic, cerebellar, pallidal, and hypothalamic inputs. Table 8-1 presents the relay and other groups of nuclei.

There are now known to be additional afferent fiber systems, conveying visual information from the tectum to the lateral posterior nucleus (LP) and

Table 8-1. Classification of Principal Nuclei of Human Thalamus Based on Their Connections

Subdivisions	Nucleus	Afferent connections	Efferent connections
"Relay" nuclei	Medial geniculate (MG) Lateral geniculate (LG) Ventral posterolateral (VPl) Ventral posteromedial (VPm) Ventral lateral (VL) Ventral anterior (VA) Anterior group (AV, AD, AM)	Brachium of inferior colliculus Optic nerve/tract Medial and spinal lemnisci Trigeminal lemniscus Dentatorubrothalamic tract Pallidothalamic fibers Mammillothalamic tract	Transverse temporal gyri (area 41) Striate occipital cortex (area 17) Postcentral gyrus (areas 3, 1, and 2) Postcentral gyrus (areas 3, 1, and 2) Motor/premotor cortex (areas 4, 6) Widespread frontal connections Cingulate gyrus
Association nuclei	Pulvinar Lateral posterior (LP) Lateral dorsal (LD) Medial dorsal (MD) Medial large-celled part Lateral small-celled part	Posterior association cortex, pretectal area Posterior association cortex, tectum (superior colliculus) Not worked out; probably from precuneus in part Amygdala, temporal neocortex Intrathalamic, hypothalamic	Posterior association cortex (parietal, temporal, occipital) Posterior association cortex Parietal association and adjacent posterior cingulate cortex Posterior orbitofrontal cortex Granular prefrontal cortex
Nuclei with widespread connections	Midline group (six or seven) Intralaminar (numerous; two largest as follows) Centromedian (CM) Parafascicular (Pf)	Hypothalamus, reticular formation (complex, poorly known) Reticular formation, intrathalamic (complex, poorly known) Motor cortex (area 4), pallidum Premotor cortex (area 6)	Hypothalamic and intrathalamic; limbic lobe, part of hippocampus Widespread, collateralizing; to striatum, cortex, & within thalamus Intrathalamic, striatum (putamen) Intrathalamic, striatum (putamen)
	Posterior	Direct and indirect spinothalamic fibers	Caudate, putamen, association cortex
Special category	Reticular (a thin screen of cells about the dorsal and lateral thalamic surfaces)*	Collaterals of thalamocortical fibers; neocortex and reticular formation; intrinsic thalamic afferents (complex network)	Feedback system of axons to most thalamic nuclei and to rostral brainstem reticular formation (mesencephalic tegmentum)

*Not to be confused with the reticular formation of the brainstem, although it does have connections with same.

from the pretectal area to the pulvinar, and still others providing auditory and somesthetic inputs from the reticular formation to the midline, intralaminar, and posterior nuclei (see below). The study of these so-called "nonlemniscal" routes is very important to a full understanding of sensory mechanisms.

Association Nuclei

Another group of thalamic nuclei does not receive as evident an afferent input as the lemniscal nuclei, although, as just described, we know that important ancillary or nonlemniscal afferent systems terminate in them. These nuclei project to and from, and thereby interrelate, the so-called "association" areas of the cerebral cortex, areas which apparently have sensory inputs of their own, as well as associative connections. We classify these thalamic cell masses as association nuclei, because their association functions are more evident than their sensory activities. The association nuclei include the extremely large pulvinar (cushion), which appears to tie together the vast parietal, occipital, and temporal association areas via reciprocal connections, and the somewhat smaller lateral posterior (LP) and lateral dorsal (LD) nuclei. These latter nuclei have similar, if more limited functions (see Table 8-1). A very important association nucleus is the medial dorsal nucleus (MD or DM), which projects in a spatially well-organized manner upon frontal association cortex. The medial dorsal nucleus is noteworthy for its integration of somatic and visceral influences (it has connections with the amygdala and hypothalamus), and may be thought of as a thalamic component of the limbic system (Chap. 12). By contrast, the pulvinar (enormously increased in primates and man; refer to Fig. 5-5) is essential to the cortex's language and gnostic functions (see Chap. 13), and also provides a "relay function" in bringing visual information from the pretectal area to the cortex, as mentioned above. Figure 8-3 shows the cortical projection areas of the relay and association thalamic nuclei.

Nuclei with Widespread Connections

These generally small clusters or thin sheets of cells, which include the midline, intralaminar, and posterior subgroupings (illustrated in Fig. 8-1), are probably older components of the thalamus that now lie buried amongst or beneath the elaborated nuclei just described. In an intricate and poorly understood manner, they connect mainly with other thalamic nu-

clei, the basal ganglia, hypothalamus, subthalamus, and reticular formation. They have important functions in integrating intrinsic thalamic activity and in tying the brainstem reticular formation and hypothalamus into
the overall activity of the forebrain. Those that project to the cortex seem to
have diffuse connections that are established by collaterals of axons ending
in the basal ganglia. The centromedian (CM) and parafascicular (Pf) nuclei
are the largest members of the intralaminar group, and the CM–Pf complex
has important connections related to motor control circuits. The midline
nuclei lie scattered just beneath the lining of the third ventricle, particularly
in the region of the interthalamic adhesion. One of them (nucleus reuniens) is now known to project to the entire limbic lobe, including a part of
the hippocampus. The posterior nuclei are a group of very small cell clusters beneath the pulvinar; they are implicated in somesthesis (see Table
8-1).

Reticular Nucleus

Surrounding the lateral and ventral surface of the thalamus, forming a thin
sheet of sprawling, octopuslike neurons, is the reticular nucleus (Fig. 8-3).
It is not to be confused with the reticular formation, even though connections and similarities between the two similarly named structures exist.
Almost all thalamocortical and corticothalamic traffic must pass through
this nuclear shell, and collaterals of these projection fibers make connections with the dendrites of reticular neurons. The reticular cells direct their
axons back to the thalamus and rostral reticular formation, thus apparently
providing feedback inhibition of thalamic output and tegmentothalamic
input. The reticular nucleus also seems to modulate and integrate intrathalamic activities. Lacking cortical connections, it is perhaps less a part
of the brainstem reticular–thalamocortical activating system than are the
midline and intralaminar nuclei, which are heavily infiltrated with core-
derived afferents and which project, at least in part, to cortex. But the
reticular nucleus does receive inputs from mesencephalic regions of the
reticular core that may be critically important to neural mechanisms of
self-awareness (see Chap. 11).

Functional Characteristics of Thalamocortical Projections

Overlap and Fusion of Modalities

In the thalamus, sometimes in a single thalamic nucleus, sensations coming together are integrated with a broader range of afferent information.

Such blending continues in the cerebral cortex, but is already notable at the thalamic level. This integrative function is evidenced in studies of the avian forebrain, which has little cortex as we know it. In the human brain, however, the feature analysis that depends on the cortex overshadows the work of the thalamus. Consider, for example, how the various somesthetic submodalities of pain, temperature, touch, pressure, and position sense must, at least crudely, be put together for a given part of the body (say, the hand or little finger) in a particular region of the ventrobasal complex. Lesions of such regions (as by a thalamic infarct) may greatly alter the discriminative and affective quality of this "mix" and also lead to abnormal positions and postures of the body part involved through impairment of position sense and possibly muscle sensibility.

Orderly Representation of Sensory Surfaces

As we have seen, orderly "maps" of the retina, cochlea, and cutaneous surface of the body are preserved in the visual, auditory, and somesthetic pathways to the thalamus, in the thalamic nuclei themselves, and in their cortical projections. Although all parts of the various sensory fields are represented, these maps may be distorted. For example, the retinotopic maps at the thalamic and cortical levels greatly exaggerate the macula, as we have noted in Chapter 5. Similarly, the somatotopic maps in the ventrobasal complex and in the inferior part of the postcentral gyrus greatly magnify the important sensory surfaces of the hand and face. The tonotopic map of the auditory system is not as well known in man, although it has been well studied in cats and monkeys. Where it has been demonstrated, it seems to present less distortion, following the frequency spectrum precisely. The essential point, however, is that there can be no cortical map without a corresponding thalamic map underneath.

Multiple Representation of Sensory Surfaces

If we pursue the preceding topic, we find that the thalamus and the cortex each contain not just one but several maps of each sensory modality. For example, somesthetic information is mapped, in varying degrees of precision and bilaterality, not only in VPl, but also in the posterior and intralaminar nuclei. Multiple representation, or parallel processing, is now recognized as an organizing principle of the CNS (see Chap. 6). Although the functional contributions of each distinctive thalamocortical network are far from clear, the sensory surfaces of the body are mapped, over and over

— for different purposes, perhaps alertness to new stimuli vs. selective analysis — in the thalamus and cortex.

Specificity of Thalamic Neurons

As in the case of cortical neurons and their functional columns, each thalamic cell or group of cells analyzes a certain feature in the pattern of sensory information, and only that feature. Such precision of information processing goes far beyond the orderly projections mentioned above. This neuronal specificity was first discovered in the visual system, where single cells were found to respond selectively to certain features. The prerequisites for individual cellular response become more and more stringent as information flashes from periphery to thalamus and on to cortex. Such progressive feature analysis illustrates the interdependent, orderly, and hierarchical design of the CNS.

Reciprocity of Thalamic and Cortical Function

Although we have not indicated so in Table 8-1, corticothalamic projections reciprocate the thalamocortical ones in almost equal numbers and in corresponding precise order. Such connections seem to modulate thalamic activity, inhibiting and/or facilitating specific thalamic neurons or groups of neurons. It is thought that these connections might offer an attention mechanism, as well as a means of refining sensory input.

FIG. 8–4. *Thalamocortical projection systems.* Fibers emanating from the thalamus form a more or less continuous fan, the thalamic radiation. Five subsidiary radiations are recognized: posteroinferior, posterior, superior, anterior, and inferior. (The inferior is compact, and is often termed a peduncle; unlike the other radiations, it does not enter the internal capsule, but descends medial to it en route to the basal forebrain.) The foregoing sectors are made up of axons coursing from the various thalamic nuclei to their cortical projection areas, as indicated by identical stippling or hatching on the lower (thalamus) and upper (cortex) diagrams.

The lower diagram is a simplified version of Fig. 8-3 in which most of the major afferent tracts have been cut away to better expose the nuclei. Can you now identify these nuclei?

The two top diagrams are maps of the cerebral cortex adapted from Economo and Koskinas, 1925. Although less well known than those of Brodmann (see Fig. 13-3), these maps have two useful features: they show the entire cortical surface, including the superior and inferior margins of the hemisphere, and they illustrate the general fissural pattern of the human cerebrum.

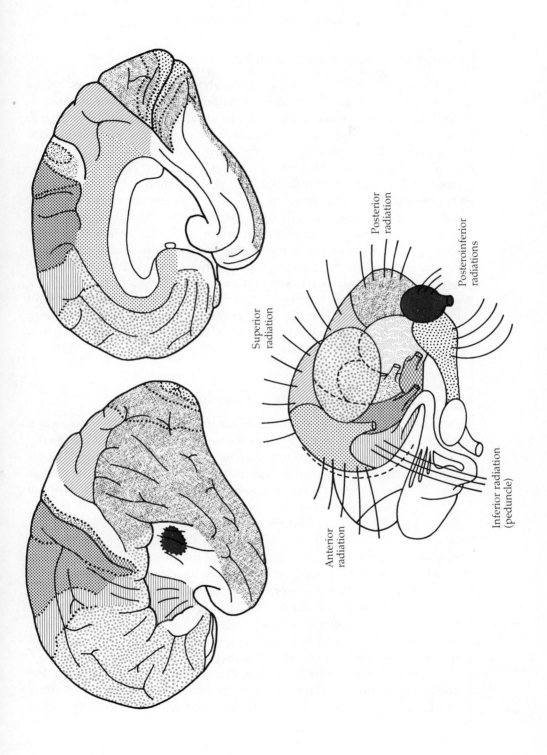

Superior
radiation

Posterior
radiation

Posteroinferior
radiations

Anterior
radiation

Inferior radiation
(peduncle)

Chemical Asymmetry of the Thalamus?

Recently, an example of chemical asymmetry has been discovered in the distribution of a particular neurotransmitter in the human thalamus. In several individuals studied postmortem, thalamic norepinephrine was found to be strongly lateralized — richly distributed in the left pulvinar and in the right VB complex. The functional or pathological significance of these findings is subject to further investigation. It may be that this chemical asymmetry relates to handedness, or perhaps merely reflects the presence of a prevalently one-sided vascular lesion. Such correlations were not possible in this pathologic study of elderly patients with case histories that did not contain this information. But whatever the explanation of these findings, it is reasonable to wonder whether association and somatosensory functions might be discharged in perhaps different ways and with possibly different transmitter systems in the two halves of the thalamus. We know that there is functional asymmetry in the two cerebral hemispheres of which the thalamic halves are central parts. Thus these findings prompt us to look for chemical dimensions to concepts of laterality and hemispheric dominance in the CNS.

Effects of Localized Thalamic Lesions in Humans

The thalamus can fall prey to injury, through vascular insults (strokes and hemorrhages), cell loss in aging, trauma, and tumor, among other causes. Of all these dangers, vascular accidents perhaps give the most useful perspective on the structure and function of the thalamus, because a small infarct or hemorrhage can interrupt with surgical precision one or more circuits in which the thalamus is a key link.

The thalamus receives blood from the internal carotid and vertebral systems of arteries (see Chap. 15). It is supplied mainly by branches of the posterior cerebral artery. The vasculature of the human thalamus is complicated and (as one might expect) variable in its layout from one person to another. But focal vascular lesions may have profound consequences.

In general, lesions of thalamic nuclei produce deficits in the functions subserved by these nuclei. There are some peculiar features, however, that seem to derive from damage to the integrative machinery of the thalamus and from interruption of circuits involving extrathalamic structures.

Vascular occlusion (embolic or thrombotic) of posterior thalamic territories leads to predominately sensory defects, the exact nature of which depends on which nucleus or nuclei are infarcted (LG, MG, VPl, etc.).

Abnormal or exaggerated sensations (paresthesias or hyperesthesias, respectively) and abnormal postures ("thalamic hand") may be present as lasting effects, along with a contralateral spastic hemiparesis (weakness) that usually clears within a short time. The paresis is likely due to transient edema in the adjacent posterior limb of the internal capsule that impairs transmission in the corticospinal tract for a relatively brief period.

Such a combination of persistent sensory deficits, distortions of sensory affect, and curious postures with a transient hemiparesis is called a thalamic syndrome (of Dejerine-Roussy). To some individuals with this syndrome, a stimulus we would consider innocuous or pleasant, such as the touch of a wisp of cotton wool, can be horribly painful — to a degree apparently so far from normal that we cannot even begin to appreciate it. Even the suggestion of a stimulus can be terrifying; a patient known to one of us (J.B.A.), with a clearly diagnosed residuum of a thalamic infarct resulting from posterior cerebral artery insufficiency, clearly illustrated this point. She suffered anguish from an ice cube placed in her palm, and became visibly agitated at the mere sight of one. She explained, "That cold . . . it feels like death itself." The thalamus, together with the brainstem reticular formation, has much to do with making such affective judgments.

In contrast, occlusion of anterior regions of the thalamus may produce a variety of nonsensory deficits, depending again on which nucleus or group of nuclei is involved. Motor disturbances may occur with infarcts of the VL and VA nuclei, through which the cerebellar and basal ganglia pathways pass. Often, however, other structures (such as the globus pallidus) are involved in these lesions, and hence the pathophysiology of the resulting disorder is complicated.

Generalized deficits may also result from thalamic lesions. Disorders of consciousness, similar to those encountered in brainstem injuries, probably reflect damage to the diffuse thalamocortical activating system — which includes the midline and intralaminar nuclei plus parts of VA. Alterations of behavior, not unlike those seen in frontal lobotomy patients, are sometimes associated with damage to the MD/anterior nuclear complex.

General Concepts

The thalamus receives not only sensory information, but also data not directly related to sensory events, e.g., cerebellar, pallidal, and limbic inputs. The information it processes is important to discriminative and affective aspects of sensation and to the coordinated activity of widely separated structures implicated in motor control and emotion.

The thalamus, sensory gateway to the cerebral cortex, admits messages, sensory and otherwise, that activate the cortex. Within this pattern of diffuse activation, specific neural images arrive, over the great lemnisci, including the optic nerve and other afferent cables such as the superior cerebellar peduncle, fields of Forel, and the mammillothalamic tract. By admitting the latter inputs, the thalamus provides key communications links for three major parts of the brain: the cerebellum, basal ganglia, and limbic lobe. By providing such links (VL and VA nuclei) between the cere-bellum and basal ganglia on one hand and the cerebral cortex on the other, the thalamus plays a key role in the organization of movement. Similarly, by providing limbic system connections, such as those between amygdala and frontal lobe (MD nucleus) or between hypothalamus and cingulate gyrus (anterior nuclei), the thalamus plays a role in mediating activities important to behavioral and endocrine states.

But the thalamus does more than collect and analyze messages and route them to the cerebral cortex. It joins the cortex and reticular activating sys-tem in maintaining and regulating consciousness, alertness, and attention. Thus, it is much more than a gateway to a higher region; it is a partner to the cortex in coordinating the teamwork between many specialized parts of the brain.

Glossary

Anterior nuclear group: the three nuclei (AV, AM, and AD) beneath the anterior thalamic tubercle; their connections (see Table 8-1) make them important components of the limbic system.

Brachium of inferior colliculus: the main auditory channel of the thalamus, terminating in the medial geniculate nucleus (body).

Centromedian nucleus: largest of the thalamic intralaminar nuclei; has fiber connections with the motor system (see Table 8-1), and is important to intrathalamic integration.

Dentatorubrothalamic tract: the main cerebellar channel of the thalamus, terminating principally in the ventral lateral nucleus.

Fields of Forel: compact, prominent fascicles of pallidal efferent fibers, first directed caudomedially toward the mesencephalic tegmentum, then mak-ing a hairpin turn up into the overlying ventral anterior nucleus; the main input of the basal ganglia to the thalamus.

Internal medullary lamina: a conspicuous, curvilinear band of myelinated axons that divides the thalamus into a medial and a lateral compartment; forks anteriorly into a compartment for the anterior nuclear group.

Intralaminar nuclei: numerous small clusters of neurons within the internal medullary lamina of the thalamus; have widespread cortical and subcortical connections.

Lateral dorsal nucleus: a small association nucleus of the thalamus, just behind the anterior tubercle, with connections to posterior association cortex and limbic system affiliations.

Lateral geniculate nucleus (body):   the principal visual sensory nucleus of the thalamus, with retinotopically organized projections to calcarine (primary visual) cortex.

Lateral posterior nucleus: one of the association nuclei of the thalamus; has important visual inputs, and projects to posterior association cortex.

Lemniscal channels: the major, grossly visible inputs to the thalamus, e.g., the optic tract, medial lemniscus, fields of Forel, etc.

Mammillothalamic tract: a conspicuous hypothalamic input to the thalamus; a key connection in the limbic system.

Medial dorsal nucleus: a major association nucleus of the thalamus; intimately related, through reciprocal fiber connections, to the cortex of the frontal lobes.

Medial geniculate nucleus (body):   the principal auditory sensory nucleus of the thalamus, with tonotopically organized projections to the supratemporal plane (primary auditory cortex).

Medial lemniscus: a major somesthetic input for bodily sensations to the thalamus; terminates in the ventral posterolateral nucleus in a somatotopically organized, laminar pattern.

Midline nuclei: numerous small clusters of neurons immediately beneath the ependymal lining of the third ventricle; have widespread cortical and subcortical connections.

Nonlemniscal channels: sensory inputs to the thalamus which are less obvious than the lemniscal channels and hence only recently discovered; exemplify the principle of parallel sensory processing.

Nucleus reuniens: a midline nucleus of the thalamus which projects to the entire limbic lobe, including a part of the hippocampus.

Parafascicular nucleus: an intralaminar nucleus immediately medial to the centromedian nucleus and with similar motor connections; these two juxtaposed nuclei form the so-called "CM-Pf complex."

Posterior nuclear group: very small nuclei beneath the pulvinar; implicated in somatic sensation, especially in pain pathways to cortex and elsewhere in thalamus.

Pulvinar: largest of the thalamic association nuclei and largest thalamic nucleus overall; the key subcortical organizer of the vast posterior association cortex in the parietal, occipital, and temporal lobes.

Reticular nucleus: a thin sheet of neurons surrounding the lateral and ventral surfaces of the thalamus (blends with the zona incerta); apparently provides for feedback inhibition of thalamic output and tegmentothalamic input.

Spinothalamic tracts: major somesthetic inputs for bodily sensations to the thalamus; terminate in the ventral posterolateral nucleus in a diffuse, net-like pattern of arborization.

Trigeminothalamic tract: a major somesthetic input for facial sensations to the thalamus; terminates in the ventral posteromedial nucleus.

Ventral anterior nucleus: the pallidal recipient zone of the thalamus; a key link in basal ganglia circuits to frontal motor and premotor cortex. Also the largest component of the generalized thalamocortical system (see p. 168).

Ventral lateral nucleus: the dentatorubral recipient zone of the thalamus; a key link in cerebellar circuits to frontal motor and premotor cortex.

Ventral posterior nucleus: the major somesthetic region of the thalamus, also commonly known as the ventrobasal complex; its lateral and medial divisions (VPl and VPm) mediate sensations from the body and face, respectively.

The Motor System

9

"Muscles move the world" (Granit, 1978), and it is the motor system that moves muscles. Talking, smiling, writing, reading, walking, looking, and so forth, from the simplest to most complex act, the motor system is our means of contact, our way to move our world.

In a pure characterization, one that excludes sensory components important to motility, the basic elements of the motor system are the motor cortex, basal ganglia, cerebellum, and various brainstem and spinal cord motor nuclei. Except for certain reflexes, almost every movement is the result of an interaction between these far-flung parts of the motor system.

Voluntary movement is directed by the motor cortex. It receives signals from the basal ganglia, cerebellum, and other cortical areas; it integrates them and passes the commands down to brainstem spinal motor neurons (usually through adjacent local interneurons) for execution. Conventionally, the motor cortex is said to be the "highest" level of motor integration, and the spinal cord the "lowest." In reality, however, the task of synthesizing innumerable signals into patterns of action is common to both regions, and to the basal ganglia and cerebellum as well. The latter two structures, in fact, seem to play decisive roles in early stages of motor programming.

Skeletal muscles are activated by brainstem and spinal cord motor neurons, which by the peripheral distribution of their terminally branched axons command specialized teams of muscle fibers (motor units; see Chap. 10). These neurons are the "final common pathway" (Sherrington) through which all neural activity converges before it becomes behavior. The various functional kinds of muscles (flexors and extensors) are rigged

185

by tendons to the skeletal system, thus providing the means to move bones in various ways at their joints. Extensor muscles are in major part antigravity muscles; flexors, which oppose the action of extensors, are important in manipulating the environment. Whenever we move, our skeleton moves by the contraction of muscles, individually and in synergistic ensembles, and by the synchronized relaxation of their antagonists.

Some movements are reflexive, others voluntary, and still others read out automatically by central motor programs which we may or may not consciously turn on. A great many of our movements are under the watchful supervision of the somesthetic cortex (Chap. 6), which monitors the constant sensory input from the muscles and joints and also, through thalamocortical association systems, from the other primary senses. Such movements, which depend on feedback, operate in a "closed loop" manner and derive from slowly developing, finely graded muscular contractions. Other movements operate without feedback, in an "open loop" fashion; these are the quick or "ballistic" movements resulting from rapid lengthening and shortening of muscles. Still other movements, however, such as chewing and breathing, are highly repetitive and stereotyped, and only need feedback for enhanced quality and timing. They are executed from central programs which store and play out patterns of muscle activity — like a mechanical toy soldier that struts forth in a particular way once wound up and set free. Such movements, which come out of "pattern generators" are usually operating in a "closed loop" mode, but we can "open" the loop at any time, as when we begin to talk while eating. Fortunately, because of these built-in programs, we do not have to concentrate on each and every movement.

Most of our movements, however, such as walking or reaching, are dynamic combinations of the closed and open loop modes, chiefly the latter. Most remarkable is that after all possibilities for responding are taken into account, there is only one coherent response, despite all the stimuli that could distract us from making the right moves.

We shall now examine each major component of the motor system in its turn.

The Motor Cortex

The motor cortex (Fig. 9-1) is essentially concerned with voluntary movements. It is a relatively narrow and precisely organized band of frontal gray matter adjoining the central sulcus, immediately in front of the primary somatosensory homunculus. It, too, features an inverted representation of

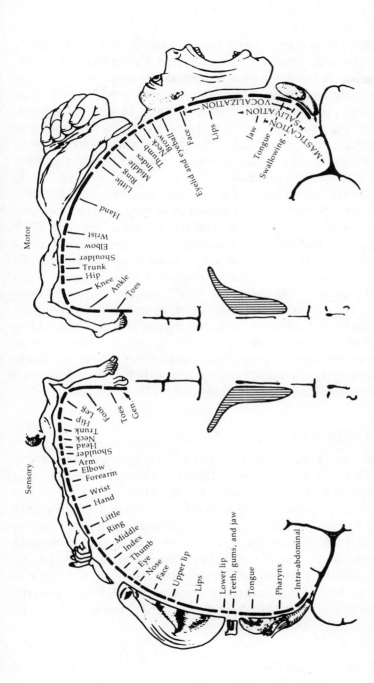

Motor

Hand
Wrist
Elbow
Shoulder
Trunk
Hip
Knee
Ankle
Toes

Little
Ring
Middle
Thumb
Neck
Brow
Eyelid and eyeball
Face
Lips
Jaw
Tongue
Swallowing

VOCALIZATION
SALIVATION
VOCALIZATION
MASTICATION

Sensory

Foot
Toes
Leg
Hip
Trunk
Neck
Head
Shoulder
Arm
Elbow
Forearm
Wrist
Hand
Little
Ring
Middle
Index
Thumb
Eye
Nose
Face
Upper lip
Lips
Lower lip
Teeth, gums, and jaw
Tongue
Pharynx
Intra-abdominal

Gen.

FIG. 9–1. *The motor cortex.* The area of cortex most immediately concerned with control of voluntary movement (right) lies just in front of the central sulcus. It features an inverted representation of the opposite half of the body, the so-called motor homunculus. Compare it to the corresponding sensory homunculus (left) which lies just behind the central sulcus. (From W. Penfield; in J. Z. Young, *Programs of the Brain*, Fig. 11, Oxford University Press, New York, 1978)

the opposite half of the body, a motor homunculus similar to its sensory twin, with which considerable overlap occurs. As with the sensory analyzing regions, this area of cortex where movement patterns are directed is organized in keeping with the functional importance of body parts. Thus the relatively large area of cortical surface devoted to the face, larynx, tongue, and hand (especially the thumb and fingers) reflects the delicacy or fineness with which their movements can be controlled and the consequent utility of these parts in facial expression, vocalization, and exploration or manipulation of the environment.

The motor homunculus was demonstrated over three decades ago by the neurosurgeon Wilder Penfield and his associates in their surgical treatment of patients with epilepsy at the Montreal Neurological Institute. They found, for example, that electrical stimulation of the exposed motor cortex at one locus in the conscious individual might bring about contraction of a muscle that adducts the thumb, while stimulation at another nearby locus might change the person's facial expression in some manner. The movements they obtained, however, were crude compared to what happens when this region of the cortex is activated by the rest of the brain in everyday life. This situation is still true today; no neurosurgeon with an electrode can hope to duplicate more than fragments of skilled movement or high-order sensory synthesis, although it is true that more-or-less intact memories and feelings can be elicited (see Chap. 13).

The Columnar Design of the Motor Cortex

Like other cortical areas, the motor cortex is built up of adjacent modules, tall columns slightly less than 1 mm in diameter. Groups of neurons in a motor column appear to drive particular segmental interneurons or clusters of motor neurons for particular muscles. Extrinsic stimulation of one part of a column, as by thalamocortical or association afferents, activates the cells in that column and inhibits activity in the adjacent columns. It is thought that cortical control of movement results from fluctuating patterns of activity in sets of columns — taking form, acting, and dissolving in the course of movement. As we stressed in discussing vision and somethesis, patterns are all important in neural activity; here the patterns direct still other patterns of neuromuscular action downstream.

Inputs and Outputs of Motor Cortex

The motor cortex receives input from other cortical areas (especially the parietal association cortex) as well as from the cerebellum and basal ganglia via the thalamus, a major center for motor and sensory interactions (Chap. 8). The outflow of the motor cortex is carried mainly by the deeply situated pyramidal cells in layer V of areas 4 and 6. Axons of these neurons project to various brainstem and spinal motor centers via the pyramidal tract, giving off collaterals to certain sensory nuclei en route (see below).

Pyramidal axons in the corticospinal tract descend in a long trajectory through many regions: the corona radiata, internal capsule, crus cerebri, pons, and medulla oblongata (Fig. 9-2). At the spinomedullary junction about 90% of the fibers cross in the pyramidal decussation and descend in the spinal cord as the lateral corticospinal tract. The uncrossed fibers form the medial corticospinal tract; generally, it does not descend below mid-thoracic levels. In contrast, the lateral corticospinal fibers terminate along the entire length of the spinal cord. A few fibers end directly, or monosynaptically, on motor neurons. Most corticospinal axons, however, synapse on nearby interneurons in the intermediate gray (Rexed's laminae VII–VIII; see Chap. 10), and these cells in turn project to motor neurons in lamina IX. In man, nearly 1 million corticospinal fibers originate from the pyramidal cells in the motor cortex. Other mammals, even primates, have fewer such fibers. The larger number of corticospinal fibers in the human neuraxis seems to be associated with the development of hand control and strength.

From careful neuronal counts in man, it is known that area 4 (primary motor cortex) contains 34,000 giant pyramidal cells of Betz. Their large-diameter axons form a corresponding number of the 1 million pyramidal tract fibers. Such thick, fast-conducting fibers probably mediate control of fine volitional movement. The remaining small-caliber fibers in the pyramidal tract originate from cortical areas 4, 3, 1, 2, and 6 (see Chap. 13). These finer, more slowly conducting axons probably are associated with control of grosser movements and muscle tone. Betz cells are big because their axons have a long way to go — up to four feet if they run to the sacral cord! But their gigantic size does not make them more important, as certain older workers thought. If anything, it is the host of small cells of our nervous system, such as the cortical stellate cells and the spinal interneurons, that achieves the miracles of feature analysis and unified response.

The Pervasiveness of "Motor" Activity

Fibers from the motor cortex also run to the reticular formation, red nucleus, pons and inferior olive, and to many other areas involved in the execution of movement. Furthermore, as indicated earlier, motor fibers pass to the nuclei of the dorsal columns — to the cells that mediate information on the sensations of touch, position, and movement of limbs. They

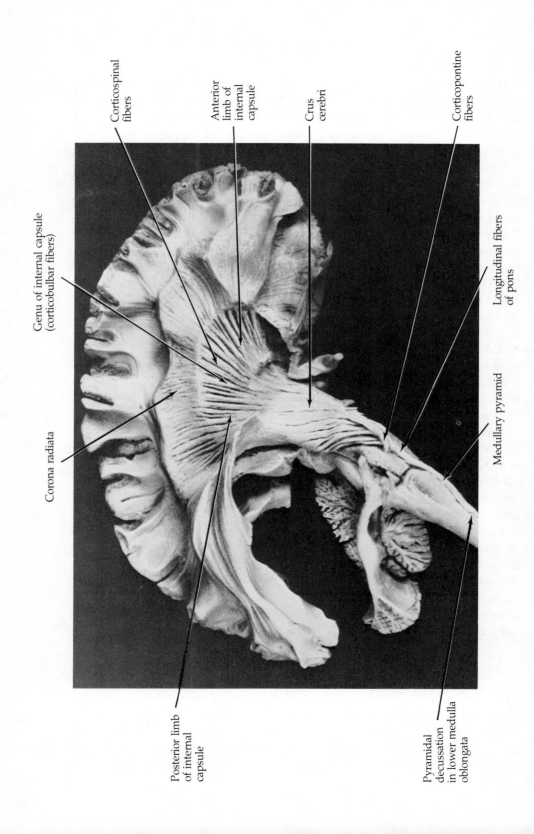

Corticospinal fibers

Anterior limb of internal capsule

Crus cerebri

Corticopontine fibers

Genu of internal capsule (corticobulbar fibers)

Longtiudinal fibers of pons

Corona radiata

Medullary pyramid

Posterior limb of internal capsule

Pyramidal decussation in lower medulla oblongata

also go to the trigeminal sensory nuclei, the nucleus proprius in the posterior horn of the spinal cord, and even to the various visceral sensory
nuclei of the brainstem and cord.

Why do motor fibers thus engage sensory and associative neurons? We
suggested the answer in Chapter 6: it appears that they exert a modulating
influence on sensory inflow. Sensory attention thus may be focused on a
smaller region, or on certain events. The motor cortex may momentarily
select the most important or relevant sensory messages and suppress the
rest.

The Basal Ganglia

The basal ganglia are massive telencephalic groupings of cells located beneath the cerebral cortex: the putamen and caudate nucleus, globus pallidus, subthalamic nucleus, and substantia nigra. The amygdala, which is
closely related to the caudate/putamen, is sometimes included. Fig. 9-3A
shows the complex relationship of the putamen, caudate, and amygdala to
each other and to the overlying hemisphere. The putamen is a large, bulging outer mass of gray matter; a more slender, inner curved piece is the
caudate. Its elongated mass curls around into the temporal lobe like the tail
of a fish. Its shape conforms to the curvature of the lateral ventricle in
which it lies. The globus pallidus lies medial to the putamen, while the
subthalamic nucleus and substantia nigra (a region containing cells deeply
pigmented with melanin) lie posteriorly and ventrally (the last two structures are not shown on the figure). We have to rotate the various ganglia in

---

FIG. 9–2. *The pyramidal tract and related cortical efferents.* This lateral view of the
dissected right hemisphere and brainstem shows the great family of cortical efferent
fibers that sweep directly in parallel fashion to diverse targets. In their graceful
descent from the cortex, these fibers form the corona radiata, internal capsule, crus
cerebri, longitudinal fibers of the pons, and medullary pyramids. The locations of
the corticospinal and corticobulbar fibers are indicated; the former lie in, the latter
just in front of, the genu of the internal capsule.

Many of the fibers shown here are corticopontine fibers arising in frontal,
parietal, occipital, and temporal lobes of the cerebral hemisphere and terminating
in the pontine nuclei. Much of these lobes, especially most of the temporal lobes,
has been cut away. Other cortical efferent fibers, which cannot be identified in this
dissection, are the corticorubral, corticonigral, corticothalamic, and corticostriate
projections — to list just a few in descending order of length. Prominently shown in
this dissection are the optic radiation and the superior and inferior cerebellar
peduncles. Can you identify them? (From E. Ludwig and J. Klingler, *Atlas Cerebri
Humani*. Little, Brown and Company, Boston, 1956, plate 26)

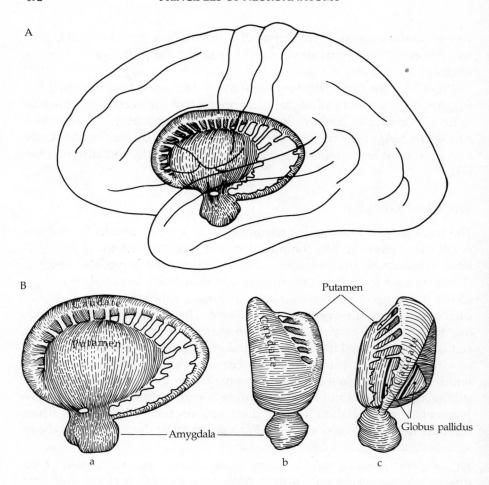

FIG. 9–3. *The basal ganglia.* (A) The basal ganglia in a "transparent" left hemisphere. The putamen, lying beneath the insula, connects rostrally with the head of the caudate nucleus. The tail of the caudate curls into the temporal lobe, following the curvature of the lateral ventricle in which it lies, and fuses with the amygdala, which in turn merges with the undersurface of the putamen. Numerous bridges of gray matter run between the caudate and putamen. Between the bridges extend the fibers of the internal capsule (not shown).

(B) The basal ganglia in lateral (a), anterior (b), and posterior (c) aspects. The posterior view shows the globus pallidus (sometimes called the pallidum). By virtue of high myelinated fiber content, it has a pallor approaching white matter in the fresh state. The globus pallidus has two divisions, as visible here.

space, as if viewing a piece of sculpture, to see all the major structures and interrelationships (Fig. 9-3B). The striatum (caudate/putamen) receives fibers from virtually every region of the cerebral cortex, as well as from the thalamus. Except for a two-way connection with the substantia nigra, its output goes entirely to the globus pallidus. The outer division of the pallidum projects to the subthalamic nucleus, which returns fibers to the inner division. The inner division, in turn, distributes fibers to the thalamus and tegmentum.

Transmitters and Transmitter Interactions

A number of neurotransmitters have a proven or probable relationship to the basal ganglia. One of the most important is dopamine, the transmitter of the dopaminergic nigrostriatal system. Cell bodies in the substantia nigra project to the striatum (a collective term for the caudate nucleus and putamen, both structures showing prominent stripes of myelinated fibers). These nigral dopamine neurons synapse with striatal cholinergic (ACh) neurons, which in turn connect with striatal GABA neurons and perhaps others. GABA (gamma-aminobutyric acid) is thus a third major transmitter in the basal ganglia. Some GABA fibers from the putamen project directly to the so-called reticulated (having a diffuse cell population) part of the substantia nigra. Other putaminal GABA fibers run to the nearby globus pallidus, while still others form local intrinsic connections in the striatum. Another chemical variety of neurons, which use the small peptide substance P as a transmitter, also apparently project to the substantia nigra. Interestingly, the globus pallidus also contains one of the highest concentrations of enkephalins in the brain.

Thus the transmitters of several of the major inputs and outputs of the basal ganglia have been tentatively identified. And, in the case of dopamine, there have already been important clinical applications. The interactions of various transmitters in the basal ganglia and elsewhere are of tremendous interest to investigators and clinicians.

Clinical Correlates of Transmitter Imbalance

The importance of the basal ganglia in movement is dramatically illustrated by the striking, often grotesque consequences of damage to them by certain types of neurologic disease processes: the tremor and shuffling gait in Parkinson's disease, the dancelike movement fragments in Huntington's chorea, the violent discus-throwing movements of hemiballismus. In all

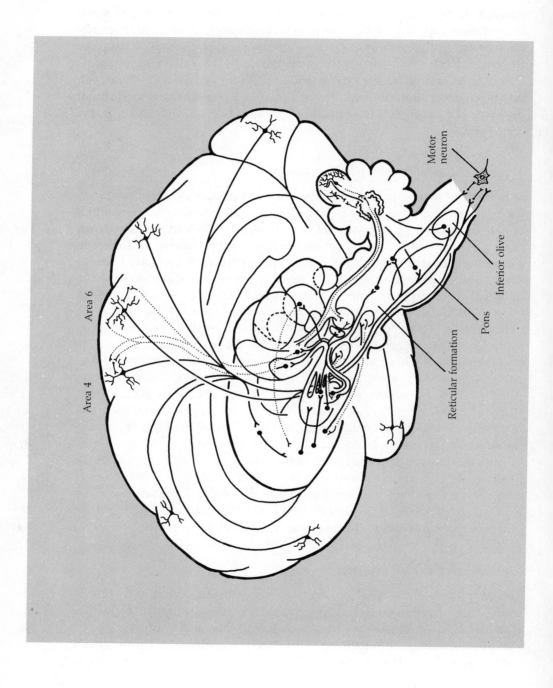

three of these disorders, we know roughly where the problem lies. Patients with Parkinson's disease suffer from a deficiency in striatal dopamine owing to loss of dopaminergic neurons in the substantia nigra. This can be relieved by administration of large quantities of L-dopa, a biosynthetic precursor of dopamine. This substance stimulates dopamine synthesis and makes more dopamine available for release by nerve impulses. Huntington's chorea, on the other hand, seems to result from a reduction in the activity of intrinsic cholinergic (and perhaps other) neurons in the basal ganglia. The neurotoxic agent kainic acid injected into the striatum in experimental animals selectively destroys these intrinsic neurons and produces a close animal model of the hyperkinetic motility of patients with Huntington's disease. The neurotransmitter implicated in hemiballismus is not yet known, but this rare and most violent of all dyskinesias, in which the limbs on one side of the body fly about continuously, usually results from a small infarct in the opposite subthalamic nucleus.

The basal ganglia work in concert with other members of the motor team. As shown in Figure 9-4, the cerebellum and basal ganglia connect, via thalamus, with the cerebral cortex in a strikingly parallel manner. Both

---

FIG. 9–4. *Circuitry of the motor system.* Major connections of primary and supplementary motor cortex (Area 4 and the medial part of Area 6, respectively). General principle of organization: the basal ganglia and cerebellum are interposed between the entire cerebral cortex and the motor cortex (via the thalamus). Thus, axons of pyramidal neurons in the orbitofrontal, frontopolar, pre-Rolandic, parietal, occipital, and temporal cortical regions project to the basal ganglia (caudate/putamen) and also to the precerebellar nuclei (pontine and inferior olivary), which effect mossy and climbing fiber terminations in the cerebellar cortex (on granule and Purkinje cells, respectively). Basal ganglia activity passes from the inner division of the globus pallidus via the ansa and fasciculus lenticularis and Forel's fields to ventral anterior and ventral lateral thalamic nuclei, and thence to the pyramidal cells and local interneurons of the primary and supplementary motor cortex (dotted lines). Similarly, cerebellar outflow (dotted lines) passes from the dentate nucleus via the superior cerebellar peduncle to the rostral thalamus and on to motor cortex.

Other connections illustrated: from external division of globus pallidus to subthalamic nucleus, then back (dotted line) to internal pallidum; from inner pallidum to prerubral and tegmental nuclei; from putamen to substantia nigra, then back (dotted line) to putamen (nigrostriatal dopaminergic system); from centromedian nucleus of thalamus to putamen; from dentate nucleus to red nucleus; from pontomedullary reticular formation via reticulospinal tracts to spinal interneurons; and from Area 4 via pyramidal tract to spinal interneurons or directly to the motor neuron.

For clarity, we left this figure virtually unlabeled; refer to Figs. 8–3 and 9–3.

receive inputs from virtually all regions of the cerebral cortex, and, through the VA–VL thalamic nuclear complex, affect the output of the motor cortex. In the case of the basal ganglia, the thalamic-bound connections originate in the globus pallidus, while cerebellothalamic fibers emanate from the deep cerebellar nuclei (chiefly the dentate).

A Neural Model of Unperformed Movement

The contributions of the basal ganglia to motor control and to other aspects of brain function are still somewhat cloudy, though an understanding of their function is rapidly developing. Many ideas have come forward: e.g., they provide the "postural background" for movements, insure the "pertinence" of movements, or act as automated "function generators" for slowly building contractions ("ramp movements"). It now appears, however, that persons with damaged basal ganglia are somehow deficient in tracking their own actions or in foreshadowing their coming movements. This curious deficiency makes it difficult for them to generate movements spontaneously and to control them predictably. A person with Parkinson's disease for example, if asked to hold out his arm, can do so easily, but if his eyes are closed the arm falls without his knowledge. Once having started, the patient can walk normally at first, but the steps become shorter and shorter, until progression stops. The individual's laughter may be similar; the "ha, ha, ha's" become faster and faster, sounding like a bouncing ping-pong ball coming to rest.

Persons with Parkinson's disease thus seem to lack a dynamic internal model of their own movements upon which to base and control such movements. Instead, they must depend solely on sensory input, which they respond to; they are not able to anticipate their movements. Unlike the normal individual, they are not "acting according to plan" — because they have no plan. Continuous movements that normally require very little corrective monitoring (e.g., gait, bodily postures, facial expressions) are particularly affected. As we mentioned earlier, central programs are necessary for such "open loop" movements. It seems, then, that damage to the basal ganglia, which are definitely involved in creating a neural image of body motion and reading out or perhaps synthesizing central movement programs, disrupts execution of such movements, but has far less effect on cortically supervised "closed loop" performances such as writing or catching a ball.

The Importance of Neural Teamwork

We must keep in mind that the distorted features of disordered motility we see in patients with basal ganglia disease — or with cerebellar disease — are the pathophysiological expressions of the anatomically intact but circuit-deprived remainder of the motor system trying to get along as best it can (see comments in next section). That it is only partly successful is heart-breaking for individuals, but the ability to carry out some movement, however affected, testifies to the resilience of the motor system and its interdependent design.

The Cerebellum

The cerebellum is tucked neatly behind and beneath the cerebral cortex, strapped to the medulla and pons by the three pairs of cerebellar peduncles (see Chap. 2). There are two cerebellar hemispheres, separated by a midline vermis (Fig. 9-5). Anatomically, the cerebellum is divided into three

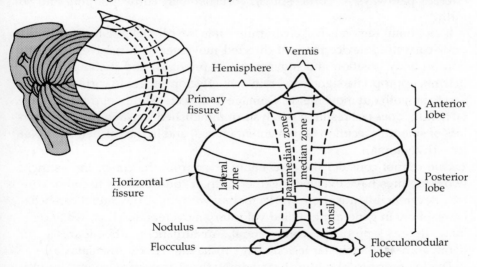

FIG. 9–5. *The concept of three longitudinal cerebellar zones.* Based on output connections, three longitudinal zones of the cerebellar cortex are recognized: a median zone, which includes the flocculonodular lobe and the rest of the vermis; a paramedian zone, which includes the more medial regions of the anterior and posterior lobes; and a lateral zone, which comprises the greatly elaborated regions of the hemispheres. These three zones make distinctively different functional contributions to motor control. (Redrawn from C. R. Noback and R. J. Demarest, *The Human Nervous System*, 2nd Ed. McGraw-Hill, New York, 1975)

transversely oriented lobes: the anterior lobe (associated with the spinal cord and serving gross movements of the head and body), the posterior lobe (associated with the neocortex and involved in finer movements of the limbs), and the flocculonodular lobe (associated with the vestibular system and thus important to equilibrium and balance).

A more recent functional scheme of subdivision emphasizes the output connections of different cortical regions to the deep cerebellar nuclei and the projections from those nuclei to various brainstem targets. Three longitudinal zones are recognized; surprisingly, these sectors fit well with the transverse anatomical subdivisions. The median zone (Fig. 9-5) is concerned with equilibrium and postural control; it facilitates tone in extensor muscles. The paramedian zone deals with posture too, but also with progression, i.e., with gait. It facilitates ipsilateral flexor muscle tone, but clinically is not as well understood as the other two zones in humans. The lateral zone participates in coordination of skilled movements involving the distal limb muscles. Its activity ultimately influences the various cerebral efferent pathways — corticospinal, corticobulbar, corticopontine, and so forth.

If any brain region is like a computer, it is the cerebellum: it serves as an error-correcting device for goal-directed movements. It receives information on body position and movements in progress, and it computes and delivers appropriate signals to brainstem effector centers to correct posture and to smooth out movements. Damage to the cerebellum, or developmental failure, does not result in paralysis or diminished sensation but rather in loss of smooth execution of movement (ataxia) and in diminished muscular tone (hypotonia).

One cannot consider the cerebellum apart from the cerebrum, as these two structures have evolved together in their contributions to motor control. A cerebral hemisphere works mainly with the contralateral cerebellar hemisphere in generating skilled voluntary movements. Thus, while cerebral lesions produce contralateral disturbances (hemiparesis or hemiparalysis), cerebellar lesions have ipsilateral effects (hemiataxia).

The long reciprocal routes that underlie these important axioms are visible in Figure 9-6. Cerebral input to cerebellum follows a corticopontocerebellar pathway. Cerebellar output returns to cerebrum via the dentato(rubro)thalamocortical pathway. The entire round trip is long — from the cerebral cortex down through the pontine nuclei to the contralateral cerebellar hemisphere, and back up through the dentate nucleus, contralateral red nucleus, and thalamus (VL nucleus) to the motor cortex on the original side.

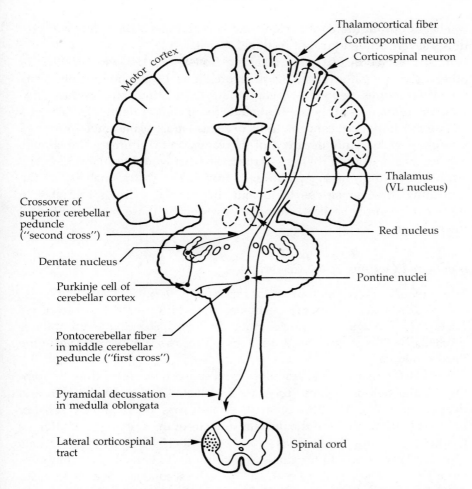

FIG. 9–6. *The "double-cross"*. In motor control, the cerebrum and cerebellum engage in a long-range crossed and recrossed teamplay. The corticospinal connection represents a third crossing of the midline.

Clinically, this loop is very important. If the circuit is broken anywhere, the smooth and orderly sequence of muscular contraction in skillful voluntary movements will noticeably suffer.

Thus cerebellar functions involve intimately related functions of many other brain components, some of which lie at a great distance from the cerebellum. As might be expected, disturbances of cerebellar function can result from many types of interruptions of this teamplay. The clinical symptoms usually become less severe with time, although damage to the cerebellar output (dentate nucleus and superior cerebellar peduncle) produces severe and enduring functional deficits.

In any event, disturbances resulting from brain lesions, cerebellar or otherwise, are pathophysiological expressions of the remaining intact neural structures deprived of controlling, regulating, and mutually interacting influences. This is a cardinal tenet of clinical neurology. To get a feel for this important concept, think of a small musical ensemble, such as a jazz quintet, suddenly deprived of its pianist and drummer. The strange harmonics and drifting rhythms of the music that would result could not be attributed to the missing piano and drums, but to the inability of the remaining three musicians to fill out the chordal voicings and stay in proper relation to the beat normally provided by these instruments and their players.

Inputs and Outputs of the Cerebellum

The cerebellum receives four major inputs (Fig. 9-7):

1. *Vestibular fibers.* Primary vestibular fibers of CN VIII and secondary fibers from the vestibular nuclei enter via a medial region of the inferior cerebellar peduncle (juxtarestiform body). These terminate primarily in the flocculonodular lobe.

2. *Ascending spinal fibers.* Impulses from sensory receptors (muscle spindles, Golgi tendon organs, pressure and tactile organs in the skin and deeper tissues) enter the spinal cord and pass to secondary sensory neurons (such as those in the nucleus dorsalis of the spinal gray matter, or Clarke's column). From these neurons, fibers ascend over various spinocerebellar tracts to terminate primarily in the anterior lobe and posterior vermis. There is also a pathway from the secondary trigeminal nuclei to certain regions of the cerebellar cortex. These fibers, which bring in information from receptors in the face, enter via the ropelike inferior cerebellar penduncle (restiform body).

3. *Pontine fibers.* Cortical fibers from all lobes of the cerebral hemisphere travel to and synapse in the pons, which in turn sends a large crossed projection to most of the cerebellar cortex. These pontine fibers enter via the middle cerebellar peduncle (brachium pontis). This cerebral input via the pontine nuclei and the resulting cerebellar output from the dentate nucleus back to the cerebral cortex are important to the clinician (Fig. 9-7).

4. *Olivary and reticular fibers.* Fibers from the contralateral inferior olivary nucleus also project to all lobules of the cerebellar cortex. The olive collects input from a variety of higher levels (motor cortex, red nucleus, and

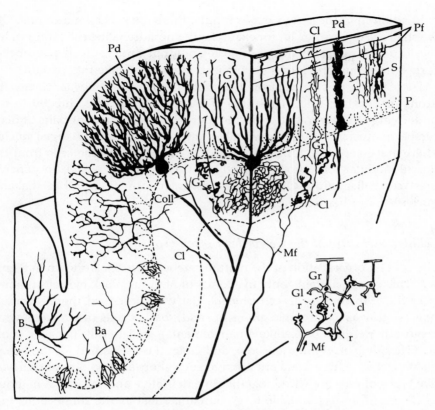

FIG. 9–7. *Block diagram of cerebellar cortex.* The five major types of intrinsic neurons, two major kinds of afferents, and single mode of output of the cerebellar cortex are shown in this diagram of part of a cerebellar convolution or folium. Purkinje cell dendrites (Pd) arborize in the transverse plane of the folium (sagittal plane of the body). Parallel fibers (Pf) extend longitudinally in the folium (transverse plane of the body), and thus intersect the Purkinje cell dendrites at right angles. Mossy fibers (Mf) synapse in glomeruli (Gl) with dendritic "claws" (cl) of granule cells (Gr; see smaller figure at lower right). Climbing fibers (Cl) arborize in a manner which faithfully follows the proximal parts of the Purkinje dendrites. Other abbreviations: (B) basket cell; (Coll) recurrent collateral of Purkinje cell axon; (G) Golgi type II cell; (P) Purkinje cell; (S) stellate cell. (From A. Brodal, *Neurologic Anatomy*, 2nd Ed. Oxford University Press, New York, 1969)

periaqueductal gray) and from the spinal cord. Fibers from the lateral reticular nucleus, which sits in the path of the nociceptive/tactile anterolateral system, also innervate the cerebellum, thus providing it with chiefly cutaneous, as opposed to musculoskeletal, information.

In addition to these four major inputs, there are several minor ones. As we shall see in Chapter 14, for example, the noradrenaline cell group called the locus coeruleus of the pontine tegmentum projects to the cerebellar cortex, and thus provides a generalized sympatheticlike innervation.

There is only one output from this multi-innervated cerebellar cortex, the axons of Purkinje cells. These fibers usually do not pass directly to the underlying brainstem, but project topographically to the four pairs of deep cerebellar nuclei: the dentate, emboliform, globose, and fastigial nuclei. There are exceptions; for example, axons of some Purkinje cells from the flocculonodular lobe project directly to the vestibular nuclei. In general, most cerebellar outflow goes to the reticular formation and to thalamic nuclei VL and VA (see Fig. 9-4D).

Cellular Structure of the Cerebellar Cortex

The cellular organization of the mature cerebellar cortex is shown in Figure 9-7. This cortex contains only five kinds of neurons: Purkinje cells (named after the 19th-century Czech physiologist who described them), granule cells (so tiny as to resemble grains of sand), basket cells (their axons wrap about other cells in basketlike entanglements), stellate cells (smaller, more superficially placed interneurons), and Golgi II cells (named for the Italian histologist who first called attention to such short-axoned neurons). These five types of cells are wired together in a definitive and invariable manner, as clear and understandable to a neuroanatomist as the connections in a light-switch are to an electrician (or perhaps we should say almost as clear).

The Purkinje cells are the key elements among these five. Largest and most impressive, they are the efferent neurons through which all the output of the cortex passes en route to the brainstem underneath. They are arranged in neat rows, with their flattened and fanlike dendritic arborizations precisely aligned in an outer cortical zone called the molecular layer. The granule cells form an incredibly dense inner zone, the granular layer, beneath the layer of Purkinje cell bodies. Great numbers of granule cells, up to 7 million of them, are found in every cubic centimeter of this inner zone. Their axons pass straight up into the molecular layer that overlies the Purkinje cell layer, where they bifurcate to form an orderly array of parallel fibers that run in both directions from the branch points of the ascending fibers. In contrast to the inhibitory effects of the other four cerebellar interneurons, the parallel fibers of the granule cells mediate excitatory influences. Among other effects, they excite the Golgi Type II neurons, thus inhibiting input (Fig. 9-8).

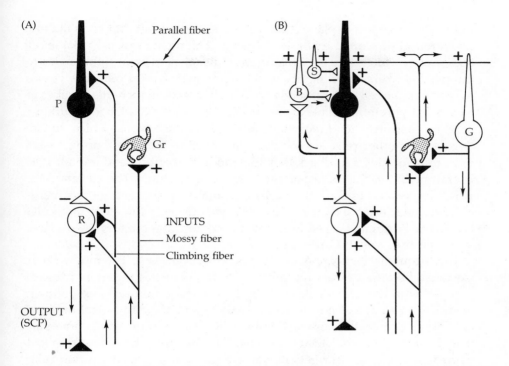

FIG. 9–8. *Representative connections of cerebellar cortical interneurons.* Excitatory connections are indicated by a (+) sign and inhibitory ones by (−). Direction of impulse conduction is shown by arrows. For simplicity, the essential circuit is shown
in (A); connections of additional interneurons are given in (B).

Many other intrinsic and extrinsic connections have recently been discovered —
for example, diffuse norepinephrine and serotonin inputs from the brainstem, and
for another, glomerular endings of climbing (as well as mossy) fibers. Nevertheless,
these diagrams show some of the major interactions of cortical interneurons. Abbreviations: (B) basket cell; (G) Golgi type II cell; (Gr) granule cell; (P) Purkinje cell;
(R) roof nucleus neuron; (S) stellate cell; (SCP) superior cerebellar peduncle.

The organization of the cerebellar cortex is strikingly geometrical. The
parallel fibers run strictly in the sagittal plane and intersect the Purkinje cell
dendrites at right angles, much as telephone lines intersect the crosspieces
on the poles. It is suspected that these excitatory fibers release glutamate.
The basket cells lie in the molecular layer, just above the Purkinje cell
bodies; their dendrites are also in this outer layer. Like the Purkinje cells,
basket cells receive input from parallel fibers. The basket cell axons run

only in the transverse plane (their collaterals branch off, but soon fall into line) around the curvature of the folium and along the row of Purkinje cell bodies over which they lie. This course thus takes them at right angles to the parallel fibers traveling above them. As each basket cell axon passes over a Purkinje cell body, it sends down a short side-branch that ramifies to form a complex terminal plexus or "basket" around that cell body. Purkinje cells, in their turn, send recurrent collaterals of their axons (which, unlike those of the other cells, leave the cortex) back to the neighboring basket cells, thus forming a feedback loop that modulates output and provides the lateral inhibition that is important to contrast function. The stellate cells, which are related to the basket cells but smaller in size and more superficially located, exert similar but less decisive effects in the outer molecular layer. The Purkinje, basket, and stellate cells are all inhibitory, as we have said, and they are all GABA neurons.

The incoming fibers are of two types, both excitatory. The mossy fibers (so-called because of their resemblance to the branches of certain mosses) synapse with the granule cells. They arise from a vast array of pontine, medullary, and spinal nuclei, and constitute an almost universal mode of entry to the cerebellar cortex. Climbing fibers, the other type, come partially from the inferior olivary nucleus, but also from the other areas just named. A climbing fiber gets its name because it singles out a particular Purkinje cell body, passes directly to it and winds its way upward over that cell body onto the principal dendrites, and then out along their finer branches as a clinging vine might ramify upon a trellis. Making multiple synapses on the mainstems and branches of the Purkinje dendritic tree, the climbing fiber is probably the most powerful excitatory cell process in the brain. Certainly it is the most thorough in making its connection; it synapses with the same target neuron over and over again.

The cerebellar cortex is constantly active. Its Purkinje cells are always firing at certain standing rates, and its parallel fibers can further excite them. Especially important, however, are the climbing fibers; they exert a great intensifying influence on the activity of Purkinje cells, one that always has some effect on their firing frequency. In contrast, the Purkinje cell recurrent collaterals, the basket and stellate cells, and the Golgi II cells all act to quell the excitation just described in some manner. Thus, within the cerebellar cortex, inhibition and excitation are continually at play and a most ingenious use of inhibition cuts away, in a kind of neural sculpturing, all but that precise activity needed from moment to moment to refine our movements and posture.

Brainstem Components of the Motor System

Various regions of the reticular core, designated as nuclei even though the distribution of their cell bodies is somewhat diffuse, send descending tracts to spinal motor neurons (Fig. 10–4). There they serve to regulate muscle tone during voluntary movement as well as postural reflexes. These medullary and pontine reticular nuclei and their descending reticulospinal tracts also participate in programmed movements: chewing, licking, and respiration.

Upstream, the giant red nucleus gives rise to the rubrospinal tract, which at least in the cat serves primarily to excite flexor motor neurons and to inhibit extensor motor neurons. In man, this tract is overshadowed by the lateral corticospinal tract just posterior to it, and has undetermined significance. Along the whole length of the spinal cord lie the better-known reticulospinal tracts, which connect with interneurons that in turn regulate motor neurons. Stimulation of caudal regions of the reticular formation generally inhibits motor neuron activity, while stimulation of rostral regions leads to excitation. These reticulospinal tracts also influence the control of vasomotor and respiratory activity, as we shall see in Chapter 11.

The vestibular nuclear complex adds important components to downstream motor control. Fibers of the lateral vestibulospinal tract, originating from the lateral vestibular (Deiter's) nucleus, extend the length of the cord to terminate on spinal interneurons. These fibers act powerfully to enhance ipsilateral extensor tone. Other vestibulospinal tracts originate in the remaining vestibular nuclei and exert varied effects on flexor and extensor activity.

These tracts illustrate the extensive and varied routes over which the brain regulates spinal cord functions. But the ability of the cord to function at least partly independently is considerable. Sometimes, as in providing the substrate of stepping mechanisms, it is of paramount importance.

General Concepts

In general, the team play in motor control is as follows. The basal ganglia are wired between nearly the entire cerebral cortex on one hand and the motor cortex, by way of the thalamus (VL-VA nuclei), on the other. The same can be said for the cerebellum. It "listens" to each lobe of the cerebral hemisphere and "reports back" via thalamus (VL-VA again) to motor cortex. Thus, with the assistance of these two members — the basal ganglia and the cerebellum — almost every region of the cerebral cortex is able to reinforce, regulate, or otherwise modulate commands from the motor homunculus.

The outputs of the cerebellum and basal ganglia are further orchestrated in the rostral thalamus and motor cortex. Evolving patterns of neural activity from the cerebellum and basal ganglia (via thalamus), as well as from sensory and association cortex, are projected upon the cortical motor homunculus, integrated in the cortical columns, and passed down as derived patterns to the brainstem and spinal cord. There, local interneurons and motor neurons play out the final score — the precise contractions and relaxations of the appropriate skeletal muscle agonists, synergists, and antagonists.

The many descending influences of the motor system accomplish a variety of things. They may facilitate or inhibit local-circuit neurons and in some instances, at least in man, motor neurons as well. Each line of command has its own goals. For examples, the corticospinal tracts primarily control fine movements of distal musculature, the reticulospinal tracts generally enhance or suppress extensor and flexor muscle tone, and the vestibulospinal tracts chiefly mediate postural reflexes.

Just as we can only think of movement as dynamic, we must envision the underlying neural activity as dynamic. Central programs are turned on, their peripheral effects monitored, and, at the proper moment, further activity damped or stopped. Movements cannot be allowed to run out of control.

A key member of the motor team that accomplishes such arrest of movement is the somesthetic cortex; it receives a continual neural picture of the body moving in space. Other programs are called into action as goals are approached and finally reached, or as our motivation changes. How much more do we have to do, and do we really want to? The information we need to answer these questions, which are posed in our brain almost every waking moment of our lives, is always there, always ready. And, as learning occurs, new programs are built into the old.

Glossary

Basket cells: inhibitory interneurons of the cerebellar cortex, located in the outermost (molecular) layer and receiving excitatory endings from parallel fibers; axon terminals form intricate "baskets" around the perikaryon and axonal region of Purkinje cells.

Betz cells: giant pyramidal cells (100–125 μm in height) in layer V of Brodmann's area 4 (motor cortex); axons pass down the neuraxis as corticospinal fibers by way of the pyramidal tract.

Caudate nucleus: see Chap. 2.

Cerebellar cortex: a thin, structurally uniform ribbon of gray matter, with three well-defined layers and five types of interneurons, covering the cerebellar folia; an ensemble of nerve cells and intrinsic circuitry of similar design in all vertebrates.

Cerebellum: see Chap. 2.

Climbing fibers: one of the two principal modes of termination of inputs to the cerebellar cortex, representing in part the endings of fibers from the inferior olivary nucleus; thin, sinuous, extensively branched fibers that follow and intertwine with the dendrites of Purkinje cells in the molecular layer, conveying powerful excitation to these key neurons.

Corticobulbar fibers: axons of neurons in the cerebral cortex that pass directly or indirectly and largely bilaterally to certain motor, sensory, or reticular nuclei of the brainstem and depart from their corticospinal counterparts at numerous points along the pyramidal tract (crus cerebri, basis pontis, medullary pyramids, etc.).

Corticospinal tract: a prominent tract from cerebral cortex to spinal cord, often called the pyramidal tract because its fibers course through the pyramid of the medulla oblongata; important to the precision and rapidity of fine, skilled movements, especially of the hand and fingers.

Dentate nucleus: largest of the four deep cerebellar nuclei; mediates cerebellar/cortical output in the long, double-crossed circuit involving the cerebral cortex, pontine nuclei, cerebellar cortex, dentate nucleus, rostral thalamus, and motor cortex.

Globus pallidus: a basal ganglion, immediately medial to the putamen; named for its content of thick, myelinated fibers, which is responsible for its pallor in fresh, unstained material. Major output component of the basal ganglia, sending fibers to rostral thalamus and tegmentum.

Glomerulus: a complex synaptic region, encapsulated by a glial sheath, in the granular layer of the cerebellar cortex; includes the mossy fiber/granule cell dendrite synapse, as well as axonal and dendritic endings of the Golgi Type II cells.

Golgi Type II cells: (1) inhibitory interneurons of the cerebellar cortex, located in the innermost (granular) layer and receiving excitatory endings of mossy fibers; axons pass to nearby cerebellar glomeruli and exert presynaptic inhibition on the mossy fiber/granule cell synapses there. (2) any CNS neuron with a short axon.

Granule cells: sole excitatory neurons of the cerebellar cortex, an enormous population (40–100 billion) of tiny, densely packed cells in the innermost (granular) layer; receive excitatory endings of mossy fibers in the glomeruli and make excitatory connections with dendrites of the four other types of cerebellar cortical interneurons (see also *Parallel fibers*).

Inferior olivary nucleus: a large, hollow nucleus in the anterolateral medulla oblongata, its crumpled layer of gray matter resembling a dried-out, pitted olive; important way station from cerebral cortex (and also spinal cord) to cerebellum.

Mossy fibers: one of the two principal modes of termination of afferents to the cerebellar cortex, representing in part the endings of spinocerebellar and pontocerebellar fibers; within a cerebellar glomerulus, each mossy fiber forms a clublike "rosette"—the presynaptic, excitatory component of the mossy fiber/granule cell dendrite synapse.

Parallel fibers: long, extremely thin (0.1 μm) fibers in the molecular layer of the cerebellar cortex, running parallel to the cerebellar folia and in both directions; formed by the T-shaped bifurcation of the upwardly directed axons of the granule cells.

Pontine nuclei: the gray matter of the pons, receiving input from corticopontine fibers and projecting, via the middle cerebellar peduncle, to the contralateral cerebellar hemisphere; the bridge between cerebral cortex and cerebellum.

Primary motor cortex: a narrow band of frontal cortex immediately anterior to the primary somesthetic cortex, from which it is separated by the central sulcus; like S I, M I features a somatotopic arrangement of body parts, here called the motor homunculus.

Purkinje cells: largest neuron and chief organizational component of the cerebellar cortex; the axons of these stately, candelabra-like cells constitute the sole output of the cortex to the underlying deep cerebellar nuclei.

Putamen: see Chap. 2.

Pyramidal cells: one of the two major types of cells in the cerebral cortex, pyramidal-shaped neurons featuring an apical dendrite and basilar dendrites extending in all directions; their axons constitute the chief output of the cerebral cortex, forming association, commissural, and projection fibers.

Pyramidal decussation: the region in the caudal medulla oblongata where numerous axons in the pyramidal tract cross the midline and pursue their further descending course in the lateral funiculus of the spinal cord.

Pyramidal tract: a long, compact bundle of some 1 million axons originating in several areas of the cerebral cortex (the primary motor and sensory cortices seem to be the most important) and leading down through the corona radiata, internal capsule, crus cerebri, base of the pons, and medullary pyramids (for which it is named) to the spinal cord.

Red nucleus: a large, well-vascularized (and hence ruddy in the fresh state) nucleus in the mesencephalic tegmentum; involved in cerebellar/ thalamocortical transactions; descending fibers from it constitute the rubrospinal tract.

Spinocerebellar tracts: four tracts (dorsal, ventral, rostral spinocerebellar, and cuneatocerebellar) carrying muscle stretch (spindle) and tension (Golgi tendon organ) information to the cerebellum, chiefly via the inferior cerebellar peduncle.

Stellate cells: (1) inhibitory neurons of the cerebellar cortex, somewhat like basket cells but located more superficially in the molecular layer and having less extensive connections with Purkinje cells; (2) one of the two main types of neurons in the cerebral cortex; an almost unlimited variety of chiefly small, starshaped, local-circuit elements.

Striatum: the putamen and caudate nucleus considered collectively; the name derives from the prominent stripes of myelinated fibers seen in both of these closely related basal ganglia.

Substantia nigra: a massive, two-layered slab of gray matter above the crus cerebri and below the tegmentum of the midbrain; neurons of the upper layer (pars compacta) contain melanin pigment, and the large cells synthesize dopamine, while neurons of the lower layer (pars reticulata) are rich in iron.

Subthalamic nucleus: a large nucleus, shaped like a biconvex lens, located beneath the thalamus and lateral to the hypothalamus; reciprocally connected to the globus pallidus and important in motor control.

Ventral anterior nucleus: see Chap. 8.

Ventral lateral nucleus: see Chap. 8.

Vestibulospinal tracts: two tracts conveying signals from the vestibular nuclei to spinal interneurons; the lateral tract (from the lateral nucleus) is important to extensor muscle tone, while the medial tract (from the medial nucleus) is an inhibitory route to cervical motor neurons involved in labyrinthine regulation of head position. *Note:* The medial tract is actually a component of the medial longitudinal fasciculus extending caudally.

The Spinal Cord

10

In its unity and widespread distribution (as described in the Introduction and Chapter 2), the nervous system is like a tree. Most of the branches of this tree of nerves spring from a slender, slightly curving trunk: the spinal cord. This segmentally almost unvarying grooved cylinder extends 43 to 45 cm from the neck to the lumbar spine; it mediates most of the sensation and motility of the body.

Basic Organization

Far below the ruling (but not omnipotent) brain, motor neurons in the spinal cord stand ready, always on duty, to dispatch orders — the considered orders of the entire nervous system. These spinal motor neurons, as well as innumerable spinal interneurons, form more or less continuous columns of cells, without evident segmentation. Nevertheless, in terms of its peripheral connections, the spinal cord is segmentally organized according to the region of the body it monitors and regulates: thus, there are said to be cervical, thoracic, lumbar, sacral, and coccygeal "segments" (Fig. 10-1).

In cross-section (Fig. 10-2), the spinal cord exhibits a butterfly-shaped core of gray matter surrounded by white matter. The no-longer patent (open) central canal — a remnant of the lumen of the embryonic neural tube — runs through the center. The posterior median sulcus and anterior median fissure partition the dorsal and ventral regions of the cord, respectively, in the sagittal plane. The sulcus is a closed seam of ependymal and glial elements that originally lined the primitive lumen, while the fissure is

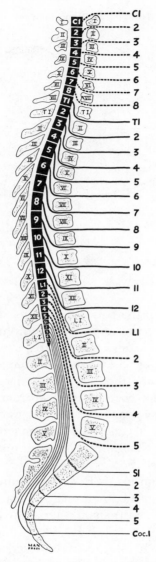

FIG. 10–1. *The spinal cord and vertebral column in sagittal section.* Alignment of spinal segments (cervical, thoracic, lumbar, sacral, and coccygeal) with vertebrae. (From W. E. Haymaker and B. Woodhall, *Peripheral Nerve Injuries: Principles of Diagnosis*, 2nd Ed. W. B. Saunders, Philadelphia, 1953)

a true indentation resulting from the burgeoning growth of the spinal gray matter on either side during embryonic development. Near the central canal, fine fibers (chiefly axons, but also some dendrites and astrocytic

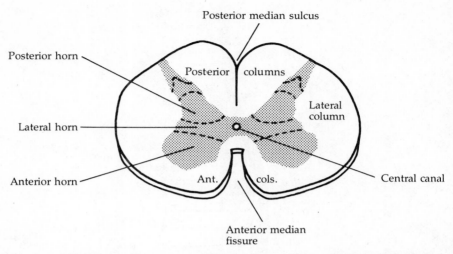

FIG. 10–2. *Subdivisions of spinal gray and white matter.* The gray matter is shaded, the white matter unshaded.

processes) pass between the two sides. Of these the anterior white commissure is most evident and important; it affords a crossing (in the strict sense, a decussation) for axons mediating pain and temperature sensation.

Various tracts, many of which we have mentioned elsewhere, are bundled and stacked here and there in more or less orderly array within the spinal white matter. The posterior (dorsal) roots, bringing in the central processes of the sensory ganglion cells, enter at the apex of the posterior gray "horn" (in reality a continuous column of cells), and the anterior (ventral) roots exit at the base of the anterior horn. The gray matter itself, which contains the cell bodies of secondary sensory neurons, interneurons, and motor neurons, is traditionally divided up into nuclei, i.e., clusters of functionally related neuronal somata, or more recently into the layers or laminae of Rexed (named after a Swedish neuroanatomist; see Fig. 10-3).

The laminae are widely used today to describe the patterns of terminal degeneration after experimentally induced lesions and to indicate discrete regions of localized function, such as pain pathways (see Chap. 6). A system of nomenclature based on this layered arrangement enables us to talk about regions of axonal and dendritic ramification and intermingling, differential distribution of incoming posterior root fibers, and a number of other important matters, just as a similar system is used to describe the cytoarchitecture of the cerebral cortex. We are not stuck with an incomplete

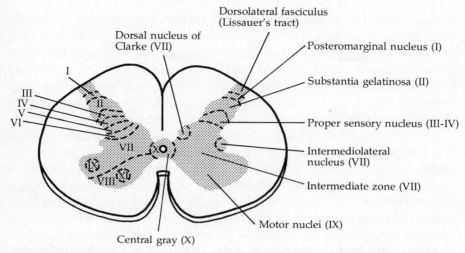

FIG. 10–3. *Structure of a typical cord segment.* The first thoracic segment (Tl) is illustrated. Major nuclei and the laminae of Rexed are shown.

map merely showing where all the different cell bodies are clustered, as with the older nuclear terminology. Instead, neuronal interactions can be considered within general subdivisions or zones. Nevertheless, the older scheme of spinal cord nuclei is important, too, especially in neurology and neuropathology.

Cellular Groupings of the Spinal Cord

Ten discrete laminae are designated by capital Roman numerals; laminae I–IX comprise various regions of the posterior, intermediate, and anterior horns, while lamina X is the central gray substance. The secondary sensory neurons are especially numerous in the upper laminae, while the majority of interneurons, together with "islands" of motor neurons, lie in the lower layers. The correlation of the laminae with the conventional nuclei is given in Figure 10-3.

Somatic Motor Neurons – The Command Cells of Skeletal Muscle

Motor neurons have long dendrites extending from the many angles of their multipolar cell bodies. These far-flung processes collect and integrate all manner of signals from near and afar. The motor neuron sends its axon through the anterior root of a spinal nerve and along that nerve to a skeletal muscle. Such efferent processes may be a matter of inches or feet in length; those to the psoas muscles, for instance, are quite short, while those that innervate the muscles of an extremity are very long. Once in the target muscle, the axon branches into many finer threads that synapse in a highly specialized manner upon a variable number of striated muscle fibers. Each thread ends in a typical neuromuscular junction; such junctions, and the motor neurons that terminate in such manner, are all cholinergic.

In some cases, such as the larger muscles of the lower extremity, several hundred muscle fibers are innervated by a single motor neuron. In other cases, as in the extraocular muscles, a motor cell may control less than a dozen fibers. A single effector neuron, then, commands a team of muscle fibers, whether it is almost a small army, or only a squad. Whether large and relatively clumsy or small and skillful, this team is a *motor unit*: the motor neuron and its set of muscle fibers. If the motor neuron in charge gives the command, all the muscle fibers in the unit will contract in unison. Within a given motor unit, these fibers will all be of a certain physiological kind: slowly contracting/fatigue resistant, fast contracting/fatigue prone, or perhaps an intermediate type combining these properties.

To avoid fatigue, motor units take turns in the activity of any muscle. One or another set of units would fire trains of impulses at the given time of its brief tour of service. The constant slight amount of tension that such fluctuating activity produces is felt as muscle tone, that little bit of contraction that is always present in normal, healthy muscle. When more powerful contractions are needed, as in maintenance of posture and locomotion, more and more motor units are called up, their number and type depending on the power, speed, and duration of effort required. A maximal contraction of the muscle puts them all to work, for as long as they can keep it up — or perhaps we should say, for as long as the CNS will let them;

FIG. 10–4. *Motor neuron in lumbosacral cord.* The nerve cell which innervates the principal (extrafusal) muscle fibers is the alpha motor neuron shown here. (The specialized intrafusal fibers of a muscle spindle are supplied by smaller gamma motor neurons.)

In the transverse plane (A) in which it is traditionally viewed, the motor neuron (shown here in a tracing after S. Ramón y Cajal, 1911) is a large, multipolar cell that differs noticeably from the presumably archaic isodendritic pattern (see Chap. 11). Its richly branched dendrites extend for considerable distances within the gray matter, even across the midline, but not into the adjoining white substance (at least not to any extent in man). The axon (a) departs more or less directly toward the anterior root of a spinal nerve, giving off a few collaterals (c) en route. Some of

(A)

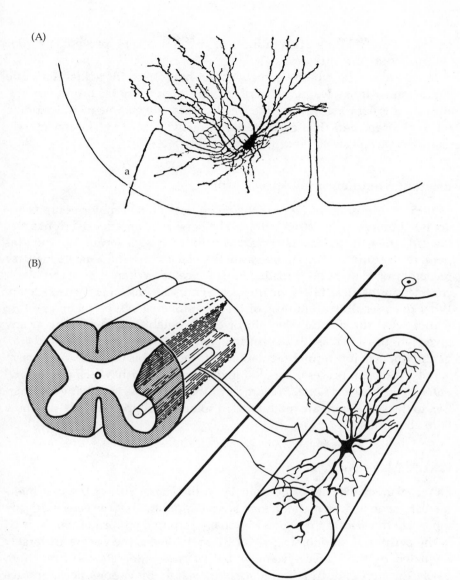

(B)

these side branches pass to nearby Renshaw interneurons, which exert feedback inhibition upon the motor neuron (see Fig. 10–8).

In the sagittal plane (B), quite a different concept of the motor neuron is seen: the radiating pattern viewed in cross-section is now seen to be only part of a larger pattern of dendritic arborization oriented along the length of the neuraxis. This pattern extends for a considerable distance in lamina IX and receives a downpour of afferent terminals from the overlying interneurons in lamina VII and from primary afferents entering the posterior columns.

central fatigue, like a system of fuses or circuit breakers, prevents us from "burning out" our muscles.

There are several types of somatic motor neurons in the spinal cord. The largest ones, those we just described with their working teams, are the alpha motor neurons. Among the smaller ones, the gamma motor neurons act to shorten, and thus regulate the sensitivity of, tiny skeletal muscle fibers that act as stretch receptors (see below).

Efferent Modulation of Spinal Input

Gamma motor neurons lie near the much larger alpha motor neurons but do not innervate the large extrafusal fibers of a muscle, as alphas do. Instead, they supply the necessary control of stretch receptors. They innervate the tiny intrafusal fibers of the muscle spindle in which these receptors or elongation transducers are located. When they bring about contractions of these fibers, no increase in muscle tension is to be expected. What does result is a tautness of the receptor that can be maintained no matter what the muscle's length, or else a heightened sensitivity at any given length — a "bias." The principle here is familiar: efferent modulation of afferent activity, central regulation of input. In this case the mechanism is not a feedback process, like that involving the Renshaw cell (see below) but a "feed-forward" one. Presumably other receptors supplying information to the spinal cord are modulated in some similar manner, but we know little about this.

Visceral Motor Neurons

Other even smaller motor neurons lie in the lateral part of the vast intermediate zone of gray matter above the anterior horn. These cells indirectly innervate the viscera through additional interposed motor neurons located in the peripheral autonomic ganglia. The activities of the viscera are largely regulated by the limbic system, hypothalamus, and reticular formation, partly through endocrine influences but mainly by various neural routes (none of which are very clear) descending through the brainstem to these tiny motor neurons.

The complex task of integrating the work of the vital organs — that of the heart, lungs, and blood vessels; the digestive and urogenital systems with all their associated glands; the skin (not to mention bringing all this into line with outward bodily activities) — is performed almost automatically by the CNS. In fact, recent evidence suggests that the autonomic ganglia, once thought to be simple relay stations (see Chap. 2), are actually outlying command posts for visceral integration and modulation. The muscles innervated by these autonomic ganglia are not skeletal, as with alpha and gamma motor neurons, but rather are the slowly contracting smooth muscles exhibiting their massagelike action in visceral and vessel walls and the specialized muscle of that tireless pump, the heart, most important of all muscles.

Spinal Interneurons

The small interneurons in the intermediate zone (between the dorsal and ventral horns) of spinal gray matter are exceedingly numerous. These local-circuit neurons receive and integrate sensory signals from the dorsal horn, conveyed by primary neurons that innervate cutaneous, muscular, and visceral regions of the body. Spinal interneurons also handle the messages from overlying control centers in the brainstem and cerebral cortex. These instructions regulate both sensory and motor activities. Very few corticospinal fibers from the motor homunculus reach a motor neuron directly, just as only certain stretch afferents on the same side of the body can influence it monosynaptically. Instead, the little cells, like aides to important public figures (i.e., the motor neurons) take care of most of the business continually being transacted in the cord. And, despite their critical role, investigations give these local-circuit neurons very little attention, especially where their constant control of visceral and viscerosomatic activities is concerned.

Were we to show even a fraction of the population of spinal interneurons, we would confront the webs of a thousand spiders — a communications network of such shocking complexity that it perhaps surpasses that seen anywhere else in the CNS, cerebral cortex included. This system contains excitatory and inhibitory cells — and largely unknown varieties of neurotransmitters — that, in addition to their visceral control function, mediate disynaptic or multisynaptic flexor and extensor reflexes on both sides of the body up and down the length of the cord with the correct timing and in every conceivable combination.

Tracts of the Spinal Cord

The principal tracts of the spinal cord fall into ascending, descending, and two-directional local-circuit categories. Although the fiber caliber and density, degree of myelination, and functional role of these tracts vary widely, such differences are not visible in routine preparations of the normal spinal cord. The white matter appears almost homogeneous in such material, and no obvious boundaries for its numerous tracts may be seen. If such boundaries were evident, one would find that many tracts blend with one another and overlap. How do we know, then, where they are? Most of our knowledge of these tracts is based on studies of specially prepared anatomical material from animals, electrophysiological investigations that include stimulation and recording of impulses, and postmortem human spinal cord tissue from individuals with a case history of specific brain or cord damage. In such material, the tracts are recognizable as preferentially stained, electrically activated, or selectively degenerated bundles of fibers. The major tracts are presented in Figure 10-5.

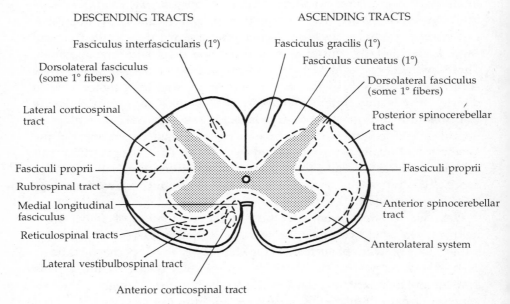

FIG. 10–5. *Tracts of the spinal cord.* Most tracts are given a compound designation of two names, the first indicating the origin of the tract (where the cell bodies lie) and the second its ending (where the axons terminate). For example, the spinothalamic tract has its cells of origin in the spinal cord — in various laminae of the gray — and its axonal terminal in the thalamus — in the ventrobasal complex.

Not all fibers in such tracts necessarily reach the stated destination; some may fall short, the number depending on the tract. Furthermore, extraneous fibers may enter a tract along the way and run with it thenceforth or depart farther on. A few tracts are named for their shape (fasciculus gracilis = a thin bundle; fasciculus cuneatus = a wedge-shaped one) or position (fasciculus interfascicularis = a fasci-

Somatotopy

The principle of somatotopic organization finds many expressions at the level of the spinal cord, both in the gray matter and in the surrounding white substance. The medial versus lateral deployment of axial versus appendicular motor neurons in the anterior horn is a good example. The general arrangement of flexor neurons above extensors is another (Fig. 10-5). Such distribution of functional elements illustrates once again the long-term adaptability and efficient modeling of the nervous system as it has evolved. Through the millennia systems are neatly preserved and reorganized as new ones evolve. We can speculate (there is no way we will ever know) that motor neurons for innervation of the limbs were added alongside the axial ones of early vertebrates, while extensor command cells might have been set in place beneath flexor neurons as exploration of the environment supplanted withdrawal — the latter a primitive but universal response almost as common in humans as in sea anemones, as any psychiatrist will confirm.

The tracts in the white matter show no less striking somatotopy (Fig. 10-6). The shortest fibers connect different levels of the cord itself (propriospinal system). These axons lead up and down from one segment to another, thus providing part of the wiring for the important spinal reflexes (see below). This heavy local traffic is handled by fibers coursing just outside the perimeter of the gray, in the fasciculi proprii or ground bundles of the cord. This arrangement exhibits a striking kind of overall intrinsic somatotopy, with local spinal circuits allocated a more expeditious inner zone than long-distance routes, which are placed more externally.

The longer spinal tracts, which may run all the way up to the brain, show a more or less distinct representation of the segmental levels of the body, including the extremities. In the posterior columns, for example, there is a medial-to-lateral stacking of sacral to cervical axons. Such order arises in the following manner: the entering primary fibers take up positions close to the posterior median septum on the same side, with the fibers that arrive

---

cle between fascicles). The location of some of the most important ascending (right side of figure) and descending (left) tracts is shown with a notation wherever the axons represent the ascending or descending branches of primary sensory fibers (e.g., the axons of dorsal root ganglion cells).

Note that fasciculus gracilis and fasciculus cuneatus collectively make up a posterior (white) column, and that the anterolateral system includes the lateral and anterior spinothalamic tracts.

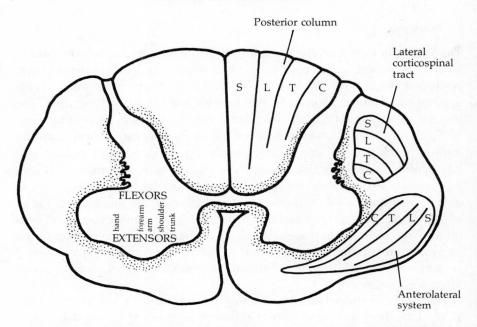

FIG. 10–6. *Somatotopy of the spinal cord.* In the gray matter, motor neurons supplying axial musculature are chiefly deployed medially to those innervating appendicular (limb) muscles, and flexor motor neurons are generally arranged posterior to extensors. The tracts of the white matter also show a more or less distinct somatotopy: sacral (S), lumbar (L), thoracic (T), and cervical (C) segments are represented in a medial-to-lateral sequence in the posterior columns and in an opposing lateral-to-medial sequence in the anterolateral system. Both of the above fiber systems are ascending tracts, with an important difference. The posterior columns consist of uncrossed primary sensory fibers, while the anterolateral system is composed of crossed second-order axons. A posterior-to-anterior sequence of sacral-to-cervical segments is claimed for the lateral corticospinal tract, which is made up of descending fibers from the contralateral motor cortex, but this arrangement is contested by some neurologists. In this regard, it is worth noting that some individual variation is apparent in the organization of certain long tracts in the human CNS, from results of neurosurgical procedures and neuroanatomical evidence.

higher up the neuraxis swinging upward alongside and displacing the fibers already present medially. Thus the leg and lower trunk (sacral, lumbar, and lower six thoracic segments) are represented in the fasciculus gracilis and the arm and upper trunk (upper six thoracic and cervical segments) in the fasciculus cuneatus. On the other hand, the anterolateral system shows just the opposite layering of fibers: a lateral-to-medial sequence of sacral to cervical axons. The explanation for this difference is that the ascending axons are not those of ipsilateral primary neurons of the dorsal root ganglia, but of secondary sensory neurons located in the spinal gray on the opposite side of the cord. As these axons cross the midline through the anterior white commissure, sacral fibers take up positions near the periphery of the cord and, as axons of higher cord levels cross to join them, the lumbar, thoracic and cervical fibers follow in turn in ever more deeply situated courses.

These two main sequences are present in other long tracts to a greater or lesser degree, depending on how many fibers are crossed and how many are uncrossed. What we stress here is the somatotopy of the spinal cables, the way such orderly arrangements come about, and their obvious clinical relevance. "Sacral sparing" — the tendency for central, space-taking lesions (such as an ependymoma) to affect the peripherally coursing sacral fibers of the anterolateral system the least — is a case in point.

Spinal Reflexes

There are a great many types of spinal reflexes — nociceptive, postural, stepping, placing, visceral, etc. A volume could be filled with their descriptions, but we have chosen to highlight only one — the stretch reflex.

Stretch Receptors and the Stretch Reflex

The primary sensory neurons of this reflex have their cell bodies in dorsal root ganglia, as usual. These cells are quick to report the need for increased activity in the muscles they innervate (Fig. 10-7). While other sensory cells may have free or encapsulated endings at the peripheral termination of their long T-shaped processes, the one illustrated is connected to a stretch receptor: it reports a change in length of a muscle and the temporal rate of that change. These clever devices consist of diminutive muscle fibers, called intrafusal fibers because they lie inside fusiform envelopes of connective tissue, the muscle spindles.

Intrafusal muscle fibers are arranged in parallel with the extrafusal muscle fibers, the powerful contractile elements that lie alongside. But the tiny fibers can contract only feebly, just enough to keep themselves taut and ready to report stretch or to heighten their normal sensitivity. If the muscle in which they lie is lengthened (as the quadriceps femoris muscle lengthens if the knee buckles or a neurologist strikes the patellar tendon with a reflex hammer), these intrafusal fibers will be stretched. The receptor transduces this change in length to sensory generator potentials which,

(1)

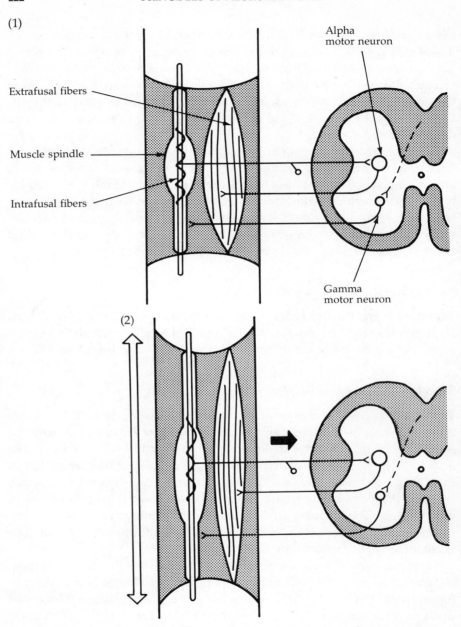

Alpha
motor neuron

Extrafusal fibers

Muscle spindle

Intrafusal fibers

Gamma
motor neuron

(2)

FIG. 10–7. *The gamma loop.* (1) The stretch receptors on the intrafusal fibers of the muscle spindle are arranged in parallel with the extrafusal muscle fibers. Gamma motor neurons innervate these intrafusal muscle fibers, while alpha motor neurons supply the extrafusals. (2) Stretch of the muscle excites the stretch receptors and

(3)

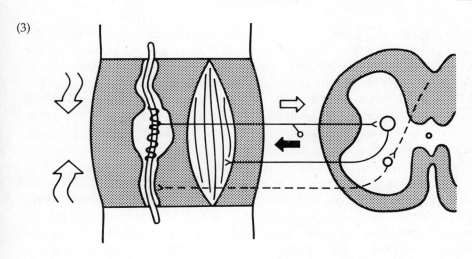

(4)

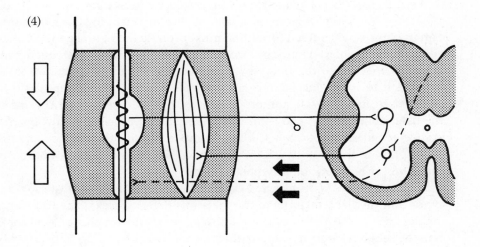

increases the sensory drive on the alpha motor neurons, thus increasing their rate of discharge. (3) The increased frequency of motor neuron discharge causes the muscle to contract. Now that the muscle length is shortened, however, the slack spindle is no longer sensitive to further stretch — an unworkable situation. (4) The gamma loop overcomes this problem. Concurrent activation by higher centers of the gamma and alpha motor neurons results in coordinated contraction of the muscle spindle, and hence continued sensitivity to muscle lengthening. This system can also work to increase the sensitivity of the muscle to stretch at any given length, i.e., to "bias" the stretch receptors.

if strong enough, trigger an action potential. The message flashes to the spinal cord, bypassing everything in its way to get the news to motor neurons as quickly as possible. The cell body of the first-order neuron is circumvented by virtue of its pseudounipolar design and the message follows a beeline along the heavily myelinated, fast-conducting (up to 100 meters per second) axon to lamina IX of the spinal gray, where the motor neurons and their companion interneurons lie. There, reports of muscle stretch have important effects on the activity of these effector elements, favoring compensatory extensor response.

Why is stretch, or increase in length, of muscles so important? Part of the answer is so simple we seldom stop to think of it. Unlike aquatic vertebrates which float when not swimming, we must continuously fight the pull of gravity. And this, of course, requires the contraction of muscle fibers to keep the skeleton upright. Thus, the stretch of extensor muscles is critical information for maintaining erect posture.

Reports about the changing length of muscles (from muscle spindles), and about the closely related tension placed by muscular contraction on tendons (from Golgi tendon organs), are essential data for the motor system in other ways. Such information must precede the neural generation of reciprocal muscular activity in locomotion and the exquisitely tuned contractions that make for fine, skilled movements. This information is so important to us, in fact, that a considerable amount of nervous tissue is devoted to its analysis: numerous groups of interneurons in the intermediate spinal gray and four separate spinocerebellar pathways for spinocerebellar computations. These components, in their effects on still other parts of the motor system, provide a largely unconscious and automatic motor feedback or servomechanism.

Some muscle/tendon afferent data are conveyed by the posterior columns and medial lemniscus to the thalamus (VB complex). The functional significance of this pathway is not known, but it appears that at least some muscle sensory data may merit thalamocortical processing and possibly reach consciousness. Perhaps such circuitry is implicated in finer motor control, in that it provides for additional sense of position and perhaps of effort.

The Remarkable Monosynaptic Extensor Reflex

More intriguing to us, however, is the extraordinary way that the nervous system deals with a small number of stretch afferents — by routing the message directly to the motor neuron, bypassing the entire circuitry of the

CNS. The incoming primary fiber leads directly through the gray and white matter of the spinal cord to the only cell through which neural function (no matter how exalted) can be translated into action.

This monosynaptic or two-neuron connection is not as simple, and perhaps not as effective in everyday life, as it seems. The patellar extensor reflex, for instance, is undeniably a fact, and it is fast, but tapping the tendon with a rubber hammer, which represents extremely sudden as well as synchronous activation of *all* the stretch receptors in the muscle, may not be a physiological situation. Under normal conditions, motor neurons do not respond as quickly as in the knee-jerk test to compensate for increasing load on a muscle. And their response, when it does come, probably reflects the activity of many components of the motor system: the spinal cord, the cerebellum and basal ganglia, the thalamus, and cerebral cortex.

Still, in terms of the direct connection involved, the stretch reflex is remarkable. Despite all the fast or slow routes that convey spinal sensations to the brain for feature analysis, all the parallel or serial pathways that carry response patterns down again, all the spinal or high-level interneurons that process and integrate sensory information — a single sensory cell far off in its ganglionic outpost can cut through the huge organization and teeming activity of the nervous system to instantly affect the activity of a motor neuron of a muscle under stretch—possibly biasing that cell to act against an impending fall.

Efferent Modulation of Spinal Output

A special type of local-circuit interneuron, the Renshaw cell, lies close to the motor neuron, intercalated between its dendrites and a recurrent branch of the departing axon of that large cell. This interneuron is inhibitory; it tends to subdue, at least momentarily, the discharge frequency of the motor cell. Collaterals of the Renshaw cell axon probably reach other nearby destinations, to inhibit other motor neurons or their small satellites. What we see here should look familiar by now: the circuitry for feedback modulation of output. Such retrograde regulation provides for finely controlled neuronal response, as well as for quick arrest of high-frequency patterns of discharge when a lesser response is in order.

Many other interneurons, in the spinal cord and elsewhere, are usually involved in such delicate checks and balances on motor neuron activity. Our account is extremely oversimplified. One detail, however, deserves note: motor neurons near the midline lack recurrent axonal branches. Such neurons innervate axial muscles near the spine. These slowly and broadly acting muscles are important in posture and locomotion, but apparently do not require the rapid, precise control that appendicular muscles (those of the extremities) demand if they are to be used in fine volitional movement. Conversely, the returning axonal branches of the laterally placed motor neurons (like the one shown in Fig. 10-8) that supply the limb muscles are probably important to dexterity.

General Concepts

At the spinal level we see the two most important neurons in the nervous system. The system would be useless if primary sensory neurons did not bring information to it. No less important to survival are the motor neurons. Individually and at any given moment integrating and reconciling perhaps 10,000 signals from all sides, they bring about the quick or slow responses that keep us into things and out of trouble. These scant 2 million indispensable cells are responsible for contraction of muscle, and thus behavior and communication: secretions and contractions, postures

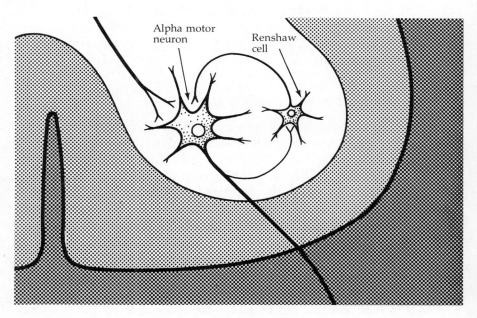

FIG. 10–8. *The Renshaw neuron.* A collateral of an alpha motor neuron activates a Renshaw cell, which in turn inhibits motor neuron discharge.

and gestures, movements and sounds — the countless outward expressions of neural function.

Glossary

Alpha motor neurons: large motor neurons in the anterior horn of the spinal cord and motor nuclei of cranial nerves; innervate the extrafusal fibers of muscles.

Anterior median fissure: a deep (3 μm) indentation of the anterior surface of the spinal cord along its entire length; caused by the burgeoning growth of the anterior gray columns during embryonic development.

Anterior roots: the ventral, motor roots of a spinal nerve, composed of a variable number of irregularly placed root filaments which emerge from the spinal cord along or near the anterolateral sulcus.

Anterior white commissure: a thin layer of decussating myelinated axons just beneath the gray commissure surrounding the central canal of the spinal cord; important to crossed spinal reflexes.

Anterolateral system: a large group of somesthetic fibers in the anterolateral region of the spinal white matter; chiefly crossed axons of secondary sensory and higher-order neurons, conveying pain, temperature, and crude tactile sensibility from the spinal cord to the reticular formation, tectum, and thalamus.

Central canal: a slender, nonfunctional remnant, lined by ependymal cells and usually blocked by epithelial debris, of the lumen of the embryonic neural tube; runs the length of the spinal cord through the center of the gray matter, contains traces of cerebrospinal fluid, and opens into the fourth ventricle at the obex of the medulla oblongata.

Extrafusal fibers: the principal, variably sized fibers of a skeletal muscle; by developing tension, perform muscular work.

Fasciculi proprii: fiber bundles coursing longitudinally just outside the perimeter of the spinal gray matter; connections "belonging" to the spinal cord that are important to local spinal reflexes.

Fasciculus: a general anatomical term for a bundle of nerve or muscle fibers.

Fasciculus cuneatus: a wedge-shaped bundle of axons that begins in the midthoracic spinal cord and makes up the lateral part of a posterior white column above that level; its heavily myelinated, fast-conducting fibers are ascending axonal branches of primary sensory neurons conveying discriminative tactile, pressure, vibration, and position sensibility of the upper part of the body to the nucleus cuneatus of the medulla oblongata.

Fasciculus gracilis: a slender bundle of axons that begins in the caudal limit of the spinal cord and makes up the medial part of a posterior white column above the level of onset of the fasciculus cuneatus; conveys sensations from the lower part of the body to the nucleus gracilis of the medulla, but otherwise is as described under fasciculus cuneatus.

Gamma motor neurons: small motor neurons in the anterior horn of the spinal cord and motor nuclei of cranial nerves; innervate the intrafusal fibers of muscles.

Golgi tendon organs: small, elongated, encapsulated receptors at the junctions of tendons and muscles (sometimes in the sheath and connective tissue partitions of a muscle); serve to detect tension produced by muscle contraction.

Intrafusal fibers: tiny, specialized muscle fibers within the spindles of a skeletal muscle that have both motor and sensory innervation; in contracting, develop no tension but instead alter their sensitivity as muscle stretch receptors.

Laminae of Rexed: a system of numbered layers (I through X) devised by a Swedish neuroanatomist in the early 1950's to describe an evident horizontal lamination pattern in the organization of neurons in the spinal gray matter.

Medial longitudinal fasciculus: a composite bundle of primarily descending axons extending from the upper midbrain into the spinal cord, where it may be traced below the upper cervical level only with difficulty; contains tectospinal, reticulospinal, and vestibulospinal fibers and is important in coordinated movements of the eyes, head, and trunk.

Motor unit: an alpha motor neuron and all the skeletal muscle fibers that are innervated by it; the basic building block of muscle tone and graded muscular contraction.

Muscle spindles: long, narrow structures arranged parallel to the extrafusal fibers of a skeletal muscle and consisting of a connective tissue capsule enclosing one or several intrafusal muscle fibers; signal the rate and extent of muscle lengthening.

Posterior columns: the longitudinally coursing shafts of white matter between the two posterior gray horns of the spinal cord; above T6, each column is subdivided into fasciculus gracilis and fasciculus cuneatus. *Note:* In the strict sense, one should use the term "posterior white columns" for this fiber region and refer to the posterior horns as "posterior gray columns," since the gray matter has longitudinal continuity, too. But in clinical practice, "column" is used only to indicate white matter.

Posterior median sulcus: a shallow, often imperceptible indentation of the posterior surface of the spinal cord along its entire length, from which a septum of glial and ependymal cells extends downward toward the central canal as a fused remnant of the opposing walls of the neural tube.

Posterior roots: the dorsal, sensory roots of a spinal nerve, composed of a variable number of regularly spaced root filaments which enter the spinal cord along the posterolateral sulcus.

Propriospinal fibers: axons of spinal interneurons which pass to other levels of the spinal cord; interconnect different cord levels (see *Fasciculi proprii*).

Renshaw cells: small, local-circuit neurons near alpha motor neurons; excited by recurrent collaterals of motor axons and, by means of axodendritic synapses, inhibitory to the activity of the motor cells.

Spinal interneurons: small, local-circuit neurons, found in great numbers in the intermediate region of the spinal gray matter (between the dorsal and ventral horns; Rexed's lamina VII) and also in the gray columns; regulate sensory, integrative, and motor activities of the spinal cord.

Stretch receptors: see *Intrafusal fibers* and *Muscle spindles*.

Visceral motor neurons: small cells in the intermediolateral nucleus of the spinal cord (lateral part of Rexed's lamina VII) which indirectly innervate the smooth muscle of visceral organs through interposed cells of the autonomic ganglia; the central elements are designated *preganglionic* visceral motor neurons, the peripheral elements *postganglionic* motor neurons.

11

The Reticular Formation and Core Mechanisms of Integration

At the core of the rostral CNS is a region that acts to unify brain function, the brainstem reticular (netlike) formation. Even in comparison with other brain regions, its variety of inputs and widespread distribution of outputs are extraordinary. Reticular neurons interrelate all kinds of neurally coded information and organize generalized responses — in the visceral realm, in posture and locomotion, in global functions, such as sleep and wakefulness, and possibly even in self-awareness. Their remarkable plan of connectivity allows the cells to be as nearly "omniscient" and "omnipotent" as any neurons are.

FIG. 11–1. *Microscopic appearance of reticular formation.* Photomicrograph (A) and matching labeled drawing (B) of a cross-section of the human brainstem; intermingled nerve fibers and cell bodies impart a reticulated appearance to the formation. Section (through medulla oblongata; mid-region of inferior olivary nuclei) stained for myelin by Loyez variant of Weigert's method. Fibers appear dark, due to staining of their myelin sheaths by hematoxylin after mordanting the lipid by potassium dichromate, and as strands or dots, depending on whether they are cut longitudinally or cross-wise. The large dark areas are tracts, such as the paired pyramids ventromedially. Clear areas, relatively free of myelin, represent nuclear regions in which cell bodies are plentiful — in round clusters, such as the hypoglossal nuclei at top center, or in curvilinear sheets, notably as in the inferior olivary nuclei in lower half of section.

The reticular formation takes in a large region above the inferior olivary nuclei, extending medially to include the raphe (seam) of the midline. Blending of cell regions and fiber bundles is especially prominent here.

Several important nuclei and tracts mentioned in previous chapters are visible here. (Brain section provided by Paul I. Yakovlev, M.D., Armed Forces Institute of Pathology)

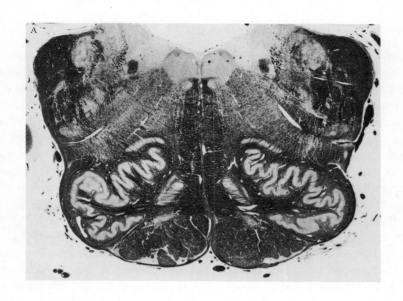

A

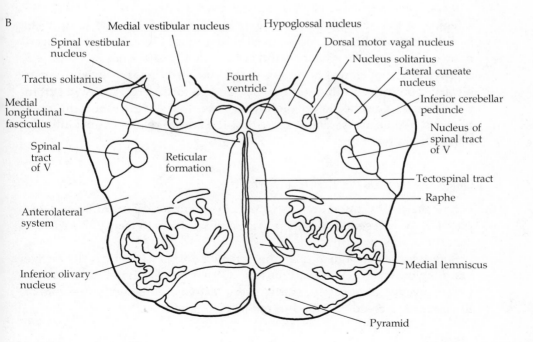

B

Medial vestibular nucleus

Hypoglossal nucleus

Spinal vestibular
nucleus

Dorsal motor vagal nucleus

Tractus solitarius

Nucleus solitarius

Lateral cuneate
nucleus

Medial
longitudinal
fasciculus

Fourth
ventricle

Inferior cerebellar
peduncle

Spinal
tract
of V

Reticular
formation

Nucleus of
spinal tract
of V

Tectospinal tract

Raphe

Anterolateral
system

Medial lemniscus

Inferior olivary
nucleus

Pyramid

Location and Basic Characteristics

The reticular formation is an extensive central region of the upper neuraxis which in routine myelin preparations displays a weave of cell bodies and interlacing fibers. It is neither pure gray matter nor pure white matter, but a mixture of both (Fig. 11-1). This reticulated or tweedlike fabric begins lateral to the posterior gray horn of the upper cervical spinal cord (reticular process) and continues rostrally through the medullary, pontine, and mesencephalic tegmentum of the lower brainstem. (The brainstem is said to have gotten its name from 19th century German anatomists, who used it as a handle to lift the brain from a jar!) Rostrally the formation may be followed into the diencephalon, especially into the subthalamic and hypothalamic regions.

Generally, the nerve cell bodies and fibers of the reticular formation are not aggregated in well-defined nuclei and tracts, although certain cell clusters and groups of axons are obvious (the lateral reticular nucleus and reticulospinal tracts). Instead, cell bodies of various sizes lie in a meshwork of their own dendrites and axons, processes which have many different sources of input and destinations, respectively. Arborizations of axon collaterals from tracts passing alongside the reticular formation further complicate this neuropil.

It was once popular to say that the reticular formation was a "residue" — a region of the neuraxis left over after the discrete nuclei and long tracts had differentiated in the course of evolution (Fig. 11-2). The uncataloged neurons in the region obviously did not fit into the categories of motor and sensory nuclei of cranial nerves or of the so-called "relay" nuclei (inferior olivary, pontine, and trapezoid nuclei, and so forth). Yet, today, far from regarding it as a collection of "leftovers," we now see the reticular formation as a neural subsystem designed for the crucial role of overall integration of brain function.

Older Concepts of the Reticular Formation

Before the 1960's, three notions of the brainstem reticular formation were popular. We present and criticize these older ideas to clarify the current concept of this structure.

Some scientists argued that the reticular formation was a distinctive brain region with cellular features found nowhere else in the nervous system. However, after careful study, every histological feature in the core of the brainstem could be found in other regions of the CNS.

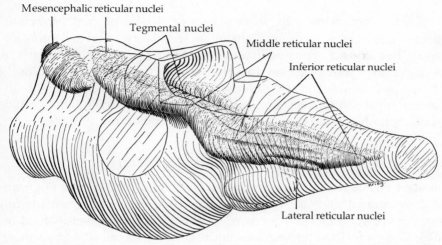

Mesencephalic reticular nuclei

Tegmental nuclei

Middle reticular nuclei

Inferior reticular nuclei

Lateral reticular nuclei

FIG. 11–2. *Three-dimensional view of human brainstem reticular formation.* Drawing shows core position of reticular formation. The various cranial nerves and relay nuclei, as well as the long tracts, lie largely outside this core. Although regions of discontinuity are indicated rostrally, the formation actually makes up a largely continuous core extending downward through tegmentum of midbrain, pons, and medulla oblongata and terminating lateral to posterior horn of cervical spinal cord. Names are given for regions that may include numerous specific nuclei. For example, the ventral tegmental nucleus of the midbrain would be found in the region labeled "mesencephalic reticular nucleus," and the raphe nuclei would lie medially in "tegmental nuclei." This diagram gives an excellent idea of the relatively large size, continuity, and core location of this important integrative region of the brain. (From W. J. S. Krieg, *Functional Neuroanatomy*, 3rd Ed. Brain Books, Evanston, Ill, 1966)

Other scientists viewed the core as a disorganized collection of neurons. The word "reticular" itself seemed to them an admission of ignorance that discouraged analysis of this network of cells and fibers and thwarted conceptualization of functional roles for these components. Those who took this view had good reasons. Electrophysiological studies yielded highly variable mixtures of visceral and somatic responses — so inconsistent, in fact, that the region became known as a "neuronal swamp." Moreover, no regional subdivisions of the core were apparent. Continued analysis, however, finally showed that the core was not a trackless waste.

Still other scientists viewed the "reticular formation" as a well-defined, useful physiological construct, but an ill-defined anatomical entity. Neurophysiologists could show that the core provided generalized control functions with respect to the major subsystems — sensory, motor, and associative. Part of the core, in fact, became known as the "ascending reticular activating system" in light of its facilitatory effect on forebrain activity. But for many years neuroanatomists could provide no comparable definition; they could only say that the reticular formation was "diffuse" and its boundaries and characteristics "indefinite." Searching for an anatomical pattern to elucidate the physiological observations, they could see no more than a disorganized tangle of cell bodies and processes.

A Unitary Anatomical Concept of the Reticular Formation

A unitary anatomical concept finally emerged. Strangely, it came not from the development and use of ultramodern techniques, but from careful inspection of brain material prepared by the old chrome silver method of Golgi. Golgi's method impregnates entire neurons (somewhat by chance) and demonstrates the courses of their fibrous processes in a beautiful and interpretable manner.

FIG. 11–3. *Input to reticular formation.* Transverse section through upper third of medulla oblongata that shows cells of the reticular formation (see text) and the relation of afferent axon collaterals from major long tracts to dendrites of core neurons.

(A) Overlapping of core dendrites and intermingling of preterminal axons with them.

(B) Convergence and overlapping of terminating afferent fibers in core. At left, a few axons from each major tract are shown, together with their complex terminal arborizations. At right, core sectors covered by these afferents are indicated. Note that no afferents enter core from the medial lemniscus; apparently its high locus/ mode specificity of sensory signaling is not important for the activity of the core. (After A. B. Scheibel, and M. E. Scheibel, *Anatomical Basis of Attention Mechanisms in Vertebrate Brains.* In *The Neurosciences: A Study Program,* G. C. Quarton, T. Melnechuk, and F. O. Schmitt, eds. Rockefeller University Press, New York, 1967, pp. 577-602)

Note: Although the original figures were of the newborn kitten, we altered the outline of the brainstem to conform with that of the human; we emphasize that these features seen with Golgi's method have not been worked out in the human brain, and represent only reasonable inferences from study of nonhuman material.

Abbreviations:

ALS = anterolateral system	MLF = medial longitudinal fasciculus
DLF = dorsal longitudinal fasciculus	Pyr = pyramidal tract
ICP = inferior cerebellar peduncle	VII = vestibular complex
ML = medial lemniscus	V sp = spinal tract of nerve V

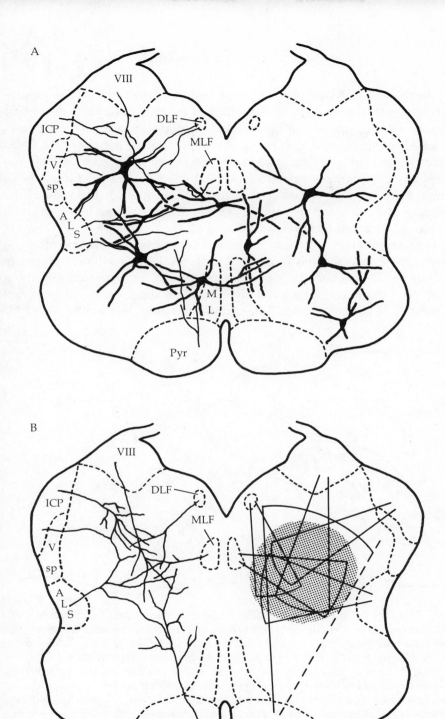

A

VIII

ICP

DLF

MLF

V
sp

A
L
S

M
L

Pyr

B

VIII

ICP

DLF

MLF

V
sp

A
L
S

Pyr

From studies of Golgi-impregnated material (mostly from the mouse, rat, and cat), we now know that there is no special hidden anatomical feature which explains the generalized integrative functions of the brain core. All its histological features can be found in other regions of the CNS. What we have finally recognized is the particular *combination* of such features that characterizes the reticular formation. What are these features? In brief, there are five attributes that together distinguish the cells of the reticular formation and enable us to define different regions of the neuraxis as part of that formation (Figs. 11-3 and 11-4):

First, the neurons — whose cell bodies vary widely in size and shape — have simple and relatively large dendritic trees. Long, rectilinear processes radiate in all directions in a plane transverse to the neuraxis, branching such that distal segments are longer than proximal ones. No recurrent ("wavy") or stubby ("tufted") dendrites are found, nor are the dendritic

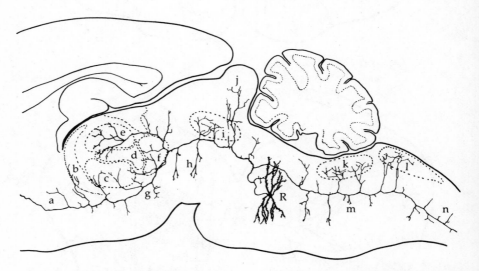

FIG. 11–4. *Output of reticular formation.* Sagittal section through rat brain to show cellular aspects of core (see text) and to illustrate the axonal ramification of a single neuron in the gigantocellular nucleus of medullary reticular formation. Axon bifurcates, like the letter T, into ascending and descending main branches.

In this instance, ascending branch sends collaterals into inferior colliculus (j), oculomotor and trochlear nuclei (i), mesencephalic reticular core (h), specific (c, e), nonspecific (d, f), and reticular (b) nuclei of thalamus, hypothalamus (g), and basal forebrain (a). Descending main branch sends collaterals into medullary core (m), hypoglossal nucleus (k), nucleus gracilis (l), and intermediate spinal gray (n). (From Scheibel and Scheibel; see credit for Fig. 11-3)

arborizations confined to one side of the cell body — as they are in more specialized cells, such as secondary sensory neurons. Long, hairy spines are present, but are unevenly distributed on the dendritic surface.

Second, the long, straight or slightly crooked dendrites of the scattered cell bodies overlap considerably. They thus form an impressive continuum of overlapping fields extending across the long axis of the brainstem. No axon (extrinsic or intrinsic) passing through can circumvent this thicket.

Third, the collaterals or terminals of myelinated and unmyelinated axons traversing the region (fibers of passage) freely intermingle with the dendrites of the resident cells. This feature, so reminiscent of vines climbing an arbor, is a radical difference from the arrangement in most other regions of the CNS. Still, it can be found elsewhere; the intimate entwinement of the cerebellar climbing fiber with the Purkinje cell dendrite is a notable example.

Fourth, the variety of inputs is great: visceral and somatic, sensory and motor, ascending and descending, local circuits and long-distance projections. The reticular formation receives a very broad sampling of the activity going on throughout the nervous system. Each reticular neuron may receive input from over 4000 other nerve cells, many of which lie at a great distance along the neuraxis. Thus, little escapes its notice.

Fifth and finally, the output of reticular neurons is correspondingly widespread, almost global. The long axons and numerous axonal collaterals of these cells achieve a massive, redundant, and far-reaching distribution up and down the length of the CNS, from spinal cord to olfactory bulb. By means of profuse collateralization of such an axon, one reticular neuron may synapse on more than 25,000 other neurons throughout the neuraxis.

Thus, the picture of the reticular formation that anatomists have finally provided is that of a mosaic of neurons with greatly overlapping dendrites extending in all directions across (not along) the brainstem and with profusely branched axonal networks running rostrally and caudally.

Plan of Connectivity in the Reticular Formation

With a few exceptions — such as the cells of the lateral reticular nucleus in the path of the anterolateral system — most neurons of the core have simple yet far-reaching dendrites and long axons (Golgi Type I variety of nerve cell) that branch in a complex manner. Few, if any, short-axon (Golgi Type II) cells are found. If impulses show long latencies (take a long time to get from one place to another), it is probably because the staggered side-branches of the long axons provide a wide range of synaptic delays — as well as much divergence of information (Fig. 11-5).

As mentioned, the maximal dendritic arborization of reticular neurons is in the transverse plane, perpendicular to the neuraxis (Fig. 11-6). In the medial two-thirds of the core, most cells show little or no dendritic spread rostrocaudally, but impressive ramification transversely. The result is a series of flattened dendritic domains, arranged alongside one another in the brainstem like so many pennies in a wrapper. The dendrites extend toward and intermingle with collaterals emanating from the various long ascending and descending tracts that surround or pass through the brainstem core — as if in quest of input. Each dendritic shaft shows a

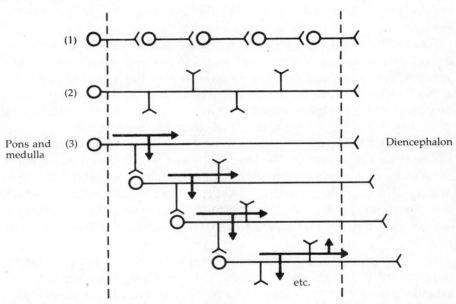

FIG. 11–5. *Impulse conduction in the reticular formation.* Diagram to show possible circuits through core; the third type is thought to be most representative.
(1) In-series chaining of short-axon neurons, as once postulated from the long delays required for stimuli to reach thalamus from brainstem and spinal cord.
(2) Neuron with single long axon reaching up or down, or in both directions, through the core; this is the type of cell (not one with a short axon) seen in the core when Golgi's method is used.
(3) In-parallel chaining of such long-axon neurons; this kind of circuitry allows lateral dispersion of signals throughout the core, and also accounts for the observed long and staggered latencies of impulses filtering up the reticular formation. (Redrawn from Scheibel and Scheibel, 1967; see credit for Fig. 11-3)

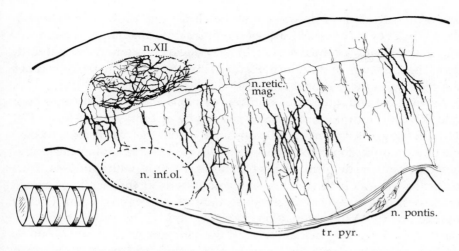

FIG. 11–6. *Integrative design of reticular formation.* Sagittal section through pon-tomedullary region of brainstem of a young rat. Dendrites of core neurons extend dorsoventrally, with marked compression rostrocaudally. Such orientation places dendrites parallel to incoming axon collaterals from long tracts, such as those of pyramidal tract as shown, and also alongside intrinsic core axons, as exemplified by an axon of a neuron in the gigantocellular nucleus of medulla oblongata (n. retic. mag.).

Contrast this "poker-chip" orientation of essentially two-dimensional dendritic fields of core neurons with the shrublike or "tumbleweed" pattern in the adjacent hypoglossal nucleus (n. XII). n. inf. ol. = inferior olivary nucleus; n. pontis = pontine nuclei; tr. pyr. = pyramidal tract. (From Scheibel and Scheibel, 1967; see credit for Fig. 11-3)

marked predominance of input mode, depending on which passing tract or tracts it "reaches for." One shaft may be loaded with corticospinal tract synapses, another with collaterals of the anterolateral system, still another with inputs from spinal tract of cranial nerve V, and so forth. Thus, these "inquisitive" reticular neurons monitor the traffic in the busy thoroughfares of the brain.

A typical reticular neuron has an axon that branches near the perikaryon like the letter T (see Fig. 11-4). Such branches, particularly those of neurons in the medial part of the core, may run far up and down the neuraxis. (The lateral part of the core gives rise to shorter projections.) Some neurons send forth an axon that runs in one direction only, rostrally or caudally. In any case, many collaterals are given off — near the cell of origin, in transit, and terminally. Where do these branches lead? Just about everywhere in the CNS. They go to other parts of the reticular formation, to the sensory and motor nuclei of cranial nerves, to relay nuclei, down to the spinal cord, up to the forebrain, and so forth. Hardly a structure in the neuraxis escapes the probing of these axonal ramifications.

As we have said, enormous numbers of axons and axon collaterals pour into the core from the many tracts passing by or through it (refer to Fig. 11-3). Even greater numbers of axons arise within the core itself, and they too show a profusion of axon collaterals. These extrinsic and intrinsic afferents sprinkle the dendritic shafts of reticular neurons with synapses. Thus each dendrite, as it threads its way among tens of thousands of axonal processes, has many heterogeneous afferents converging upon it, even though one type of input may predominate. If, in Golgi preparations, one traces these afferents back to their sources, one can see that no two shafts receive quite the same "mix" of extrareticular and core inputs. Thus, each shaft is uniquely, as well as widely, informed.

Similarly, each reticular neuron is uniquely and widely informed by virtue of its position in the core — dorsal or ventral, medial or lateral, rostral or caudal, and so forth. A reticular neuron in one location, say, adjacent to the anterolateral system, will receive a different mix of extrinsic and intrinsic inputs than will another neuron near the raphe of the midline. No two cells monitor the same events (receive the same mix of afferents), just as no two persons see the same things unless they stand in the same place.

In integrating all these afferent signals, it appears that specific informational content is lost by the neurons in the reticular mosaic. The neurons probably read the amount of activity passing up and down the major tracts and keep track of the local traffic in the core, but the inputs are so diverse that the cells apparently respond only to the degree of activity, not to its specific detail. Thus, the output of each cell seems to represent only the intensity of current events. But for certain purposes, such as promoting alertness, this is all that is necessary.

General alerting and arousal are known to be associated with the intensity, as well as the suddenness, novelty, or biologically compelling nature, of events. We can think of everyday examples: a splash of ice-cold water or a slap in the face, the sound of a snapping twig (or perhaps a gun shot), the discomfort of a full bladder, or the awful feeling that one is going to throw up. Such perturbations markedly alter the input to the core from the trigeminal, auditory, and visceral sensory pathways, all three of which send rich axon collateral arborizations into the domain of reticular neurons.

Functions that Depend on the Reticular Formation

Since the output of reticular neurons is so wide-reaching, it is no wonder that so many functions of the nervous system are affected by it (Fig. 11-7). Reticular "alerting bulletins" are delivered to the sensory and relay nuclei of the brainstem, where raw data receive initial analysis and projection upward. These influences pass also to tectal, thalamic, and even cortical regions, where information is differentiated and compared. They are further dispatched to downstream effector centers — including the motor neurons of the craniospinal nerves. And finally, these messages are directed back into the core, further regulating its teeming activity. The effects of this activity will be described in the following sections.

Establishment and Maintenance of Arousal and Alerting States

These key functions are facilitated by way of reticulothalamic connections leading to the diffuse thalamocortical activating system. Stimulation of the

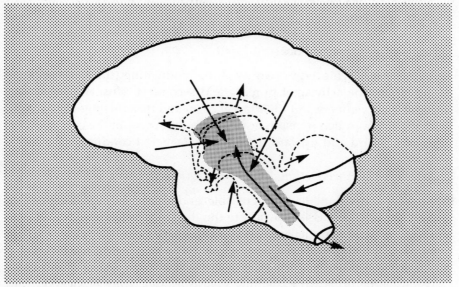

FIG. 11–7. *The reticular formation in core mechanisms of integration.* Diagram shows relationship of core to other neural subsystems. Collaterals of axons descending from cerebral cortex and of various ascending tracts allow impulses of all kinds — motor and sensory — to percolate into the core. In turn, the core acts broadly — on cerebral and cerebellar cortices, on central relays of many kinds, and on the spinal cord. (After R. B. Livingston, *Brain Circuitry Relating to Complex Behavior.* In *The Neurosciences: A Study Program.* G. C. Quarton, T. Melnechuk and F. O. Schmitt, eds. Rockefeller University Press, New York, 1967, pp. 490-515)

core in sleeping animals, or of sensory nerve fibers in the craniospinal nerves (I, II, V, VII, VIII, IX and X, sciatic, etc.), results in a change from the synchronous EEG sleep pattern to the desynchronized pattern of arousal. Through the midline, intralaminar, and VA nuclei of the thalamus, the reticular formation activates the cerebral cortex.

Regulation of Spinal Motor Activity

Through the medial and lateral reticulospinal tracts, excitatory and inhibitory effects are exerted by the reticular formation on both reflex and voluntary movements. For example, a bulbar extensor-inhibitory area is found in the medial medulla oblongata; electrical stimulation of this region brings about marked inhibition of extensor muscle activity. Similarly, an extensor-facilitatory area extends through the lateral medulla and pons into the medial region of the midbrain. Both alpha and gamma motor neurons are influenced by these control centers, and, although stimulation of either area has bilateral effects downstream, the effects are more pronounced ipsilaterally.

Regulation of Peripheral Sensory Input

This function is achieved in two ways, by modulating (through excitation or inhibition) the activity of primary and secondary sensory components (incoming nerve fibers and their target cells) and by adjusting (by synaptic "gating" or controlled transmission) the amount of input the core allows to percolate inward and upward through its staggered conductors.

Contribution to Affective Qualities of Sensation

Information important to the agreeable and disagreeable colorations of sensory experience passes upward to the thalamus (VB complex and posterior group) and hypothalamus (via mammillary peduncle, etc.). Parts of these diencephalic structures show some of the histological features noted earlier for the reticular formation itself — the presence of presumably archaic-type neurons with far-flung dendrites and richly branched axons distributing over wide areas in the basal ganglia and cerebral cortex.

Activation of Sleep and Sleeplike States

Sleep is an active process, not just the absence of wakefulness. It consists of several states. Serotonergic neurons in the raphe (seam or midline) nuclei of the pons, the most medial part of the reticular formation at that level, seem to be involved in slow-wave high-voltage sleep. They also activate certain noradrenergic neurons in the lateral pontine tegmentum (locus coeruleus) which appear to trigger fast-wave low-voltage (paradoxical or REM) sleep. Accordingly, inhibition of serotonin synthesis (or destruction of raphe neurons) leads to total insomnia, while bilateral lesions of the locus coeruleus selectively suppress paradoxical sleep. Lesions in caudal parts of the raphe nuclei diminish paradoxical sleep relative to slow-wave sleep.

In this connection, it is interesting to note that certain of the raphe nuclei have distinct and highly specialized relationships to the arterioles in this midline region. Dendrites of raphe neurons which lie near the course of paramedian vessels form skeinlike arborizations about the vessel walls, and seem to make contact with the vascular basal lamina — or at least come very close to it. This intimate neurovascular arrangement suggests a chemosensory function. Any such ability of raphe neurons to monitor and react to amounts of blood-borne substances (circulating hormones and biologically active peptides) could be very important to the genesis of sleep, a set of states that we know depends on these cells. The raphe neurons thus may transduce circadian or shorter rhythms of variation in the internal medium into particular states of neural activity that in turn could affect the activity of almost every part of the CNS: midbrain and forebrain, cerebellum and lower brainstem. Thus, as we indicated in Chapter 6, even the brain itself has receptors, devices to monitor the internal milieu of the body.

Contribution to Vital Functions

The convergent, multimodal inputs and divergent, multiaddressed outputs of the reticular formation are important connections for the control of respiratory, cardiac, vasomotor, and splanchnic activities. Although these activities draw upon many regions of the neuraxis, and may be affected by electrical stimulation of many neural structures, the brainstem reticular formation is known to contain important respiratory, cardiovascular, and visceromotor control "centers" necessary for normal discharge of these functions.

Think for a moment about the act of vomiting (we promise not to mention it again after this). Many things must be done in sequence and in perfect timing in different parts of the body: a preliminary salivation and sweating, a deep intake of breath, closure of the glottis, contraction of the skeletal musculature of the diaphragm, abdominal wall, and pelvis, relaxation of the smooth muscle of the cardiac sphincter, reverse peristalsis of the stomach and esophagus, opening of the mouth, numerous postural accommodations, and perhaps assorted gestures and grimaces expressive of distress. All this commotion is called the vomiting "reflex." Obviously, many neurons in many structures in the CNS are involved — in the autonomic ganglia, hypothalamus, and basal ganglia, to name just a few. It is clear, however, from anatomical, physiological, and clinical studies that the reticular formation provides circuits that are indispensable to the organization of such complex responses.

Awareness of Self

Certain upper mesencephalic structures — the deep layers of the superior colliculus and underlying nucleus cuneiformis of the reticular formation — receive closely interrelated sensory inputs. Like other reticular neurons, most of the neurons in these regions are typically multimodal, receiving inputs related to several sensory modalities. In this case, however, the inputs reflect congruent visual, auditory, and somatic stimuli, i.e., stimuli coming from a certain direction.

For example, a given cell in nucleus cuneiformis responds preferentially to cutaneous stimulation of the hindlimb, and may also have an auditory receptive field restricted to posterior regions of binaural space. Moreover, such a cell may lie immediately beneath, and thus be closely connected to, cells in the superior colliculus concerned with stimuli coming from the most lateral parts of the peripheral retina, i.e., of objects lying toward the rear of the animal. Other cells in this region have similar multimodal inputs of adjacent parts of the environment surrounding the organism. The grid-like placement of such cells apparently serves to neurally reconstruct the space envelope around the body in the upper midbrain (Fig. 11-8).

This closely correlated representation or "three-way" map of sights, sounds, and physical contacts emanating from the space around an animal could be important to its eye and head movements, binaural localization, body relocations, and so forth. But there are further implications. The output of this broadly informed region is directed rostrally to the thalamus, and in a comprehensive manner: to the polymodal or nonspecific (midline and intralaminar) nuclei, to the specific sensory nuclei (such as the lateral and medial geniculates and the ventrobasal complex), and even to the output-modulating reticular nucleus that screens the dorsolateral surface of the thalamus.

Through such output, the mesencephalic reticular formation could facili-

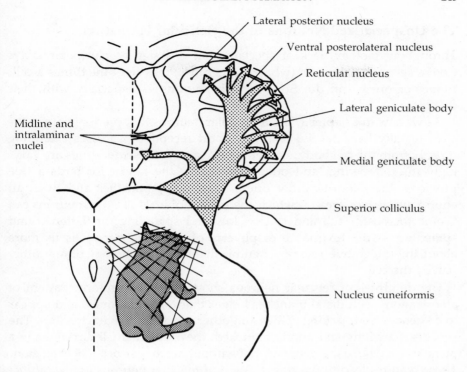

FIG. 11–8. *An anatomical substrate for awareness of self?* Diagram shows gridlike placement of multimodal tectal neurons in deep layers of superior colliculus and subjacent nucleus cuneiformis in the cat. Such neurons respond to certain combinations of visual, auditory, and somatic stimuli, with congruent receptive fields in the three-dimensional space envelope around the body. Efferent projections of this "broadly informed" region lead upward to nonspecific, specific, and reticular nuclei of thalamus — forebrain components that facilitate alertness to stimuli, enhance analysis of sensory features, and selectively gate thalamocortical interactions, respectively. Such sensory activities may give the mesencephalic core a key role in body awareness and in sustaining our image of self-entity. (From M. E. Scheibel and A. B. Scheibel, The anatomy of constancy. *Ann. N.Y. Acad. Sci. 290*: 421–435, 1977)

tate alertness to stimuli and enhanced analysis — by visual, auditory, and somatosensory thalamocortical analyzer systems — of the environmental events that produced them. The connection to the thalamic reticular nucleus could provide selective "gating" of the interaction between thalamus and cortex. Thus, the reticular formation seems to be involved in the process of providing a mental picture of the body in space and even, some think, an image of self-entity: the sense of the continuity and consistency of our existence.

The Unspecialized Neurons of the Reticular Formation

Throughout biology, lack of specialization is a sign of pluripotentiality. Conversely, specialization (whatever its cause) may limit the things a cell, tissue, or organ can do. So it is with neurons — especially with their dendrites.

As we saw in Chapter 1, the multipolar neurons that predominate in the CNS usually have several relatively short receptive processes extending directly from the cell body. Branching like a tree, these dendrites are varyingly thick, tapering, and often spiny. Like the haven for birds a tree provides, the dendritic arbor offers in its many branches and twigs an enormous surface area on which the axon terminals of other neurons can "come to roost." Tall and stately, low and spreading, or flattened and sprawling — the luxuriance or poverty of dendritic trees tells us more about the integrative role of a neuron than the morphology of any other part of the cell.

The dendrites of reticular neurons show a simple, uniform pattern of arborization, with distal branches longer than proximal ones, and appear to be generalized, lacking spines and other specialized characteristics. The processes are long and poorly branched; they radiate in all directions in a plane transverse to the neuraxis, but without much rostrocaudal extension. These features lead to the classification of reticular neurons as *isodendritic*, and such neurons are thought to be prototypical, i.e., to conform to a presumed archaic pattern (Fig. 11-9).

Most of the isodendritic neurons in the reticular formation are small, the total extent of their dendritic radiation being less than 200 μm from tip to tip. Some reticular neurons, however, (as in nucleus gigantocellularis) are quite large, and their dendrites may reach 600 μm or more in the diameter of the area explored by them.

Sensory neurons (as found in substantia gelatinosa, spinal nucleus of V, or cerebral cortex) noticeably depart from this pattern, and are therefore classified as *allodendritic*. Their dendrites show some type of specialization as to branching, orientation, and so forth — being more extensively arborized, concentrated on one side of the cell, more spiny, or combining such features. It is hypothesized that such obviously specialized neurons may have evolved from the primitive reticular cells in response to the presence of a dominant input arriving from a certain direction.

Certain neurons, particularly in laminated or cortical structures, show even more advanced dendritic specialization. Such cells can only be called peculiar, and are therefore classified as *idiodendritic*. The dendrites may be

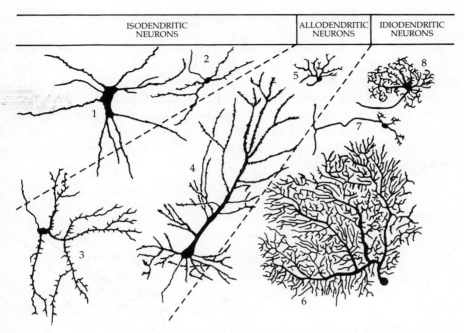

ISODENDRITIC NEURONS		ALLODENDRITIC NEURONS	IDIODENDRITIC NEURONS

FIG. 11–9. *Classification of neurons by their dendrites.* Dendritic features and patterns eloquently bespeak the integrative roles of neurons. At left (cells 1 and 2) are a large and a small reticular neuron; with long, poorly branched, radiating processes they are classified as *isodendritic.* Toward the center (cells 3, 4, and 5) we find *allodendritic* neurons, whose dendrites depart from the presumed archaic pattern by some sort of specialization. The neurons shown are a cell from the spinal nucleus of nerve V, a pyramidal cell of the cerebral cortex, and a cell from the substantia gelatinosa of the spinal cord, respectively. At right (cells 6, 7, and 8) are *idiodendritic* neurons, with such advanced dendritic specialization as to be considered peculiar. Cell 6, a Purkinje cell of the cerebellar cortex, shows a rigid confinement of its elaborately branched dendrites to one plane of space, like a Japanese fan or an espalier tree. Cell 7, a cerebellar granule cell, has small, stubby, tufted dendrites, and only a few of these. Cell 8, from the inferior olivary nucleus, has distinctively wavy dendrites, curving back upon the perikaryon. (Drawing combines delineations of individual neurons from the classical studies of S. Ramón y Cajal, Madrid, and the more recent work of the late Dr. Clement R. Fox, Wayne State University)

wavy, curving back upon the perikaryon, as seen in inferior olivary neurons. Or they may be tufted, forming short, small stubs, as in the cerebellar granule cells. They may even show both of these unusual characteristics, and also be rigidly confined to one plane of space. The Purkinje cell of the cerebellar cortex, with its sagittally oriented dendritic fan, is an example.

What does the above classification teach us about the cells of the reticular formation? Specialization of dendrites to receive certain inputs decreases the number of potential connections to that neuron, and hence curtails its functional capabilities. On the other hand, a generalized and far-reaching dendritic pattern is clearly an ideal cellular design for integrating a large number of inputs arriving in all directions. As the old saying goes, "Jack of all trades, but master of none." This could be the epigraph of a neuron in the reticular formation (Fig. 11-10).

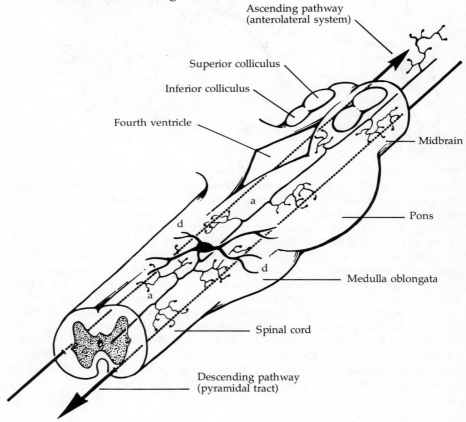

FIG. 11–10. *View of isodendritic neuron in medullary reticular formation.* Through its sprawling, "inquisitive" dendrites (d) a reticular nerve cell monitors all the information flowing up and down the neuraxis, inside and outside the core. Through its wide-ranging, profusely branching axon (a) the cell exerts its influences throughout the CNS — upward and downward, as well as on itself.

General Concepts

At first glance, the seemingly unspecialized neurons of the reticular formation and their sprawling processes convey an impression of disorder in the extreme: a thicket of neuropil that appears chaotic under the compound microscope. Yet these unruly-looking cells inhabit those parts of the brain that control homeostatic mechanisms.

It is ironic that out of this apparent anatomical disorder can come such exquisite physiological order: breathing, an appropriately varying heart rate and stroke volume, the properly changing caliber of all our small blood vessels, swallowing, digesting, waking, and sleeping — a host of elaborately timed, synchronized, and critical life functions. More than this, levels of activity in the entire neuraxis are subject to the influence of reticular neurons. Consciousness and alertness depend on their upward effects. Readiness and coordination of spinal motor neurons and effective use of spinal programs for posture, locomotion, and visceral control rely on their downward activity.

The cells and circuits of the reticular core seem remarkably similar in all vertebrates. Yet the plan could be still evolving, albeit slowly. For example, the reticular formation has acquired inputs, via axon collaterals, from the anterolateral and corticospinal fiber systems; such ascending and descending tracts, respectively, are believed to be of relatively recent origin. Moreover, some of the output connections of the core are long and direct, as seen in the reticulospinal tracts. Thus, the reticular formation seems to show, no less than the thalamus and cerebral cortex, the ever-present adaptability that characterizes the nervous system.

Glossary

Allodendritic neurons: nerve cells with dendrites that noticeably depart from the simple, uniform mode of branching thought to be prototypical (compare *Isodendritic neuron*).

Ascending reticular activating system: the neurophysiological concept that part of the brainstem, corresponding in large measure to the reticular formation as defined neuroanatomically, exerts powerful facilitatory effects (EEG desynchronization and behavioral arousal) on forebrain activity.

Axon collaterals: side branches, tending to depart at right angles, of the axon of a neuron; as exemplified by cells of the reticular formation, a neuron may have an extensive system of axon collaterals, running in different directions and dividing repeatedly into subsidiary collaterals. Such offshoots spread the influences of the parent cell around to many other neurons and target regions.

Bulbar extensor-facilitatory area: a region of the bulb (medulla oblongata) in which electrical stimulation brings about marked enhancement of spinal extensor neuromuscular activity.

Bulbar extensor-inhibitory area: a region of the bulb (medulla oblongata) in which electrical stimulation brings about marked inhibition of spinal extensor neuromuscular activity.

Diffuse thalamocortical activating system: the neurophysiological concept that part of the thalamus, chiefly the midline, intralaminar, and ventral anterior nuclei, exerts widespread, bilateral, long latency, and progressive ("recruiting") effects on electrocortical activity, particularly in association areas and most powerfully in frontal association cortex. Anatomically, a richly collateralizing projection of these nuclei, that spreads across the midline (interthalamic adhesion), mediates these influences.

Golgi Type I cell: one of the two major types of neurons as classified by the Italian histologist Camillo Golgi at the turn of the century and a term still widely used; a cell with a *long* axon, that thereby suits the neuron for long-distance signaling (examples are motor neurons, cerebellar Purkinje cells, and cerebral pyramidal cells).

Golgi Type II cell: the other main type of neuron according to Golgi; a cell with a *short* axon, thus adapted for short-range integrative functions (the Golgi Type II cell of the cerebellar cortex was the first of this type that Golgi noted, but in fact the entire CNS teems with such cells). *Note:* While it is possible in many instances to equate these two types, as defined on the basis of axonal length, with other classifications (large cells vs. small ones, projection neurons vs. local-circuit neurons, etc.), these correlations do not necessarily hold true.

Idiodendritic neurons: nerve cells with dendrites that depart in great degree from the simple, uniform mode of branching thought to be prototypical (compare *Isodendritic* and *Allodendritic neurons*).

Isodendritic neurons: nerve cells with a simple, uniformly radiating mode of dendritic arborization, in which distal segments of the long, poorly branching processes are longer than proximal ones; found in the reticular formation, nonspecific thalamic nuclei, and hypothalamus, they are thought to represent a primitive unspecialized vertebrate interneuron (compare *Allodendritic* and *Idiodendritic neurons*).

Lateral reticular nucleus: one of many named groups of cell bodies in the reticular formation, in the zone of the medulla occupied by fibers of the anterolateral system; somewhat more specialized and concentrated than in other reticular nuclei, its cells transmit exteroceptive influences to the cerebellum.

Locus coeruleus: a distinct, pigmented area near the central gray of the rostral pons that distributes norepinephrine axon terminals directly (with thalamic intermediation) to wide regions and most layers of the cerebral cortex, as well as to the cerebellar cortex. A traditionally enigmatic reticular nucleus now seen as simultaneously influencing activity in almost all cortical areas of the brain.

Neuropil: the complex, tangled web of dendritic, axonal, and glial processes in the CNS and some parts of the PNS; characterized by one contemporary neuroanatomist (W. J. H. Nauta) as the "marketplace" of neuronal interaction.

Nonspecific thalamic nuclei: nuclei, such as the midline, intralaminar, and reticular, with widespread, non-modality-specific cortical and subcortical connections; mediate influences of the brainstem reticular formation upon the cortex.

Nucleus gigantocellularis: a large reticular nucleus, occupying the medial two-thirds of the rostral medullary reticular formation, containing giant neurons, most (if not all) of which give rise to reticulospinal fibers; similar cells, projecting both caudally and rostrally, are found in the pontine reticular formation.

Raphe nuclei: various nuclei, generally small, in the median seam or raphe of myelinated fibers in the medullary, pontine, and mesencephalic levels of the reticular formation; contain serotonergic neurons, and have distinctive functions, including involvement in sleep mechanisms (see also Chap. 6).

Reticular formation: classically, an extensive central region of the brainstem which in routine material shows a netlike arrangement of cell bodies and interwoven fibers; contemporaneously, any part of the brain which contains isodendritic neurons and displays a distinctive combination of neuronal features, such as widespread, overlapping dendrites and profusely collateralizing axons running rostrally and caudally. *Note:* Annexation of regions of the thalamus, hypothalamus, and other forebrain structures has recently taken place in maps of the extent of the formation by some neuroanatomists, since these regions meet the requirements of the newer definition. (See also Chap. 2).

Reticular nucleus: see Chap. 8.

Reticulospinal tracts: two tracts, both largely uncrossed, conveying signals from the reticular formation to spinal interneurons; the lateral tract originates chiefly from nucleus gigantocellularis in the medulla and facilitates activity of flexor muscles, while the medial tract arises more rostrally (from medial pontine tegmentum) and enhances extensor muscle activity.

Specific thalamic nuclei: nuclei, such as the geniculate bodies and ventral nuclei, with sharply directed, modality-specific cortical connections; mediate the features of sensory and other systems analysis to the cerebral cortex.

Tegmentum: a "covering" of gray matter above the basal structures of the brainstem; a continuous core of gray matter surmounting the crura cerebri and substantia nigra of the midbrain, longitudinal fibers and nuclei of the pons, and pyramids and olives of the medulla oblongata. *Note:* Includes the reticular formation, but also takes in the nuclei of the cranial nerves, brainstem relay nuclei, and the various brainstem tracts. (See also Chap. 2).

The Limbic System and Hypothalamus

12

The limbic system is a complex group of closely interrelated forebrain and midbrain structures that has a broad influence on brain function and behavior. Anatomically, it features multimodal inputs — sensory and associative — and dual outputs — neural and endocrine. Functionally, it mediates memories, drives, and rewards crucial to motivational states, affects visceral functions central to emotional expression, and even influences sensory and associative mechanisms that are essential ingredients of perceptions and perhaps thoughts.

At the outset, we emphasize that the limbic system is the most controversial of all the systems discussed in this book. Unlike the other systems, it does not belong to one sensory modality, nor to one effector mode. Moreover, not everyone agrees on its components. Some, in fact, dispute its very existence and prefer to consider its parts individually or as components of other subsystems.

There is, however, a distinct advantage to giving all these structures status as a CNS subsystem. It provides a construct of a forebrain-midbrain continuum in which a variety of separate neural regions achieve functional unity through heavy and reciprocal connections.

What are the parts to this system? Though there is some debate, almost everyone includes the limbic lobe (cingulate and parahippocampal gyri), hippocampus, amygdala, septal area, and habenula. Also encompassed in most schemes is a group of paramedian midbrain nuclei. Some investigators include the hypothalamus and certain nuclei of the thalamus; whether they do or not, all acknowledge that these regions are closely tied into limbic circuitry. Several authors attach importance to the frontal lobes,

and recently the nucleus accumbens has apparently been granted member-
ship. But much of all this is arbitrary — a matter of tradition, preference, or
bias. The important issue is to understand the functional roles of the various structures and their connections. To this end, the concept of a limbic
system is not only useful, but a virtual necessity.

In order to understand the system it is appropriate to trace its roots and
see where it arose. The Latin word "limbus" means a border distinguished
by color or structure. In 1878, Pierre Paul Broca, a French surgeon and
scholar, used the term "le grand lobe limbique" to describe the large arcuate convolution, formed by the cingulate and parahippocampal gyri, that
borders the corpus callosum and underlying rostral brainstem on the medial aspect of the cerebral hemisphere. The cortical areas of the limbic lobe
have obvious anatomical continuity, as Broca noted a century ago. He was
not the first, however, to see this. Thomas Willis, for whom the circle of
Willis is named, delineated this region of the brain and referred to it as the
limbus in 1664. And many other anatomists were to recognize this cortical
"borderland" before Broca.

These were the beginnings of the limbic system concept. In 1937, the
neurologist/neuroanatomist James Wenceslas Papez published his classic
paper, "A Proposed Mechanism for Emotion." He emphasized the circular
flow of impulses from the hippocampus via fornix, hypothalamus,
thalamus, and limbic lobe back to hippocampus and hypothesized that this
cerebral ring served as the neural substrate of emotion. Could a substrate
exist for emotion in the way the visual system does for vision? Many
sensed that the hypothalamus was related to emotion, but it was also
obvious that emotion depended on thalamocortical activity. These early
theories have been modified, but the premise that forebrain structures are
connected to certain midbrain ones by fibers that course through and play
upon the hypothalamus is incontestable.

The term "limbic *system*" was introduced by Paul MacLean, a neurologist strongly influenced by Papez and interested in knowing where emotions came from. At first he used the term "visceral brain" because in its
original 16th century sense "visceral" denoted strong, inward feelings. This
term, though, met with objection: it sounded like a system for the viscera
only. Accordingly, MacLean substituted "limbic system," as he said, ". . .
hoping that the neutral, descriptive word would not give people—especially my colleagues—unpleasant 'visceral' feelings!"

Figure 12-1 gives an overview of the structures and main interconnections of the limbic system. The first section of this chapter deals with the

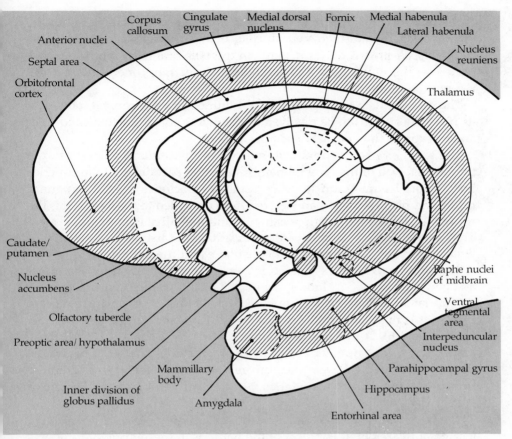

FIG. 12–1. *Sagittal schematic of the limbic system.* The location of major limbic structures and the hypothalamus is shown. (After W. J. H. Nauta and V. B. Domesick, in
Neural Substrates of Behavior, A. Beckman, ed. Spectrum, New York and London,
1980)

parts of the system individually and then describes their interconnections.
The second section focuses on the hypothalamus, its parts, connections,
and functions.

Components of the Limbic System

Among its many components and maze of interconnections, several parts
of the limbic system stand out in importance (see Fig. 12-1):

The *limbic lobe* is a ring of cortex, shaped like a tennis racket (its "handle" is the olfactory bulb and tract), forming a border or "limbus" around the corpus callosum and brainstem. It collects a vast range of cortical inputs.

The *hippocampus* is a buried gyrus in the temporal lobe, intimately connected to the limbic lobe and implicated in learning, memory, and the recognition of novelty.

The *amygdala* is a basal ganglion, also buried in the temporal lobe (near its pole), that seems to be involved in regulating somatic activities to meet and/or express the internal needs of the body.

The *septal area* is a ventral continuation of the septum pellucidum, the thin medial wall of the cerebral hemisphere that partitions off the superior horn at the lateral ventricle. The septal area includes several important nuclei and fiber tracts that are derived from or related to the fornix. It is the main link between the hippocampus and hypothalamic-preoptic area. Thus it is a part of a neural continuum extending between the medial or limbic structures of the cerebral hemisphere and the brainstem.

The *orbitofrontal cortex* is the large cerebral region in front of the motor and premotor cortex, including the frontal pole. It contains a high proportion of small stellate cells to pyramidal cells and a very wide range of inputs. It is made up of all the cortical fields in front of the motor cortex (areas 4 and 6). It includes Brodmann's areas 8–12 and 44–47. All these areas show a large number of stellate or granule cells in layer IV (as will be discussed in Chap. 14), and thus this region is also referred to as granular frontal cortex. It has no boundaries, just the feature of high cell density or granularity.

The *raphe nuclei* (Latin, "seam") are a group of nuclei in the brainstem located at the midline. For most of the neurons in these nuclei serotonin is the transmitter.

The *tegmental area* (Latin, "covering") is located immediately posterior to the hypothalamus. It is closely related to the substantia nigra.

The *hypothalamus*, a part of the diencephalon, extends from the region of the optic chiasm to the caudal tip of the mammillary bodies. It controls hormone release from the pituitary, regulates autonomic activity, and modulates the function of limbic structures.

The *preoptic area* is immediately in front of the optic chiasm. Though technically a telencephalic region, it is closely related to the hypothalamic zone of the diencephalon.

The *habenula* (Latin, "reins"), a midline diencephalic structure, is located medial to the pulvinar of the thalamus, near the roof of the third ventricle. It is an important link between forebrain and midbrain structures.

Limbic Interconnections

In overview, the limbic forebrain (limbic lobe, orbitofrontal cortex, hippocampus, amygdala) is seen to be reciprocally connected with a continuum of subcortical gray matter that begins with the septum, continues caudally over the preoptic region and hypothalamus, and extends as far as the pontine tegmentum. The midbrain part of the continuum is called the limbic midbrain area. It contains the ventral tegmental area, a region of central gray substance that includes the raphe nuclei and interpeduncular nucleus. It is a common distribution area for direct and indirect projections

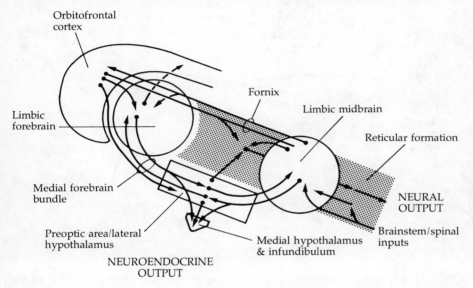

FIG. 12–2. *General scheme of limbic circuitry as related to hypothalamus.* The limbic system is conceptualized as a neural dipole, in which the limbic forebrain (limbic lobe, hippocampus, septal area, amygdala, etc.) and limbic midbrain (ventral tegmental area, central gray, raphe, interpeduncular nucleus) form the two poles. The preoptic area and lateral hypothalamus sit between the two poles, and their activity is regulated by impulse traffic in the dipole circuit. Two major influences determine the amount and nature of this traffic. The orbitofrontal cortex has direct connections to the hypothalamus and both poles of the circuit, while ascending spinothalamic/ reticulothalamic inputs (chiefly nociceptive and stressful) pass through the limbic midbrain. These influences exert powerful effects on dipole activity.

Thus modulated, the activity of the limbic dipole is expressed in two ways: through neuroendocrine output mediated by the medial hypothalamus and hypophysis, and through neural output via multisynaptic descending pathways in the reticular formation (central tegmental tract, comma tract of Schütz, etc.).

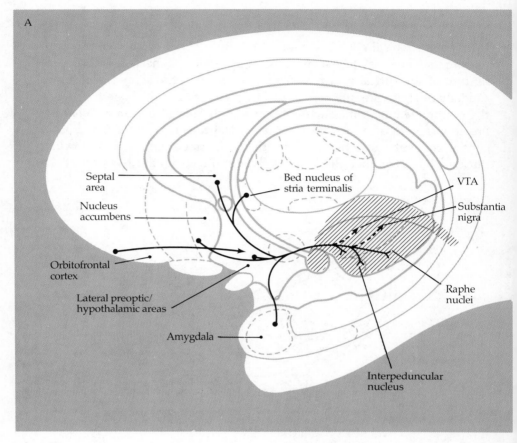

FIG. 12–3. *The two major descending projections of the limbic system.* (A) The medial
forebrain bundle (MFB) route. The most prominent sources that contribute to the
MFB are certain cell groups of the septal and lateral preoptic/hypothalamic areas.
Other structures that send fibers into it are the nucleus accumbens (limbic
striatum), amygdala, bed nucleus of the stria terminalis, and orbitofrontal cortex.
Hippocampal influences reach it indirectly, via septum and nucleus accumbens.
MFB axons fan out upon entering the limbic midbrain, (shaded area) passing to
VTA, substantia nigra, interpeduncular nucleus, the raphe nuclei, locus coeruleus,
and other structures. The MFB does not extend past the locus coeruleus. (B) The
stria medullaris/fasciculus retroflexus route includes three distinct subsidiary
routes. One of these originates from the dorsal septal area and leads via the stria to

from the septum, preoptic region, and hypothalamus. Moreover, the limbic midbrain area gives rise to an ascending projection joining those from
the anterior hypothalamus and septum that courses back to the amygdala
and hippocampus. This set of connections is known as the limbic

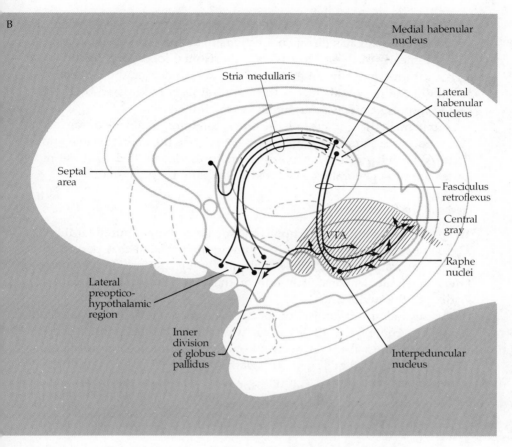

B

Medial habenular
nucleus

Stria medullaris

Lateral
habenular
nucleus

Septal
area

Fasciculus
retroflexus

Central
gray

VTA

Raphe
nuclei

Lateral
preoptico-
hypothalamic
region

Inner
division
of globus
pallidus

Interpeduncular
nucleus

the medial habenular nucleus, and then through the core of the fasciculus to the interpeduncular nucleus. From there, fibers run to the raphe nuclei and periaqueductal gray matter (central gray). The second route begins in the lateral preoptic/hypothalamic region and leads to the lateral habenula. It is joined by fibers from the inner division of the globus pallidus, this contingent making up the third route. Axons of the lateral habenula go directly to the raphe nuclei via an outer zone of the fasciculus retroflexus. Side-branches spread laterally to VTA and substantia nigra, as well as rostrally into hypothalamus and basal forebrain. Although transmitters for all these routes are being worked out, it is known that the medial habenula/interpeduncular connection is a major cholinergic system in the brain. (After Nauta and Domesick, 1980; see credit for Fig. 12-1)

forebrain–limbic midbrain circuit. It is the central concept of limbic system organization.

The key relationships of the above parts are summarized in Figure 12-2. The limbic forebrain and limbic midbrain form the two poles of limbic system circuitry. The hypothalamus lies between these poles, while the orbitofrontal cortex has direct connections to all three of the above ensembles. By means of these "hot lines," the frontal lobes presumably exert higher control over the interplay of the remainder of the system, and activity of the hypothalamus is thus continuously modulated by the prevailing impulse traffic in the dipole in which it sits.

Certain major fiber tracts link the limbic forebrain–limbic midbrain areas. These tracts are so prominent, in fact, as to define the limbic system and its circuitry for all practical purposes. Structures closely tied to these main routes are now generally considered to be parts of the system.

Descending Projections

The major descending projection is the medial forebrain bundle (MFB; Fig. 12-3A), a complex longitudinally coursing fiber system that pervades the limbic forebrain/hypothalamus/limbic midbrain continuum with myriad finely myelinated axons. It is one of the two primary limbic pathways leading to the midbrain.

The second major projection is the stria medullaris thalami/fasciculus retroflexus route (Fig. 12-3B). This two-stage connection runs over the thalamus to the habenular nuclear complex, then descends precipitously into the paramedian midbrain. This pathway, which has several subsidiary routes as shown in the figure, is a sort of "high road" linking the mediobasal forebrain and the midbrain, the "low road" being the MFB.

Ascending Projections

Several well-studied projections with known transmitters form important ascending components of the limbic forebrain–limbic midbrain circuit. Most of these ascending fibers travel over the MFB, and achieve widespread distribution among limbic system components. Two systems stand out: dopamine projections from the ventral tegmental area (VTA), a small group of neurons between and closely related to the paired masses of the substantia nigra, and serotonin projections from the mesencephalic raphe nuclei. These projections are illustrated in Figures 12-4A and 12-4B, respectively.

The Papez Circuit

The most widely known limbic pathway is the so-called Papez circuit (Fig. 12-5). Its name commemorates the neuroanatomist who first noted the main elements of the route and the tremendous impact that these observations had on the development of the limbic system concept. This circuit, now somewhat modified from the original, reflects the connecting role of the thalamus (see Chap. 8). In essence, it leads from the hippocampus and related structures to the hypothalamus, by way of the fornix, and thence to the thalamus via the mammillothalamic tract. Thalamic projections lead to the cortex of the limbic lobe, and impulses from this cortical borderland eventually pass back into the hippocampus over various intervening connections and structures. In a very real sense, the circular pathway outlined above represents "the great beltway" of the limbic system, a preeminent loop of fibers encircling the corpus callosum and underlying brainstem and linking the various major limbic structures, including parts of the thalamus and hypothalamus, in an integrated perimeter of action.

In summary, by way of both MFB and stria medullaris/fasciculus retroflexus routes, the limbic forebrain influences the limbic midbrain, as we indicated early on in Figure 12-2. Reciprocal routes, including dopamine and serotonin projections from VTA and raphe nuclei, respectively, of the limbic midbrain, innervate most components of the limbic forebrain. The Papez circuit ties all these together.

Overview of Limbic System Function

The classic notion that the limbic system is tied to emotional or motivational aspects of behavior is as accurate as a simple generalization can be. But it is too generalized to be truly instructive. Motivation for what kinds of behavior or actions, over what precise circuits, and to what ends?

Some investigators (including the authors, we might add) think the hippocampus holds the secret to limbic system functions, or at least a large part of it. This structure seems to be involved in encoding memories, particularly those relating to place in the environment. Lesions of the hippocampus, for example, make it more difficult for an animal to identify where it has been previously, as in a T maze. Moreover, hippocampal neurons dramatically increase their firing rate when, upon exploring the environment, the animal locates the place it intends to go. Such findings have led to the hypothesis that the hippocampus acts as a "cognitive map."

But it is clear that the hippocampus is involved in more than just memory. Lesions of the hippocampus in experimental animals make it more difficult for those animals to change an ingrained response to a new one. Furthermore, hippocampal neurons are sensitive to changing levels of bodily hormones, and the hippocampus receives direct neural feedback from

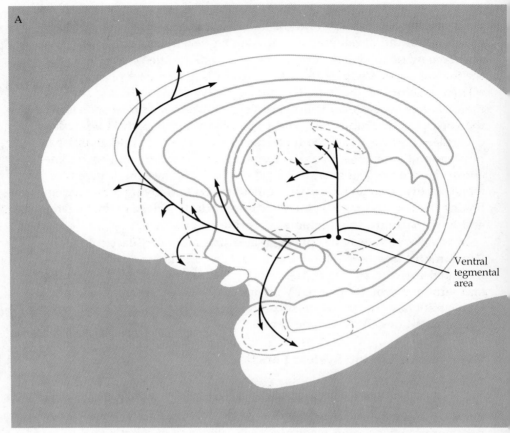

FIG. 12–4. *The two major ascending projections of the limbic system.* (A) The ventral tegmental area projection. Dopamine neurons in VTA project to nucleus accumbens, olfactory tubercle, amygdala, septum, and frontocingulate cortex. Other VTA fibers, probably also dopaminergic, pass to caudate/putamen, thalamus (MD nucleus), epithalamus (lateral habenular nucleus), and limbic midbrain.
(B) Raphe nuclei projections. Serotonin neurons in the mesencephalic raphe nuclei project widely to limbic structures of the cerebral hemisphere: the caudate/

the hypothalamus. It also collects messages from entorhinal cortex, septum, raphe nuclei, locus coeruleus, nucleus accumbens, and numerous other centers. Many of these connections have impressive plasticity: lesions to them induce reactive synapse formation, and brief stimulation can change their output properties for days. This so-called "long-term potentiation" may be a synaptic analogue of short-term memory. These features

B

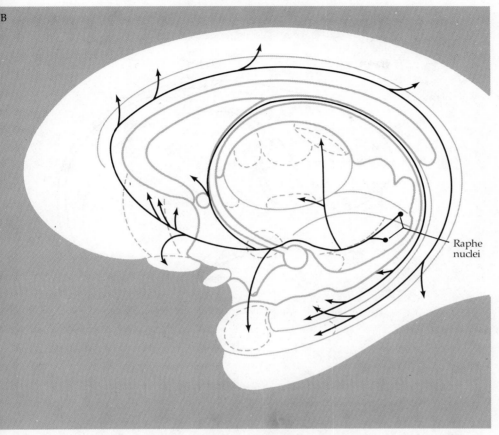

Raphe
nuclei

putamen, amygdala, entire limbic lobe (including the entorhinal area), and septum.
Other fibers, probably also serotonergic, pass to the diencephalon (nucleus reuniens thalami and lateral habenula) as in the case of the VTA projection. The raphe
nucleus projections are much more extensive than those of the VTA, as comparison
of the above figures will show. (After Nauta and Domesick, 1980; see credit for Fig.
12-1)

suggest that the hippocampus is well suited to meet and direct changing
programs of limbic activity.

Understanding the functions of the limbic system is difficult because its
inputs and outputs are not as simple to control experimentally, even to
identify, as those for sensory or motor systems. We have noted that the
limbic system has several outputs. It clearly influences hypothalamic function and thus hormonal secretions from the pituitary. It also influences the
activity of preganglionic motor neurons of the brainstem and spinal cord

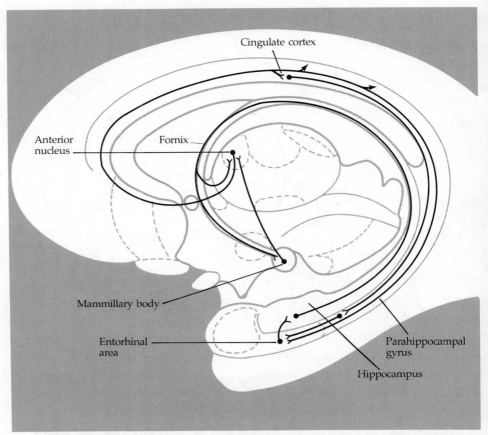

FIG. 12–5. *The Papez circuit.* Hippocampal projections (originating primarily from the subiculum, a neighboring cortical structure) pass by way of the fornix to the mammillary body of the hypothalamus. Projections from the mammillary body then lead to the anterior nuclei of the thalamus (to which some hippocampal fibers are now known to project directly). Fibers from cell bodies in the anterior nuclei extend via the thalamic radiation (see Chap. 8) to the cingulate gyrus; recent studies show that this projection is more widespread, including the more inferior regions of the limbic lobe as shown in the figure. These projections travel by way of the cingulum, the major association bundle of the limbic lobe; they are probably reinforced by contributions from the cingulate and parahippocampal gyri en route. Eventually, the limbic lobe projects back into the hippocampus, through several complex cortical formations and fiber tracts (e.g., presubiculum and perforant path; not illustrated). Thus, information in this circuit has gone full circle — from hippocampus to diencephalon to limbic lobe and back to hippocampus. As first suggested by Papez, this circuit was hypothesized to provide an anatomical substrate for emotion; to a degree, this interpretation still holds appeal, in light of the immense amount of sensory and nonsensory information that the circuit pulls together and integrates.

and thus visceral motor functions. It can influence the midbrain reticular formation via the MFB and the more dorsal habenular route and thus the many generalized brain functions dependent on the reticular core (see Chap. 11). Many of the reticular nuclei in the more lateral forebrain-midbrain circuits receive direct projections from the nucleus of the solitary tract, a prominent link in the gustatory pathway. Such circuits, which involve the amygdala prominently, may serve visceral and motivational mechanisms underlying the selection and intake of food. Thus, the limbic system has pervasive influence on visceral processes. But where does the access to skeletal movement take place?

Traditionally the limbic system and basal ganglia (striatum and globus pallidus) have been viewed as separate neural systems, the projections of which do not seem to overlap. Recently, however, points of convergence ("crossroads") between limbic and striatal efferent systems have been identified. We have discussed two of them already: the lateral habenular nucleus and the nucleus accumbens. As Figure 12-6 shows, these centers receive and send forth connections which link the two systems together, thus providing interfaces between brain regions involved in motivation and movement. Recently it has also been found that the primate cingulate cortex projects directly to the pons and the entire limbic lobe projects directly to the striatum, thereby further increasing motor limbic interactions. To what ends? Food procurement, postures and actions of attack and fear, mating behavior, and all the other outward expressions of internal state.

By virtue of its far-reaching cortical connections, the limbic system also appears to monitor sensory processes of the cerebral cortex and to intervene in them. Two limbic areas (amygdala and nucleus of diagonal band) project widely to the cerebral cortex, particularly to orbitofrontal and inferior temporal cortex. These two regions are reciprocally connected by the uncinate and inferior front-occipital fasciculus on the lateral aspect of the brain and by the cingulum medially. This orbitofrontal-temporal alliance has direct connections over which it could affect the function and interplay of other limbic structures, perhaps modifying hippocampal activity, regulating upward traffic from limbic midbrain areas, and modulating the neural and endocrine output of the hypothalamus. The frontotemporal cortex receives input from each primary sensory area and projects directly or indirectly to the amygdala and entorhinal area, the major portal to the hippocampus. Thus, it appears that there are reciprocal projections involved in the flow of multisensory information between the cerebral cortex and the limbic system. However, the frontal cortex, if not the temporal, lies at a great distance from the sensory cortical areas, and it is considerably

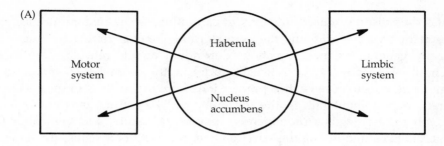

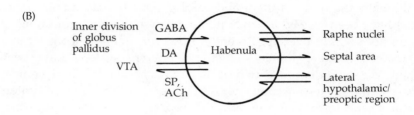

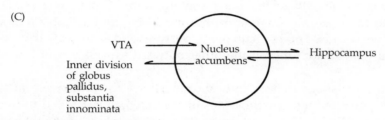

FIG. 12–6. *Limbic–motor interactions.*
(A) "Crossroads" between motor and limbic systems: the habenular nuclei and the nucleus accumbens (limbic striatum).
(B) Details of the connections comprising the habenular "crossroads."
(C) Details of the connections comprising the accumbens "crossroads." (The substantia innominata is a region of atypical cortex just caudal to the anterior perforated substance on the base of the frontal lobe, immediately beneath and apparently related to the basal ganglia.)

removed from association cortex as well. Thus we could say that the frontal lobes are not close to the sensory business of the CNS, even though they have very direct output connections. When their influence is lost through bilateral damage or destruction (see Chap. 14), short-term behavior, long range planning, goal-directed activity, and even moral character are greatly disturbed.

The Hypothalamus

The hypothalamus is at the heart of the limbic system and plays a cardinal role in both the short-term and long-range homeostasis of the body. Its output is both neural and endocrine. The hypothalamus plays key roles in vital vegetative functions, such as control of body temperature, caloric input, water-osmolar balance, sleep and wakefulness; and it serves to both select and integrate autonomic responses. It also controls the release of pituitary hormones that have far-ranging effects on body function. Let us turn now to its specific location, general subdivisions, and incoming and outgoing connections.

Location, Boundaries, and Major Subdivisions

The hypothalamus, as its name indicates, lies immediately below the thalamus in the adult human brain (during development, a so-called ventral thalamus intervenes). It is a small region that makes up only about 1/300th to 1/400th of the total brain weight. It is packed with tiny clusters of cell bodies and less well-defined zones (over 18 discrete nuclei or areas are recognized) amidst a fine network of fibers, which incorporate the major known neurotransmitter systems of the CNS, including dopamine, norepinephrine, and acetylcholine, as well as virtually every peptide identified in the CNS (see Chap. 14).

The boundaries of the hypothalamus are mostly clear, or at least well-defined by convention (see Figs. 12-1 and 12-6). They extend from the optic chiasm to the caudal edge of the mammillary bodies. The region immediately in front of the chiasm is the preoptic area. The lateral boundary is indistinct, probably because certain neuronal groups migrate away during embryonic development to form other structures, such as the globus pallidus and entopeduncular nuclei. For practical purposes, this boundary is just medial to the internal capsule, where cortical fibers are descending to the brainstem and spinal cord.

Below the hypothalamus, the pituitary gland (or hypophysis) literally dangles from the ventral surface of the diencephalic brainstem. The pituitary contains many hormones which are released into the bloodstream only upon hypothalamic command. Its two major subdivisions, the adenohypophysis and neurohypophysis, each store and release particular groups of hormones (Table 12-1).

Overall, three main nuclear regions and three concentric zones of the hypothalamus are recognized (Fig. 12-7). It is subdivided from front to back into supraoptic, middle (or tuberal), and mammillary groups of nu-

Table 12-1. Anterior and Posterior Pituitary Hormones and their Main Target
Tissues

Hormone	Target	Effects
a. Anterior lobe (adenohypophysis)		
Adrenocorticotrophin (ACTH)	Adrenal cortex	Synthesis and release of glucocorticoids
Luteinizing hormone (LH)	Ovary, Leydig cells of testis	Ovulation and testosterone production
Follicle-stimulating hormone (FSH)	Ovary, testis	Follicular growth and spermatogenesis
Thyroid-stimulating hormone (TSH)	Thyroid gland	Thyroxine secretion Lipolysis
Growth hormone (GH)	All tissues	Growth of tissues
Prolactin	Mammary glands	Milk production
Melanocyte-stimulating hormone (MSH)	Melanocytes	Darkening of skin
Beta-lipotrophin (beta-LPH)	Adipose tissue	Fat metabolism
b. Posterior lobe (neurohypophysis)		
Oxytocin	Uterus, myoepithelial cells of mammary glands	Contraction of smooth muscle Milk ejection
Vasopressin	Kidneys Arteries	Reabsorption of water Contraction of smooth muscle

clei, and from the midline laterally into periventricular, medial, and lateral
zones (the column of the fornix separates the latter two).

Supraoptic group. Five nuclei are recognized at the rostrocaudal level of the
optic chiasm, above which they lie in various positions in one or another of
the three concentric zones just mentioned.

The most well known of these are the supraoptic nucleus, paraventricular nucleus, and periventricular nucleus. The supraoptic nucleus consists
of several well-defined clusters of nerve cell bodies (which stain deeply

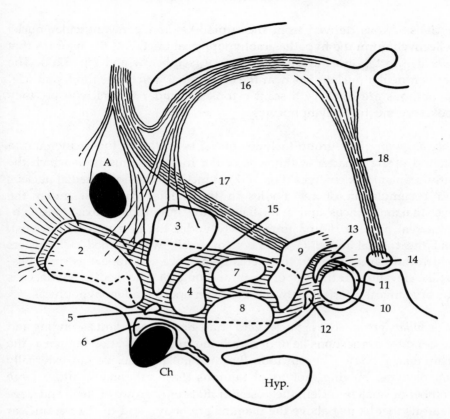

FIG. 12–7. *Major nuclei and fiber connections of the hypothalamus*. Key to abbreviations:
(A) anterior commissure; (Ch) optic chiasm; (Hyp) hypophysis; (1) lateral preoptic
nucleus (permeated by medial forebrain bundle); (2) medial preoptic nucleus; (3)
paraventricular nucleus; (4) anterior hypothalamic area; (5) suprachiasmatic nucleus; (6) supraoptic nucleus; (7) dorsomedial nucleus; (8) ventromedial nucleus; (9)
posterior hypothalamic nucleus; (10) medial mammillary nucleus; (11) lateral
mammillary nucleus; (12) premammillary nucleus; (13) supramammillary nucleus;
(14) interpeduncular nucleus of midbrain; (15) lateral hypothalamic area (also permeated by medial forebrain bundle); (16) stria medullaris thalami; (17) fornix (note
that many fibers do not end in the mammillary nucleus); (18) fasciculus retroflexus.
(From W. E. Le G. Clark, J. Beattie, G. Riddoch, and N. Dott, *The Hypothalamus*.
Oliver and Boyd, London, 1938)

with organic dyes) that are found immediately above the junction of the
optic chiasm and optic tract, all within the medial zone. The paraventricular nucleus is a similar group of large cell bodies just behind the anterior
commissure, again within the medial zone but well above the supraoptic

nucleus. Axons derived from the supraoptic and paraventricular nuclei collectively form the hypothalamohypophysial tract, and the neurons that give rise to this tract are neurosecretory (see below and Fig. 12-1). The periventricular nucleus lies near the ependymal wall of the third ventricle. Its neurons are small with scant cytoplasm; under the microscope, they look very much like lymphocytes.

Tuberal group. This group includes nuclei beneath the tuber cinereum, a mound of gray matter at the base of the hypothalamus from which the infundibular stalk emerges (Fig. 12-7). It includes the dorsomedial nucleus (an accumulation of cell bodies in the medial zone just under the hypothalamic sulcus and a bit behind the infundibular axis), the ventromedial nucleus (found immediately under the dorsomedial nucleus), and the tuberal nuclei (a collection of small, well-defined cell clusters which form and surround the median eminence and appear as small blisterlike elevations at the root of the infundibulum). The median eminence is the anatomical interface between the brain and the adenohypophysis.

Mammillary group. These nuclei with strategically important ascending and descending connections lie underneath the surface elevation known as the mammillary body. They include the mammillary nucleus (an externally conspicuous, bulging mound of neurons itself subdivided into a large number of smaller nuclei), the posterior nucleus (a group of small and large neurons that lie just above the mammillary body), and the lateral nuclear area (a lateral zone component that extends through all three rostrocaudal nuclear groups of the hypothalamus).

Hypothalamic Control of Pituitary Hormone Release

There are two classical neurosecretory pathways between the hypothalamus and the pituitary: the hypothalamohypophysial or neurohypophysial tract and the tuberoinfundibular tract (Fig. 12-8).

The *neurohypophysial tract* originates from the magnocellular paraventricular and supraoptic neurons. Axons from these neurons pass through the infundibular stalk of the pituitary to innervate the pars nervosa of the neurohypophysis. These neurons release two closely related hormones, oxytocin and vasopressin, into the capillaries of the pars nervosa. Oxytocin stimulates smooth muscle in the mammary glands and uterus to contract, while vasopressin has an antidiuretic effect, promoting reabsorption of water by the kidney, as well as a less important elevating (pressor) effect on blood pressure.

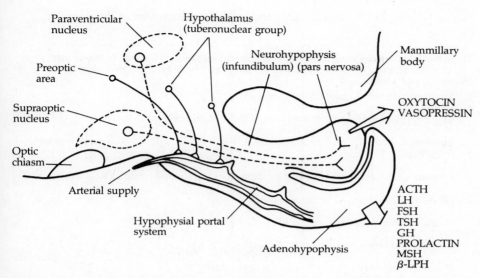

FIG. 12–8. *The two classical neurosecretory pathways*. The neurohypophysial tract and the tuberoinfundibular tract. (After J. Renaud, In *Approaches to the Cell Biology of Neurons*, W. M. Cowan and J. A. Ferrendelli, eds. Society for Neuroscience, Bethesda, Md., 1977)

The *milk ejection reflex* illustrates how this system functions. Through pathways not clearly known, the cutaneous stimuli of a suckling baby cause the supraoptic and paraventricular neurons to release oxytocin in the pars nervosa. The oxytocin is then carried by the vascular system to the mammary gland where it causes contraction of the myoepithelial cells that surround the glandular acini and consequent milk let-down. In a similar way, internal osmotic stimuli produced by dehydration lead to the secretion of vasopressin which increases the reabsorption of water in the distal convoluted tubules of the kidney.

The *tuberoinfundibular tract* originates from cells in the tuberonuclear group and preoptic area which control the secretion of hormones from the adenohypophysis. Unlike the neurohypophysial tract, however, hormonal release is not direct and there are no neural connections between the brain and the secretory cells of the adenohypophysis. Instead, release is mediated or suppressed by substances called releasing or inhibiting factors, respectively (Table 12-2). These factors, which are hormones themselves, are produced primarily in tuberal cell bodies and transported via axons in the tuberoinfundibular tract to the capillary plexus in the median eminence, where they are released into the capillary blood. The portal

Table 12-2. Hypothalamic Releasing and Inhibiting Hormones of the Anterior
Pituitary

There is at least one releasing and/or inhibiting hormone or factor for each hormone produced
in the anterior pituitary. Three hypothalamic hormones have been isolated, structurally
identified, and synthesized.

1. *Structurally Identified Hypothalamic Hormones*

    Thyrotrophin releasing hormone (TRH; a cyclic tripeptide)

    Luteinizing hormone-releasing hormone (LH-RH, LRH, GnRH; a decapeptide; releases
        FSH also)

    Growth hormone-release inhibiting hormone (GH-RIH, somatostatin; a tetradecapeptide)

2. *Unidentified Releasing and Inhibiting Factors*

    Corticotrophin releasing factor (CRF)

    Growth hormone-releasing factor (GH-RF)

    Prolactin inhibitory factor (PIF; may be dopamine)

    Prolactin releasing factor (PRF)

    Melanocyte stimulating hormone-inhibitory factor (MIF)

    Melanocyte stimulating hormone-releasing factor (MRF)

    Follicle stimulating hormone-releasing factor (FSH-RF)

---

system between these hypothalamic capillaries and those of the underlying
gland then carries these hormones to the adenohypophysis where they
stimulate or inhibit the release of pituitary hormones synthesized and
stored there. Nearly all releasing and inhibiting hormones are found in
highest concentrations in the arcuate nucleus-median eminence region (the
arcuate nucleus is a special tuberal nucleus). Releasing and inhibiting hormones are stored in small dense-core vesicles in the axon terminals of the
median eminence.

Thyrotrophin releasing hormone, the first factor identified, causes the
pituitary to secrete thyroid-stimulating hormone. Somatostatin, on the
other hand, inhibits the secretion of growth hormone. Other releasing and
inhibiting hormones of the hypothalamus regulate other adenohypophy-
sial hormones and thereby the hormonal secretions of the entire endocrine
system.

Neuronal Inputs to the Hypothalamus

The hypothalamus receives inputs from many structures of the limbic forebrain-midbrain axis, and directs its outputs mainly to the brainstem tegmentum, overlying thalamus, and pituitary. These major afferent and efferent connections are illustrated in Figures 12-9A and 12-9B, respectively.

We can see from these figures that the hypothalamus collects messages from numerous forebrain and midbrain areas, and has both neural and endocrine outputs. But perhaps more important than the total amount of input is the balance of activity reaching the various hypothalamic nuclei at any given moment. This complex mix of signals is probably the key determinant of the responsiveness of individual target neurons (see Fig. 12-10).

Vascular and Hormonal Influences on the Hypothalamus

The third major influence on the hypothalamus is neither neural nor endocrine, but vascular. The composition of the blood affects various hypothalamic nuclei in important ways.

As we have emphasized, one of the tasks of the CNS is to oversee the care and maintenance of body function. Cells in the hypothalamus monitor osmotic pressure to control water balance, blood volume to maintain blood flow within the proper range and blood glucose levels, and free fatty acids and insulin levels to regulate food intake. We will illustrate the role of the hypothalamus in water balance and food intake.

The homeostatic control of total body water and osmolarity depends on the balance between thirst drive, drinking behavior, and vasopressin release. The two most important stimuli are increased osmotic pressure of the extracellular fluid and the loss of body fluids that deprives the general circulation of water. Hypothalamic osmoreceptors detect increased osmotic pressure in the carotid blood supply. These osmoreceptors appear to be located in the perinuclear areas around the supraoptic and periventricular nuclei. They stimulate cells of the supraoptic nucleus and periventricular nucleus to release vasopressin, which, as we have mentioned, signals the kidneys to increase reabsorption of water from the dilute filtrate back into the bloodstream, thus concentrating the urine. Osmoreceptors are also located in the lateral hypothalamic area. Traditionally this area has been regarded as the "drinking center," because stimulation of it leads to thirst.

The hypothalamus also plays a central role in food intake and weight regulation. Most evidence points to the ventromedial nucleus of the

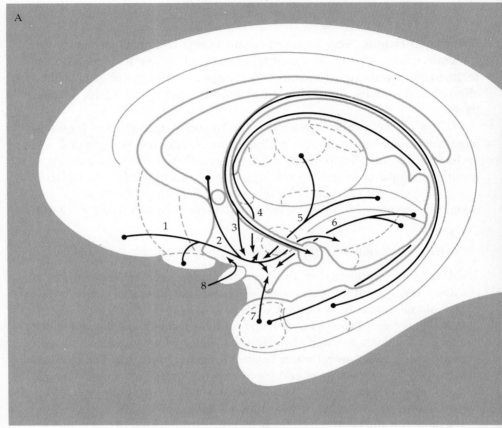

FIG. 12–9A. *Afferent connections of the hypothalamus.* Most tracts pervading the hypothalamus are two-way avenues between their stated origins and destinations; paths traced here show the prevailing direction of impulse traffic. Key: (1) corticohypothalamic fibers, from orbitofrontal cortex; (2) medial forebrain bundle, from basal olfactory and septal regions; (3) fornix, from hippocampus (subiculum) and projecting into anterior hypothalamus and mammillary body; (4) stria terminalis, from amygdala and projecting to anterior hypothalamus and ventromedial nucleus; (5) periventricular fiber system, an intricate net of fine fibers between the central gray and nearby structures of the thalamus, midbrain, and hypothalamus; (6) mammillary peduncle, from the tegmental nuclei and other brainstem structures; (7) ventral amygdalofugal pathway, from amygdala and overlying temporal cortex; (8) retinohypothalamic fibers to the suprachiasmatic nucleus (mediating diurnal and seasonal effects on pineal/hypothalamic-hypophysial function, as recent experimental studies on animals suggest). The medial forebrain bundle and periventricular fiber systems provide key substrates for the so-called "reward" and "punishment" mechanisms of the hypothalamus, respectively.

B

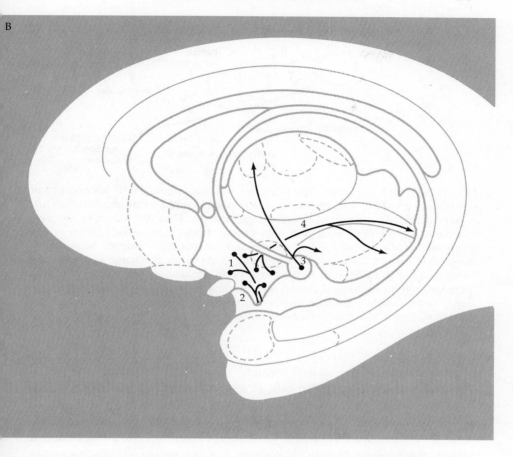

FIG. 12–9B. *Efferent connections of the hypothalamus.* The comment in (A) on the bidirectionality of hypothalamic tracts applies here only to the last connection listed. Key: (1) hypothalamohypophysial tract, from supraoptic and paraventricular nuclei; (2) tuberoinfundibular tract, chiefly from the tuberal nuclei of the median eminence; (3) principal mammillary fasciculus, from the mammillary nuclear complex and bifurcating into mammillothalamic and mammillotegmental tracts to the anterior thalamic nuclei and mesencephalic tegmentum, respectively: (4) dorsal longitudinal fasciculus (comma tract of Schütz), arising out of the periventricular fiber system (see Fig. 12-9A) and distributing to the central gray, tectal, and tegmental regions (with some fibers running as far caudally as the medulla and others peeling off into the central tegmental tract, etc.). Tracts 1 and 2 mediate the endocrine output of the hypothalamus, tract 3 is a key link in the Papez circuit (see Fig. 12-5), as well as an important part of the descending neural output, and tract 4 is an additional avenue for hypothalamic modulation of brainstem autonomic output (from Edinger-Westphal, salivatory and dorsal motor vagal nuclei, etc.).

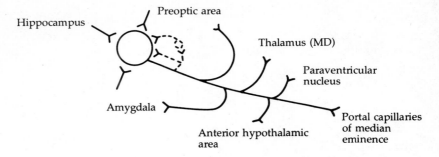

FIG. 12–10. *Inputs and outputs of a single hypothalamic neuron.* These connections of one tuberoinfundibular neuron in the mediobasal hypothalamus illustrate two important principles governing hypothalamic activity. First, the complex mix and balance of signals reaching a particular neuron from other neural centers at any given moment is probably a key determinant of that cell's output. Second, this output has many effects, not only in bringing about the discharge of a releasing factor into the hypothalamic-hypophysial portal circulation, but also by affecting (perhaps ever so slightly, but quite possibly more) the activity in many brain regions, some closely related and others not, through its seldom recognized but extensive system of axonal collaterals. (After J. Renaud, see credit for Fig. 12-8)

hypothalamus as the "satiety center." It appears to inhibit the lateral hypothalamic nucleus, the so-called "feeding center." Lesions of the ventromedial hypothalamus result in overeating and obesity. Rats so damaged may double their weight. These animals, however, gain weight until they reach a new plateau ("set point") and then even if force-fed will undereat to bring their weight back to the plateau. It is as if more weight is necessary to provide enough of the long-term satiety signal to activate the damaged hypothalamus. By contrast, lesions of the lateral hypothalamus result in undereating or hypophagia. After these lesions, animals establish a lower set point. Catecholamine pathways to the hypothalamus play a key role in the regulation of food intake.

Direct electrical stimulation of the lateral hypothalamus causes eating, which stops when the current is off. Animals will also self-stimulate, that is, activate the electrical stimulation of their own hypothalamus to some probably gratifying result.

The medial zone of the hypothalamus has glucoreceptors that respond to blood glucose and insulin levels. The firing rate of neurons in that region is increased upon application of glucose, especially glucose plus insulin. Conversely, the firing of neurons in the lateral hypothalamic zone tends to decrease under such conditions. Their receptors monitor the composition of the ventricular fluid, which reflects the composition of the blood.

The hypothalamus not only controls the output of hormones but is itself a target tissue for the peptide hormones of the adenohypophysis and other endocrine glands. For example, estradiol (the primary estrogen secreted by the ovaries) is accumulated by hypothalamic cells, as well as by other neurons in an extensive cell system running from the septum through the hypothalamus. Such hormone sensitivity probably is very important in feedback modulation of hypothalamic endocrine output.

Neuronal Outputs of the Hypothalamus.

The hypothalamus is influenced by many brain areas, and it in turn influences many others. The fibers travel in several prominent pathways. Most of these tracts are reciprocal, containing afferent and efferent fibers.

One output of the hypothalamus is endocrine, effecting control of the pituitary. However, hypothalamic cells also project to other areas of the brain, and thus mediate endocrine feedback and influence limbic transactions and activities of the autonomic nervous system. Figure 12-10 illustrates the complex feedback connections of some mediobasal hypothalamic neurons. The principal fiber terminates on median eminence portal capillaries as previously mentioned. Recurrent collaterals, however, act back on tuberoinfundibular neurons, either directly or indirectly via an interneuron. Still other collaterals project to the medial preoptic area, midline hypothalamic nuclei, and amygdala.

The main tracts that carry neural outputs from the hypothalamus are the principal mammillary fasciculus and the dorsal longitudinal fasciculus. The principal mammillary fasciculus is a thick tract, grossly visible by minimal dissection, that originates from several of the mammillary nuclei and forks into two branches, the mammillothalamic and mammillotegmental tracts, which convey synchronous activity to the anterior nuclei of the thalamus and dorsal tegmental nuclei, respectively. From the former, impulses travel over the thalamic radiation to the cingulate gyrus (limbic lobe), and from the latter nuclei impulses filter down the neuraxis.

The dorsal longitudinal fasciculus (bundle of Schütz) is a wisp of almost unmyelinated axons which arises out of the system of periventricular fibers and innervates the central gray, tectal, and tegmental regions of the midbrain. From there, reticulospinal fibers pass impulses on to the spinal cord. Some fibers (direct or indirect) reach the parasympathetic brainstem nuclei (Edinger-Westphal, salivatory, lacrimal, and dorsal motor vagal). The dorsal longitudinal fasciculus lies near the medial longitudinal fasciculus; it is a very important command pathway by which the hypothalamus regulates the activity of visceral preganglionic motor neurons.

These pathways underlie what has been clear for many years: the hypothalamus is a prominent, if not the primary, organizer of autonomic activity. Stimulation of the anterior hypothalamus generally has an inhibitory or parasympathetic effect (decreasing heart rate and blood pressure, dilating cutaneous blood vessels, etc.), while stimulation of the posterior hypothalamus chiefly brings about excitatory or sympathetic responses. Thus, the complex neural programs that lead either to rest and body renewal or to "fight or flight" depend on the hypothalamus.

General Concepts

The limbic system may be regarded as a sort of neural dipole in which the two poles are the limbic forebrain system (orbitofrontal cortex, limbic lobe, hippocampus, septal area, amygdala, and habenula) and the limbic midbrain area (medial and lateral mesencephalic reticular formation, including the periaqueductal gray). The lateral zone of the hypothalamus is interposed between these poles, and upward and downward impulses course through many tracts, of which the fornix, medial forebrain bundle, mammillothalamic/tegmental tract, and mammillary peduncle are especially prominent. The traffic in the lateral zone appears to be a critical determinant of activity in the medial and periventricular zones of the hypothalamus; these regions have important neural and neurovascular connections with the pituitary gland, and also represent the source of visceral motor control fibers that proceed downstream. A very important upstream influence on the limbic midbrain pole of the circuit is the rich blend of monoamine transmitters released by spinothalamic and reticulothalamic fibers. But even more important, at least in the primate and human brain, are direct influences exerted by the overlying frontal cortex on the dipole and its interposed lateral hypothalamic zone. This circuitry provides for cortical regulation of activity in every part of the dipole circuit. The nodal position of the hypothalamus and the comprehensive control of all limbic system components by the overlying neocortex are two of the three key elements in the layout of the limbic system. The provision of "crossroads" to the basal ganglia seems to be the third.

The hypothalamus may be thought of as the "instrument panel" of the limbic system, monitoring and regulating visceral and endocrine functions essential to homeostasis of the internal milieu of the body, trophic or defensive-offensive responses, and continued pursuit of personal long-range goals. The basal ganglia, on the other hand, involved in imaging, programming, and playing out body movements (Chap. 9), seem to be the structures through which the limbic system has access to the somatic motor system and through which motivation has access to motility.

Glossary

Adenohypophysis: the anterior lobe of the pituitary gland, embryologically derived from the roof of the oral cavity; secretes numerous trophic hormones (ACTH, TSH, etc.) which promote activity of the other endocrine glands.

Amygdala: see Chap. 2.

Anterior commissure: a small, sharply defined cable of axons crossing the midline just beneath and behind the rostrum of the corpus callosum; its rostral fibers interconnect olfactory structures, while its caudal fibers link the amygdala and adjacent temporal cortical regions of the two sides of the brain.

Anterior hypothalamic area: a diffuse region of neurons, just lateral to the supraoptic and paraventricular nuclei and caudal to the preoptic area; lies in the path of the medial forebrain bundle.

Anterior thalamic nuclei: see *Anterior nuclear group*, Chap. 8.

Arcuate nucleus: a small, but conspicuous member of the tuberal group of hypothalamic nuclei; a major source of hypothalamic/hypophysial releasing and inhibiting hormones.

Cingulate gyrus: see Chap. 2.

Cingulum: association fiber tract of the cingulate and parahippocampal gyri; a discrete cable of axons bringing information collected in the limbic lobe down to the entorhinal area, for subsequent passage into the hippocampus.

Diagonal band: a conspicuous, flat tract at the base of the brain, running diagonally forward from the amygdala to the septal and subcallosal gray matter; courses parallel and superior to, and slightly in front of, the optic tract.

Dorsal longitudinal fasciculus: a thin, wispy bundle of poorly myelinated axons coursing through the central gray of the midbrain, pons, and medulla; includes descending projections from the hypothalamus to the autonomic motor nuclei (Edinger-Westphal, salivatory, dorsal vagal, and possibly intermediolateral cell column of the spinal cord).

Dorsomedial nucleus: a member of the tuberal group of hypothalamic nuclei located just beneath the hypothalamic sulcus.

Entorhinal cortex: most rostral third of the parahippocampal gyrus, including several distinctive transitional zones between isocortex and allocortex; serves as olfactory association cortex and as "gateway" to the hippocampus for impulses derived from the entire limbic lobe.

Fasciculus retroflexus: the habenulointerpeduncular tract, a complex bundle of axons originating in the habenular nuclei and following a complex, curved trajectory down to the interpeduncular nucleus.

Fornix: see Chap. 2.

Habenula: a small but conspicuous triangle of gray matter on the posteromedial surface of the thalamus, immediately anterior to the pineal gland; mediates the stria medullaris thalami pathway of the limbic system (see text).

Hippocampus: a gyrus of the temporal lobe representing an involution of cerebral gray and white matter into the lateral ventricle (not the usual outwardly directed convolution); a major cortical component of the limbic system, with an almost machinelike plan of neural organization.

Hypophysis: the pituitary gland, the endocrine instrumentality of the limbic system.

Hypothalamohypophysial tract: synonym for neurohypophysial tract.

Hypothalamus: see Chap. 2.

Interpeduncular nucleus: a component of the limbic midbrain area receiving the dorsally coursing stria medullaris thalami/fasciculus retroflexus pathway and projecting into more caudal regions of the mesencephalic tegmentum.

Lateral forebrain bundle: one of the two main avenues of intercommunication between the forebrain and midbrain; includes pallidothalamic, pallidotegmental, and amygdalofugal connections, as well as the corticospinal tract and other efferent systems of the human brain.

Lateral hypothalamic area: a diffuse region of neurons, extending almost the entire length of the hypothalamus; lies in the path of the medial forebrain bundle and conveys influences from it to the other hypothalamic nuclei.

Limbic lobe: see Chap. 2.

Limbic system: see Chap. 2.

Locus coeruleus: see Chap. 11.

Mammillary bodies: a pair of grossly visible nuclei, each made up of several subsidiary cell clusters, at the posterior end of the hypothalamus; source of major hypothalamic output to tegmentum and thalamus.

Mammillary peduncle: an afferent tract of the hypothalamus, arising from the tegmental nuclei and other brainstem structures; brings visceral and gustatory input to the hypothalamus.

Mammillotegmental tract: a caudally directed offshoot of the mammillothalamic tract, many of its fibers representing collaterals of mammillothalamic axons. *Note:* These two tracts originate as a common bundle, the principal mammillary fasciculus.

Mammillothalamic tract: see Chap. 8.

Medial dorsal nucleus: see Chap. 8.

Medial forebrain bundle: one of the two major avenues of intercommunication between the forebrain and midbrain; coursing through the lateral hypothalamus, its downwardly directed olfactovisceral projections and upwardly coursing neurotransmitter systems profoundly affect the activity of that structure.

Median eminence: a small, blisterlike elevation at the root of the infundibulum containing, and surrounded by, the tuberal nuclei; anatomical interface between hypothalamus and adenohypophysis.

Neurohypophysial tract: one of the two endocrine outputs of the hypothalamus, originating from the paraventricular and supraoptic nuclei and releasing oxytocin and vasopressin into capillaries of the neurohypophysis (pars nervosa).

Neurohypophysis: the posterior lobe of the pituitary gland, embryologically derived from the floor of the diencephalon (infundibulum); receives, stores, and releases oxytocin and vasopressin, smooth-muscle-stimulating and antidiuretic hormones, respectively.

Nucleus accumbens: a large mass of gray matter immediately lateral to the septal area and lying against the head of the caudate nucleus; traditionally considered a septal structure, but now recognized as the limbic striatum (target of mesocortical dopamine system), a "crossroads" between basal ganglia and limbic circuitry.

Orbitofrontal cortex: the granular, eulaminate (distinctly six-layered) cortex characterizing all the frontal lobe anterior to the motor and supplementary motor areas; major neocortical modulator of the limbic system.

Parahippocampal gyrus: see Chap. 2.

Paraventricular nucleus: the more dorsal of the two nuclei of the supraoptic group of the hypothalamus; contains large, deeply staining neurosecretory neurons that give rise to axons of the neurohypophysial tract.

Periaqueductal gray: a narrow zone of tiny neurons and poorly myelinated fibers surrounding the mesencephalic aqueduct and comprising a part of the limbic midbrain area; a similar zone of central gray is found throughout most of the rest of the brain, representing an innermost continuum or core of primitive neuropil important to nociceptive and vasomotor functions.

Periventricular fiber system: a complex, pervasive feltwork of thinly myelinated fibers running through the central gray of the hypothalamus and interconnecting that structure with adjacent regions (preoptic area, mesencephalic tectum, etc.).

Periventricular nucleus: a zone of tiny neurons immediately beneath the ependymal wall of the third ventricle and running the length of the hypothalamus; a major source of hypophysial releasing and inhibiting hormones.

Posterior nucleus: a member of the mammillary group of hypothalamic nuclei, just above the mammillary body; gives rise to fibers projecting caudally into the tegmentum which convey hypothalamic impulses to lower centers.

Principal mammillary fasciculus: the combined stem of the mammillothalamic and mammillotegmental tracts (also known as fasciculus mammillaris princeps).

Raphe nuclei: see Chaps. 6 and 11.

Septal area: see Chap. 2.

Stria medullaris thalami: one of the two largest descending projections of the limbic system; runs from the mediobasal forebrain (including the septal area) to the habenular nuclear complex, from which the fasciculus retroflexus continues down to the interpeduncular nucleus of the midbrain.

Stria terminalis: a thin, wispy tract from the amygdala to the septal and preoptic areas and hypothalamus; courses immediately medial to the tail and body of the caudate nucleus.

Supraoptic nucleus: the more ventral of the two nuclei of the supraoptic group of the hypothalamus; comprises several clusters of large, deeply staining neurosecretory neurons that give rise to axons of the neurohypophysial tract.

Tegmental area: see *Tegmentum*, Chaps. 2 and 11.

Tuber cinereum: a prominent mound of gray matter in the mediobasal hypothalamus containing the median eminence and the root of the infundibular stalk.

Tuberoinfundibular tract: one of the two endocrine outputs of the hypothalamus, originating from cells in the preoptic, periventricular, and tuberal regions; controls hormonal output of the adenohypophysis by conveying releasing and inhibiting factors to the hypothalamic/hypophysial portal system.

Uncinate fasciculus: a large band of association fibers curving beneath the stem of the lateral fissure; interconnects the orbitofrontal and anterior temporal cortex.

Ventral tegmental area: a region of the mesencephalic tegmentum between the two halves of the substantia nigra and containing dopamine neurons; source of the mesocortical dopamine system.

Ventromedial nucleus: a member of the tuberal group of hypothalamic nuclei, located immediately beneath the dorsomedial nucleus.

The Cerebral Cortex
and the Lobes of the Brain

13

The cerebral cortex, by virtue of its progressive arrangement of circuits, provides a degree of sensory feature analysis unequaled by other parts of the brain. The fine qualities of sensation that depend on it, as we have seen in previous chapters, include the spatial, temporal, and associative aspects of sights, sounds, bodily sensations, tastes, and smells. The cortex also acts to organize skilled responses. Together with deeper structures, such as the basal ganglia, and in the presence of constant sensory feedback, it synthesizes patterns of response that are often intricate, as in the performance of fine movements. The cortex provides for memory, particularly through interactions between the hippocampus and the extensive, widely connected cortical regions that cover it. Finally, the cortex acts to reduce and combine sensory and motor data; the association cortex, with the help of the thalamus, weaves things together in broad tapestries of reference — of our environment and of our selves within that environment.

Anatomy of the Cerebral Cortex

The longitudinal cerebral fissure divides the cerebrum almost completely into two hemispheres that are joined centrally by the corpus callosum, the most massive fiber tract in the brain. Each of these hemispheres is covered by that stratified mantle of gray matter, the cerebral cortex. Viewed from without, this cortex appears rumpled; it is, in fact, intricately and deeply folded. Its topography is defined by fissures and sulci which divide it into six lobes: frontal, parietal, occipital, central, temporal, and limbic (Fig. 13-1). The central sulcus (of Rolando) and the lateral fissure (of Sylvius) are

(A)

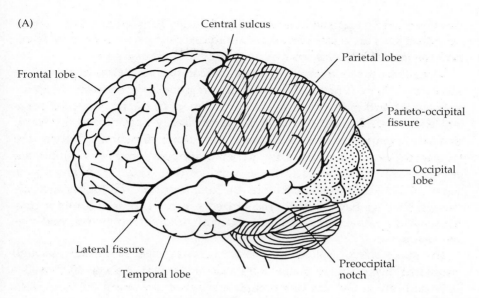

(B)

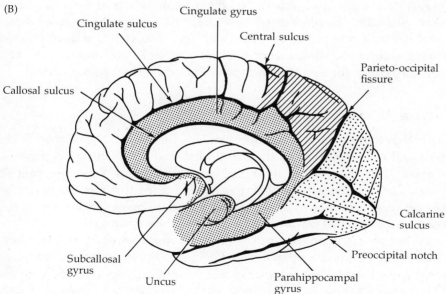

FIG. 13–1. *Lobes of the cerebrum.* (A) The frontal, parietal (hatched area), occipital (stippled), and temporal lobes are indicated on the lateral surface of the cerebral hemisphere. The central lobe (insula) lies deep within the lateral (Sylvian) fissure, and hence cannot be seen (see Fig. 13-8). (B) The limbic lobe (cingulate, parahippocampal, and subcallosal gyri; shaded region) is delineated on the medial surface.

the major infoldings and boundary lines in each hemisphere. The numerous other sulci are remarkably constant in essential pattern, if not in detail, and are important landmarks in neurology and neurosurgery.

Large areas of the human cortex are difficult to characterize in physiological terms. These functionally ambivalent regions lie in between the clearcut sensory and motor areas in the cortical map. In the rat, this problem is not encountered: most of the cortex is obviously apportioned to visual, auditory, somatosensory, olfactory, and motor functions. But in the human cortex, large areas of the parietal, temporal, and frontal lobes are not obviously constrained to these activities (Fig. 13-2). Such areas have been characterized as "association" or "uncommitted" cortex because, although they do have recently recognized sensory inputs and motor connections, they have even more important associative, integrative, and cognitive functions.

The sheer size of the cerebral cortex is impressive. It is a thin (though laminated) layer of gray matter with a surface extent of about 4000 cm² — unfolded, about the size of a complete sheet of newsprint (left and right pages). It contains upwards of 50 billion neurons and at least five times more glial cells. The phylogenetically recent and uniformly six-layered cerebral cortex is referred to as "neocortex" or "isocortex," to distinguish it from the older and dissimilar cortical areas, such as the hippocampus and olfactory cortex (uncus), that comprise the "allocortex" (other cortex).

Cortical Areas

Although the isocortex is basically similar everywhere, the relative thickness and cell density of its six layers vary, and so do the arrangements, shapes, sizes, and types of cortical neurons present. Over the past 75 years, such local structural characteristics have led to a number of similar but progressively more detailed cytoarchitectonic maps. At the turn of the century, perhaps 20 distinctive cortical areas were recognized in the human, but shortly thereafter nearly 50 areas were described in a monkey. Before long, certain investigators had delineated (with letters, numbers, or other labels) nearly 250 supposedly recognizable patches of human cortex! Other workers, however, remained skeptical, seeing only eight obviously different zones.

Clearly, such parcellations of the essentially similar isocortex were overzealous, occasionally becoming almost as ridiculous as the phrenology charts of a century ago. But this passion for mapping the cortex for regional

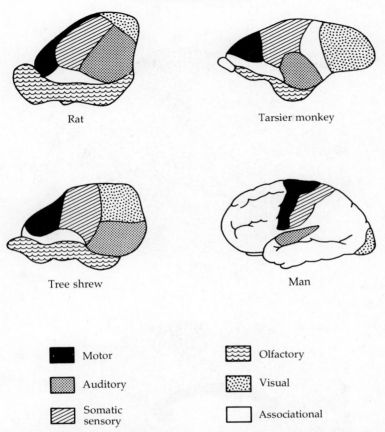

Rat

Tarsier monkey

Tree shrew

Man

Motor

Auditory

Somatic
sensory

Olfactory

Visual

Associational

FIG. 13–2. *Functional map of cerebral cortex in certain mammals.* The white area indicates the extent of association cortex, i.e., cortex transcending sensory/motor function, in the cerebral hemispheres of several well-studied mammals. The rat is in a
distinctly different evolutionary line from that leading to man, but the tree shrew
and tarsier (a small insectivorous monkey) are believed to lie in the primate family
tree. (Redrawn from W. Penfield, *The Mystery of the Mind.* Princeton University
Press, Princeton, N.J., 1975)

differences shown by routine dye stains uncovered many structural features and functional correlates which remain valid.

Brodmann's scheme (1909) of 52 numbered areas is still in clinical use
(Fig. 13-3). To some extent, structural specialization reflects functional
specialization, and some of Brodmann's areas correspond to primary sensory and motor areas. Other areas, however, do not have obvious
physiological significance, and the numbers for them are chiefly useful for

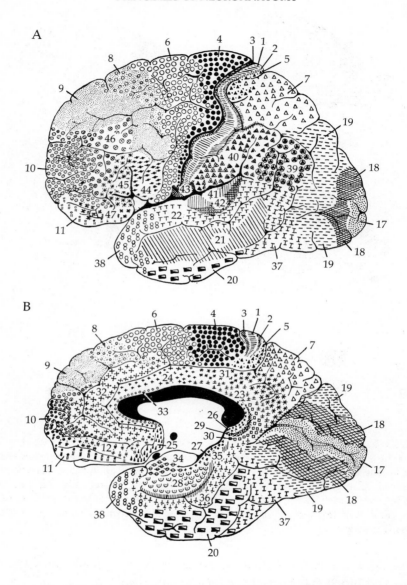

FIG. 13–3. *Cytoarchitectonic areas according to Brodmann (1909).* This scheme, originally worked out for the *Cercopithecus* monkey, remains the most popular (if not the
best) cytoarchitectonic map. It is widely used in clinical accounts of cerebral territories. The numbers themselves mean nothing; they merely reflect the order in
which tissue sections were cut from several large blocks of the original brain. (From
K. Brodmann, *Vergleichende Lokalisationslehre der Grosshirrinde.* Barth, Leipzig, 1909)

reference purposes. Little did the mapmakers dream, however, that functional individuality could extend down to the level of a single cortical nerve cell, or at least to a functional column of such cells, as microelectrode studies have clearly shown in recent years. That it does is a consequence of the integrative design of neurons and neuronal groups.

Primary Neuronal Types

The neurons of the cerebral cortex are organized in horizontal planes or layers and in vertical modules or small, functional columns. Such laminar and columnar modes of organization, as we have emphasized in previous chapters, are expressions of central organizing principles, and the cerebral cortex offers the supreme illustrations of these principles. Before describing these two modes of organization, we shall briefly examine the neurons of the neocortex.

The cerebral cortex is a showcase of neuronal design. Some of its cells are familiar types, while others are so specialized as to appear exotic. Cortical neurons, like other neurons, are classified on the basis of size and shape. There are two main types, pyramidal cells and stellate cells, but within these types there is great variety in size, structure, and connectivity.

Pyramidal cells. The cell body has the form of a pyramid (Fig. 13-4). Some pyramidal cells (in area 4 and other regions) give rise to the pyramidal tract, but this is only a coincidence; the tract gets its name from the pyramids of the medulla oblongata it passes through en route to the spinal cord. The apical dendrite of a pyramidal cell extends upward, the numerous basal dendrites project radially and horizontally, and the axon emerges from the base of the ·perikaryon. Pyramidal cells have prominent Nissl substance (rough-surfaced endoplasmic reticulum). Their perikarya vary in size from small (10 μm) to large (50 μm). A Betz cell in area 4 is a giant in height (100–125 μm).

Stellate cells. The cell body has the form of a star or polygon (Fig. 13-4), and is usually much smaller than that of a pyramidal cell. These generally tiny cells greatly outnumber the pyramidal cells. In certain areas, they are so numerous that they resemble a cloud of dust particles. Such a region is called *koniocortex* (the Greek word for dust is *konios*) or, more commonly, granular cortex. Many short dendrites reach out in all directions from the stellate cells, and a short axon extends from the small (4–8 μm) cell body,

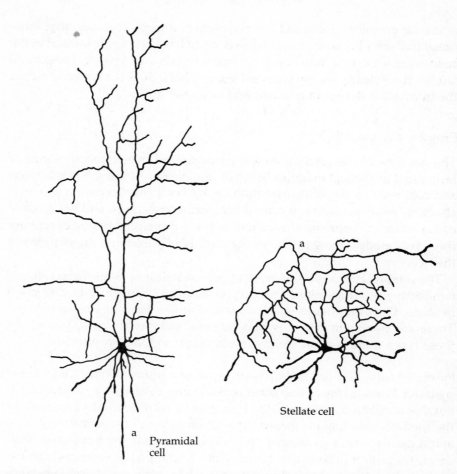

Stellate cell

a
Pyramidal
cell

FIG. 13–4. *The two main types of cortical neurons.* Despite their variety, all cortical neurons may be classified as pyramidal or stellate cells. In general, pyramidal cells are the projection neurons of the cortex, while the much smaller and more numerous stellate cells serve local-circuit functions. Pyramidal cells are especially abundant in cortical layers III and V, whereas stellate cells abound in layers II and IV. Axon of each cell is indicated by an (a). (Neurons patterned after cells originally drawn from the microscope by S. Ramón y Cajal and R. Lorente de Nó)

which has scant cytoplasm and inconspicuous Nissl bodies. Stellate cells are found in all the layers and areas of cortex, but are especially numerous in layer IV (see below) and in the primary sensory areas (such as areas 17, 41, 3, 1, and 2).

The axons of most cortical neurons have collaterals that greatly extend the cell's sphere of influence. Pyramidal cells, for example, have upward, diagonally coursing recurrent axon collaterals as well as horizontal ones, while stellate cells may have extremely complex axonal arborizations that form nets, baskets, or showers. If the stellate cell has a triangular shape and an ascending axon destined for some overlying layer, it is called a Martinotti cell; such upward signaling elements are found in all layers of the cortex.

Such wealth of collaterals and ascending/descending connections permits extremely extensive interaction of cortical neurons, much as in the cerebellar cortex. Here, however, the interplay involves many more kinds of cells and local circuits than we find in the cerebellum, as well as a much more complex and less evident circuit geometry.

Laminar Organization

Within any given cortical area, the cortical neurons are organized in six layers, usually designated by Roman numerals. The various cortical areas, on the other hand, are designated by Arabic numerals, according to Brodmann. The general plan and nomenclature are shown in Figure 13-5.

Layer I is called the molecular layer (because the few specklike cell bodies scattered there looked like "molecules" to 19th century anatomists). It contains small, isolated neurons (horizontal cells of Cajal) lying amidst tangential axonal and dendritic plexuses.

Layer II is the external granular layer. It contains many densely packed small pyramidal cells, whose dendrites ramify in layer I and whose axons pass down to deeper layers.

Layer III is the external pyramidal layer. It features a population of medium-size pyramidal cells, the deeper ones tending to be larger. Dendrites reach toward layer I; axons descend to the white matter as associational and commissural fibers.

Layer IV is the internal granular layer. It varies greatly in different cortical areas, but generally shows a high cell density — extremely high in some areas. Stellate cells predominate, with axons ramifying in this layer and extending into deeper areas. Myelinated fibers are prominent, forming the outer band of Baillarger. In this layer, the terminal ramifications of specific thalamic afferents articulate with the dendrites of a horde of small stellate cells for initial cortical information processing. For example, as we noted in Chapter 5, lateral geniculate fibers terminate primarily in this layer of area 17, where the prominent outer band of Baillarger is otherwise known as the stripe of Gennari.

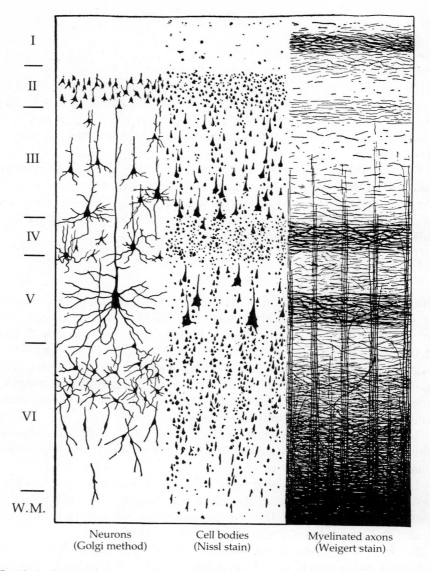

I			
II			
III			
IV			
V			
VI			
W.M.			

Neurons (Golgi method)	Cell bodies (Nissl stain)	Myelinated axons (Weigert stain)

FIG. 13–5. *Layers of the neocortex.* Cortical neurons are arranged in six principal layers designated by Roman numerals. (Sublayers are also recognized, but are not shown here.) W. M. = underlying white matter. While horizontal lamination is evident, especially in some areas (association cortex), there is also a prominent vertical plan of organization (see text and Fig. 13-6). Note pyramidal and stellate cells; the multiform (many-shaped) cells in layer VI fall into both pyramidal and stellate categories, depending on the size and length of their axons. (From S. W. Ranson, *The Anatomy of the Nervous System.* W. B. Saunders, Philadelphia, 1959)

Layer V is the internal pyramidal layer. Most of its cells are medium-size to large pyramidal neurons whose apical dendrites often reach up to layer I. Axons leaving this layer are mainly projection fibers, but some association fibers also originate here. This layer contains abundant vertically directed fibers; in area 4 (primary motor cortex), for instance, some 34,000 giant pyramidal cells of Betz contribute a corresponding number of large-caliber, fast-conducting axons to the pyramidal tract.

Layer VI is the multiform layer. Small pyramidal cells and a variety of stellate cells are present. As in layer V, many cortical efferent fibers originate here. Taken together and considered apart from the remainder of the cortical mantle, layers V and VI represent the principal efferent component of the cortex. In this respect, these two layers could be thought of as "motor cortex" even though that term is usually reserved for the primary motor areas 4 and 6.

As one might expect from the cortical map-making activities mentioned above, there is considerable variation in lamination between cortical areas. The isocortex is not actually of uniform structure, although its overall similarity is much more important than its regional differences. The local variations pertain to thickness of layers, cell density, neuronal types, cell sizes, etc. Two main types of isocortex (neocortex) are recognized:

1. *Homotypical cortex:* the six layers are easily seen. Association cortex is generally of this type.
2. *Heterotypical cortex:* the cortex shows granular or agranular specialization (an abundance or paucity of stellate cells), departures from the usual pattern. In either case, the layers are usually less distinct than those of homotypical cortex.
   a. *Granular or koniocortex:* a high density of stellate cells, especially in layer IV. Examples are the primary sensory areas: 17, 41, 3, 1, and 2.
   b. *Agranular cortex:* a paucity of stellate cells, especially in layer IV. Examples are the primary motor areas: 4, 44, and 6.

Vertical Columnar Organization

In the 1940's Lorente de Nó, a student of the great neurohistologist Ramón y Cajal, made a great discovery. He found, in addition to the evident horizontal lamination, "vertical chains" of neurons in the cortex. Such chains of intracortical interneurons are arranged perpendicular to the layers, in a cylindrical module of cortex called a functional column. Each column contains about 100–300 neurons, heavily interconnected up and down between cortical layers, but with only weak horizontal connections. These columns turn out to be input/output data processing ensembles that comprise the elementary working units of the cortex. It is estimated that the cortex consists of about 500 million such columns. These modules are activated by different modes of stimulation (cutaneous stimuli, movement of joints, activation of periosteal or fascial receptors, etc.), inputs which they process in a more or less similar manner and then distribute through their distinctive output channels. An interesting feature is that activation of a column tends to inhibit neural activity in adjacent ones.

The cellular structure of a column is similar in design throughout the cortex (Fig. 13-6). The columns of motor, somatosensory, and temporal homotypical cortices in the mouse, rat, rhesus monkey, and man (no evolutionary sequence intended in such an assortment of diverse species) are virtually identical, a 30 μm cylinder containing about 110 neurons. There are, however, variations in columnar structure and population, and they seem to be important to the functional specialization of regions. In the visual or striate cortex, for example, the number of cells doubles, and intercolumnar connectivities may vary. The key features, nonetheless, are the common functional unit and the widely varied inputs and outputs.

Cortical columns, in turn, form larger columnar structures called macrocolumns. These vary in width from 100–500 μm in different areas, and in cross section may be round, oval, or of other configuration. In the visual cortex, macrocolumns are slablike and serve to plot ocular dominance and orientation preference. In the auditory cortex, sound frequency and binaural representation of sound in space are the parameters defined. And in the somatosensory cortex, the macrocolumns represent particular places on the body surface and particular submodalities of somatic sensation (touch, temperature, joint movement, etc.).

Inputs and Outputs of the Cortex

There are three major sources of input to the cortex:

1.. *Projection fibers* come to the cortex from specific thalamic nuclei (such as the geniculate bodies and ventrobasal complex) and end in specific cortical areas (such as area 17). These fibers terminate primarily in cortical layers III and IV.
2.. *Association fibers* originate from other cortical areas of the same hemisphere. Within a hemisphere, there is a distinct stepping-stone or cascadelike progression of corticocortical pathways from primary sensory

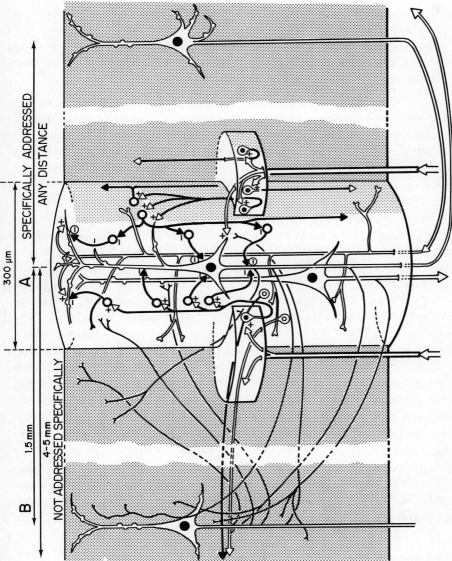

FIG. 13–6. *Columnar organization of the cerebral cortex.* In addition to the obvious layers of cells (I–VI, as shown in Fig. 13-5), there are vertical chains of neurons in the cortex arranged in cylindrical columns. These columns are the basic functional units of the cortex. A specific afferent fiber from the thalamus and several varieties of stellate and star-pyramidal cells are labeled. (Redrawn from J. Szentágothai, *Advan. Physiol. Sci. 1, 14*, 1980)

areas (visual, acoustic, and somesthetic) forward to parietal and temporal cortices (see below).

3.. *Commissural fibers* come from homologous or mirror-image cortical regions of the opposite hemisphere, by way of the corpus callosum. The striate area of the occipital cortex and hand region of the somatosensory cortex are exceptions, in that they do not receive commissural connections. All other areas do, apparently.

In addition, diffuse projections to the entire cortex arise from the nonspecific thalamic nuclei (such as the ventral anterior, midline, and intralaminar), certain basal forebrain areas, and the various monoaminergic pathways. The locus coeruleus (a pigmented nucleus near the central gray of the rostral pons) gives rise to a very large ascending noradrenergic axonal system that terminates diffusely over all cortical layers.

Cortical efferents arise chiefly from pyramidal cells (a few come from stellate cells) of the deeper layers, especially V and VI, and project extensively throughout the brain and spinal cord. The longest projection of the human cortex is the pyramidal tract, many fibers of which extend into the spinal cord. It originates primarily in precentral motor cortex (including areas 4, 6, and 44), but also comes from postcentral somatosensory regions. Corticothalamic fibers project topographically to the thalamus, in a reciprocal relation with thalamocortical fibers. For example, the ventral posterior nucleus (VP) of the thalamus projects somatotopically to the primary somatosensory cortex (areas 3, 1, and 2) which, in turn, projects back onto VP. Other major efferent systems include the corticopontine tracts, as well as projections to the caudate nucleus and putamen, the red nucleus, and the brainstem reticular formation. There are minor projections to the dorsal column nuclei, inferior olive, substantia nigra, and the subthalamic nucleus. In general, cortical efferents project to nearly all subcortical gray masses (refer to Fig. 9-2). This direct, in-parallel arrangement enables the cortex to exercise direct effects on the activity of almost every other region of the CNS, expeditiously and selectively, thus giving it even greater means of influence than its vast and ordered cell populations already confer upon it.

The Lobes of the Brain: an Overview of Higher Functions

A good way to get some idea of the higher functions of the cortex is by a regional consideration — "lobe by lobe." We shall briefly characterize the occipital, temporal, parietal, central, and frontal lobes, touching here and there upon the association cortex. (The limbic lobe was described in Chap. 12.)

The Occipital Lobe—Vision and Dependent Functions

The most notable feature of the occipital lobes is the beautifully organized visual cortex. Visual images are transmitted retinotopically from the neural retina to Brodmann's area 17, then on to area 18, the secondary visual cortex, and from there to still other cortical fields (Fig. 13-7).

In the dominant hemisphere, a large region anterior to the visual cortex and including the posterior parts of the parietal and temporal lobes is critically important for language functions: reading, writing, and speech. This language area includes the auditory association cortex or Wernicke's area, which lies in the superior temporal gyrus, and a part of the adjacent middle temporal gyrus just posterior to the primary auditory cortex. Injury here can cause striking language defects of many types, depending on the location of the lesion. Word finding difficulties (*anomia*), word blindness or inability to read (*alexia*), and a variety of speech disorders (*aphasias*) result from damage to this meeting ground of occipital, temporal, and parietal lobes and their association fibers.

Contrary to what we might expect from its precise wiring, epileptic discharge or electrical stimulation (during surgery to remove an epileptic focus) of the occipital cortex produces imprecise effects: the patient experiences sensations in the contralateral field of vision which are rudimentary in character — lights, shadows, colors with movements. The images are not familiar, but the color and general nature of what is seen may be described. An interesting negative effect is that the patient may become partially or totally blind during the seizure or stimulation.

Surprisingly large lesions of occipital cortex may not abolish effective vision as long as macular vision (allotted a large territory at the occipital pole) is spared. Such macular sparing is frequently observed in clinical practice. But the macular zone is not immune to damage, and so much visual analysis takes place in it that a person is virtually blind after its destruction or removal.

As described in Chapter 5, the visual cortex displays striking precision in its organization: the columnar plan is especially noticeable here, and the neurons concerned with one aspect of sensory information (such as orientation of the edges of visualized objects) lie stacked in one column, while neurons dealing with some other aspect (ocular dominance) lie in another.

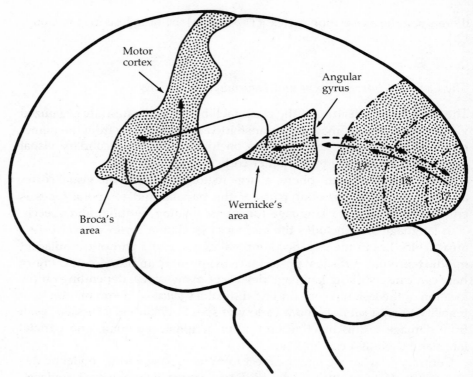

FIG. 13–7. *Progressive sensory processing from primary visual cortex.* The output of area 17 proceeds forward via short association fibers to area 18, and from area 18 to 19. From these points of departure, several routes are possible, leading to temporal and frontal cortical areas (see also Fig. 13-9). Many, if not all, of these connections are reciprocal (as indicated by smaller arrows). Some connections lead to the angular gyrus of the parietal lobe, which is important in associating the visual appearance of a word with the neural representation of its sound in the auditory area nearby. Powerful systems of fibers course between Wernicke's speech area and Broca's motor speech area (via the superior longitudinal fasciculus; see also Fig. 2-9). In this way, visual sensory processing becomes part of the greater pattern of cortical activity involved in verbal communication.

The Temporal Lobe—Audition and Related Functions, Memory, and Retrieval

The temporal lobe processes sounds, vestibular sensations, sights, smells, and other experiences in a complex manner. Evidently perception, recording, and retrieval of events depend on this large, anatomically diversified lobe. The temporal lobe is also important in the emotional coloration of experience, as we pointed out in Chapter 12.

The auditory cortex is a small region of the temporal lobe that could be covered by a thumbprint. It lies on the lower bank of the Sylvian fissure, toward the rear of the lobe — on the transverse temporal gyri that comprise Brodmann's areas 41 and 42. Adjoining the auditory cortex anteriorly is a region of the superior temporal gyrus that appears to represent the projection field of the vestibular system. Here, movements and positions of the head, as signaled by the hair cells of the inner ear, receive further study.

Auditory impressions following epileptic discharge or stimulation of primary acoustic cortex have the same elementary quality (clicks, roaring) noted for the visual cortex. Again there is a negative effect: the patient experiences some deafness as the stimulation takes place. Stimulation of the nearby vestibular cortex may produce dizziness and vertigo (the subjective sense of rotation when rotation is not actually taking place).

Unilateral injury to auditory cortex may seriously impair certain qualities of hearing, such as short-term memory storage, identification of novel stimuli, retaining the temporal order of auditory events, and localization of sounds in space. It will not cause complete deafness, however, since messages from each ear go to both sides of the brain and are extensively processed by numerous subcortical centers.

Striking emotional, hallucinatory, and memory disturbances follow destructive or irritative insults to the more anterior temporal lobe encompassing the uncus and amygdaloid region:

1. *The Klüver-Bucy syndrome* features a combination of five symptoms — visual agnosia, hyperphagia, hypersexuality, docility, and stimulus-bound behavior. Damage to the amygdala and its cortical affiliations is the usual cause of such dramatic behavioral alterations.

2. *Uncinate fits* are seizures or hallucinations consisting of the experience of an odor (usually foul), a period of oral motility, and a fearful feeling of unreality. As in the case of the Klüver-Bucy syndrome, these epileptiform attacks are usually due to a tumor or other irritative lesion near the uncus and underlying amygdala.

3. *Loss of recent memory* involves a complete inability to store any events occurring after its onset — with preservation, however, of long-term memory and intellect. Usually damage to both sides of the brain is necessary to produce such a deficit: a bilateral surgical ablation of temporal cortex (to remove seizure foci) or bilateral infarcts in the amygdaloid-hippocampas region/fornix system. Such man-made or natural lesions impair the functions of what we might think of as a pair of "temporal tape recorders" — running and recording most of what happens to us during our wakeful hours.

In keeping with these clinical findings, stimulation of particular regions of the temporal lobe during brain surgery may call forth psychic phenomena of a high order, in fact, complete memories and the emotions associated with them. Such coherent responses cannot be evoked from other parts of the cortex, only fragments. As an electrode probes the occipitotemporal meeting ground, however, hallucinations and illusions unfold dramatically — like a motion picture of past events with sound and color, based on the person's memories or dreams, capable of being stopped and restarted at various points by the surgeon. For example, a mother undergoing electrical stimulation of the temporal lobe in the operating room felt that she was standing in her kitchen, listening to the voice of her little boy playing in the backyard. She experienced déjà vu, and probably felt sad as the illusion faded away.

Thus the temporal lobe is involved in recording and storing events, in the affect of these experiences, and in their retrieval. The "replay" circuits for experiences already "on tape" may survive damage to the temporal lobe. But with larger or more generalized types of brain damage, long-term memory loss is an expected consequence.

Information storage probably does not take place in the temporal lobe alone, even though auditory and olfactory memories appear to rely heavily on its neurons and connections. As we have stressed, such high functions as memory or consciousness almost certainly are responsibilities of many brain regions working together. Particularly involved in such functions are the thalamus and its many upstream and downstream affiliates.

The Parietal Lobe—Somesthesis, Sensory Integration, and Gnostic Function

The sensorimotor strip runs down the two sides of the central sulcus, including Brodmann's areas 3, 1, and 2 postcentrally and area 4 precentrally. Much overlap of sensory and motor representation occurs here, but in both functional respects the parts of the body are somatotopically arranged.

Despite the complete body layout in the primary somesthetic area (S I), only crude sensations, such as tingling of some part of the body, are evoked when a region of the sensory homunculus is stimulated or involved in a seizure. Because of the overlapping motor representation, simple motions — such as those that a baby might make — are also elicited here, as they are from the precentral convolution also. All these effects, of course, are contralateral, due to the more or less complete cross-over of the sensory and motor pathways (decussation of medial lemnisci and pyramids, respectively).

The secondary somesthetic area (S II), at the base of the postcentral gyrus, has less topographically precise, bilateral inputs, and it apparently lacks face, mouth, and throat territories. Stimulation of this less extensive area produces similar effects: numbness, tingling, a feeling of electricity, or a sense of movement. These sensations, however, may be felt bilaterally. The explanation is that S II receives input from the posterior nuclear group of the thalamus, where spinothalamic fibers of both sides of the body enter and ramify profusely.

A gustatory area is located just outside the parietal lobe: either at the base of the precentral gyrus (anterior to S II) or in the adjacent region of the insula. Stimulation or epileptic discharge here may produce hallucinations of taste, usually sour or bitter.

Thus the somesthetic cortex analyzes and combines sensations from the skin and deeper regions of the body, including its joints — where the angles between bones and changes in these angles bespeak position and movement, respectively — and from those mucous membranes that contain chemoceptors for substances in food.

The somesthetic cortex is intimately connected with more posteriorly located regions of the parietal lobe: the supramarginal and angular gyri. These regions weave body sensations together with the sights and sounds evaluated by the occipital and temporal lobes. The result is a body image or body schema — a synthesis of sensory experience in which the sense of one's own body begins to take form amidst the backdrop of one's environment.

Obviously, injury to cortical areas or their connections leads to trouble. For example, clinicians recognize numerous speech defects, or *aphasias*, and the study of aphasia is a complex topic. The problem can be mainly in comprehension of written or spoken words, i.e., receptive aphasia, due to a lesion in the posterior part of the left superior temporal gyrus (Wernicke's area). It can be chiefly in expressing what one wants to say, a so-called motor aphasia, usually produced by damage to the inferior frontal gyrus (Broca's area) and adjacent lower part of the precentral convolution. Or it can be pronounced in both comprehensive and expressive spheres — global aphasia. Massive destruction of the left frontotemporal region and the underlying superior longitudinal fasciculus is the usual cause of total aphasia. Aphasias can range from a slight, almost unnoticeable difficulty in the choice of words or cadence of speech to total incomprehension and mutism.

Different deficits result from damage to the parietal lobe or its numerous intercortical connections: losses in knowledge, or awareness, of the significance of things. These "disconnection syndromes" are called *agnosias* ("not knowings") and are of several types and degrees of severity, such as the following:

1. *Astereognosia* means not knowing solid objects; it consists of deficits in the recognition of palpated things. It is caused by damage to S I and adjoining areas of the parietal lobe posteriorly.
2. *Atopognosia* means not knowing the place; it signifies a problem in correctly and precisely localizing sensations. Again, it is caused by damage to S I and its adjoining areas.
3. *Psychic blindness and deafness* are terms that refer to deficits in recognizing or heeding visual and auditory cues. The conditions are caused by damage to visual association areas (18 and 19), especially in the dominant hemisphere, or to the auditory association area (22).
4. *Amorphosynthesis* is an interesting word that literally means an inability to "put one's body together." It is a profound deficit in a person's awareness and acceptance of an entire half of the body. The afflicted individual may fail to dress or undress one side of his or her body or attend to its cosmetic care — the person may even complain strongly about the strange unwanted presence of this half-body in bed! Usually this bizarre condition is caused by a large lesion in the superior parietal cortex on the nondominant side, where spatial relations rather than speech are among the most important functional dependencies.

Through myriad association fibers, such as the cablelike superior longitudinal fasciculus, the combined and reduced data of the parietal lobe are passed forward to the frontal lobe and also to the underlying basal ganglia. With the participation of both these regions, stratagems of response are drawn up and set in motion.

The Central Lobe—Viscerosomatic Integration

This lobe cannot easily be seen in the gross examination of the brain. Very little is known about it. Just to visualize the central lobe, we have to pry open the frontal, parietal, and temporal folds (opercula) that cover it (Fig. 13-8).

The central lobe is also called the insula or island of Reil. It derives from the lateral surface of the early telencephalic vesicle. During the fetal period,

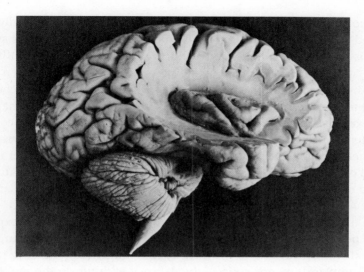

FIG. 13–8. *The insula.* This "island" of cortex derives from the lateral surface of the embryonic cerebral vesicle. It is rapidly covered over during development by the frontal, parietal, and temporal lobes. (From N. Gluhbegovic and T. Williams, *The Human Brain, A Photographic Guide.* Harper and Row, New York, 1980)

it is quickly covered up by the burgeoning growth of the frontal, parietal, and temporal lobes. In the adult, it lies buried in the Sylvian fissure, not far from the auditory, somesthetic (S II), and gustatory areas in the surrounding temporoparietal operculum. Stimulation of the human insula indicates that intra-abdominal sensation is represented here, along with some representation of visceral motility. But its concealed position and covering vasculature (middle cerebral artery) greatly limit such surgical exploration.

The Frontal Lobe—Motility, Ethical Sensitivity, Programs for Living

The frontal lobe takes in a large territory above the Sylvian fissure and in front of the central sulcus. It comprises the precentral, superior, middle, and inferior frontal gyri on the lateral aspect of the cerebral hemisphere and the orbital gyri on the basal aspect; an additional region of the superior frontal gyrus forms a broad band of cortex around the cingulate gyrus on the medial aspect.

The bulging size of the frontal lobe and tremendous number of direct connections to and from other parts of the CNS are among the most characteristically human of all aspects of man's nervous system. Through these connections, the human frontal lobes appear to be extraordinarily well-informed about what is transpiring in other regions of the nervous system, and thus in all parts of the body and its surroundings. The influences exerted by the frontal lobes are equally far-reaching. We have seen examples in the guiding and restraining effects of the granular frontal cortex on other components of the limbic system to which it belongs (Chap. 12). Other examples include the skillful functions dependent on the cortex at the posterior margin of the frontal lobe, where the primary motor area (M I, area 4) lies. As we have noted (Chap. 9), this motor cortex, a rather narrow but well organized band of gray matter in the precentral gyrus, features an inverted representation of the opposite half of the body, very similar to the primary sensory homunculus in the postcentral gyrus.

As in the sensory homunculus, the layout of the motor cortex expresses the functional importance of body parts, not their size. Thus the large area of cortical surface devoted to the face, larynx, tongue, and hand, especially to the thumb and fingers, reflects the delicacy with which the movements of these parts of the body can be controlled — and their consequent utility in facial expression, vocalization, exploration, and manipulation of the environment.

Much has been learned from the painless and prudent electrical mapping of the motor cortex during brain surgery. To obviate lasting and crippling paralysis (and loss of speech, if in the dominant hemisphere), the M I region must be spared if at all possible in the surgical removal of a blood clot, tumor, or epileptogenic focus. When the electrode current is not too great and cortical activity not overly depressed by anesthesia, faradic stimulation brings about twitchlike (phasic, not tonic) contractions, usually in groups of muscles but sometimes in individual muscles, that produce definite, if crude, movements. Changes in facial expression, swallowing or grunting, licking or smacking of the lips, twisting of the body or rotation or flexion of an extremity, abduction or adduction of the thumb — all predominately on the opposite side — are some of the effects of focal stimulation. And a negative effect, like that seen in stimulation of sensory cortical areas, is that voluntary control of muscles is lost during the period of stimulation. For example, if the person is gripping an object, the grip is relaxed when the opposite hand area is stimulated.

In considering these crude responses to electrical stimulation of the primary motor area, we must remember that the motor cortex is part of an ensemble — including the supplementary motor cortex, sensory cortex, and basal ganglia — that only the brain, not an electrode, can activate appropriately. Abnormal intrinsic activity of the motor cortex, by contrast, may bring about dramatic responses. Such activity occurs in a focal motor seizure or Jacksonian fit, named after John Hughlings Jackson (1835-1911), a London neurologist. This brilliant clinician worked out the cortical map of movement almost a century before the Canadian neurosurgeon Wilder Penfield and his associates demonstrated the motor homunculus electrically. In a Jacksonian fit, repeated muscular contractions may be restricted, in the form of sustained or twitching movements, to the face, arm, or leg. Or they may start with twitching of a finger, then spread from distal to proximal arm musculature, down one side of the body and into the lower extremity, up the opposite side of the body to its upper extremity and thence to the face. Examine a picture of the motor homunculus (refer to Fig. 9-1) and think of its contralateral counterpart as you read the preceding description. You will see how such a chain reaction or "march" of movement comes about, just as Hughlings Jackson did over 100 years ago.

If the seizure activity spreads to both sides of the brain, consciousness is usually lost, probably due to the greater havoc that such an electrical storm rains down upon the thalamus below. Cutting the corpus callosum prevents spread between the two hemispheres, and this operation (commissurotomy) may be a last resort in severe, intractable cases of epilepsy.

Anterior to the motor cortex, a larger frontal region extends to and includes the frontal pole. Part of it (Brodmann's area 6) further elaborates movement patterns. A greater part (areas 8–12 and 44–47) makes up the orbitofrontal or granular frontal cortex. As we have noted (Chap. 12), the latter region is involved in regulating emotional tone, assigning priorities to bodily and environmental demands, and stabilizing programs for meeting short-term and long-range goals.

To appreciate the human qualities that depend on the frontal lobes, consider two hallmarks of frontal lobe injury or loss: debased ethical conduct and inappropriate actions. Over a century ago, an accidental explosion of blasting powder caused a tamping iron to be blown through the cheek and forehead of a railway construction foreman, Phineas P. Gage. Gage miraculously survived this "crowbar lobotomy" (apparently losing consciousness only momentarily) but underwent a striking deterioration of personality. Previously an upright, dependable worker, he became so profane and irresponsible that he lost his job and spent the rest of his life as a drifter. While some of his personality changes may have resulted from a post-traumatic infection (meningitis), this famous incident is still considered a prime illustration of the effects of frontal lobe damage.

A major deficit noted after injury or surgical isolation of the frontal lobes is diminished anxiety and concern — a loss all too evident in the reduction of that person's ethical standards. Another striking effect is a lessening of the person's judgment and planning ability that leads to ill-timed actions or inappropriate reactions. Such unfortunate characteristics develop, apparently, because the limbic system is operating without its highest level of control. Bilateral loss of the orbitofrontal cortex diminishes a human being, without noticeably impairing intellect, memory, or consciousness. But it does lessen the capacity to meet and accommodate to changing internal and external pressures. Someone who has lost a substantial part of this region of association cortex bilaterally is less likely to persevere in an activity in the face of distraction, discomfort, or pain.

Association Cortex—The Cascade Concept

The expanse of uncommitted cortex — cortex that we have defined as not obviously devoted to some primary sensory or motor function — is so broad that it occupies over 75% of the total cerebral surface. Many of its functions have been inferred from cases of brain injury, epilepsy, and psychosurgery. From observations of soldiers who had huge parietal areas blown away by shell fragments came the idea of the "body schema" mentioned earlier. And from studies on people in whom the corpus callosum and other commissures were surgically divided came the concepts of laterality and functional asymmetry discussed below. Until recently, however, anatomical understanding of these concepts of association cortical function has been limited.

A new principle, that association cortex is progressively interconnected, has emerged from studies with powerful new neuroanatomical techniques for tracing fibers. This "cascade concept" is as important to understanding hemispheric functions as laterality and functional asymmetry have been to interhemispheric ones. In essence, it states that cortical impulses flow forward, sideways, and backward through precise sequences of cortical regions. This recognition of complex, branching, and bidirectional serial connections helps one to understand association cortex interactions. Recall the intricate and numerous cortical association fibers described in Chapter 2 (refer to Fig. 2-9); now we are beginning to learn that their origins and terminations are precisely situated among cortical layers. We illustrate the cascade concept for the somesthetic and visual systems (Fig. 13-9), but as far as we know it holds true for all sensory subsystems.

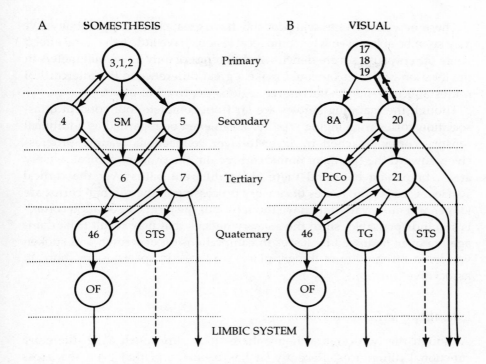

A   SOMESTHESIS   B   VISUAL

FIG. 13–9. *Cascade connections of somesthetic and visual subsystems in cortex.* In both these sensory subsystems, the sequence or "cascade" has at least four levels. At each level, signals attain a greater distance from their origin in primary sensory cortex, as well as a distinctive distribution to certain cortical regions and not to others. For example, at the secondary level some somesthetic signals reach the motor cortex and supplementary motor area, while some visual signals attain the prefrontal eye field, an area involved in eye movements. Thus at this point, movement may result or be affected, even though sensory processing is far from finished. Eventually, information filters down to the orbitofrontal cortex and into the limbic system, where emotional colorations and affect may be factored in. Both in-series and bypass connections are evident in the later steps. Most of the unidirectional connections shown are really bidirectional, and this reciprocity suggests that complex cortical feedback mechanisms are at work in the cascades, possibly acting to sharpen up feature detection and analysis — even at the periphery. Key: (3, 1, 2) primary somesthetic cortex; (4) motor cortex; (5, 7) parietal cortex; (6) premotor cortex; (46) prefrontal cortex; (STS) a polymodal area in the depths of the superior temporal sulcus; (OF) orbitofrontal cortex; (SM) supplementary motor cortex; (17, 18, 19) primary and surrounding visual cortex; (8A) prefrontal eye field; (20) inferior temporal cortex; (21) middle temporal gyrus; (PrCo) precentral agranular field; (TG) temporopolar paralimbic region. (From K. R. Popper and J. C. Eccles, *The Self and Its Brain.* Springer-Verlag. New York, 1977)

These new discoveries will probably have great clinical applicability. We may soon be able to see why some focal lesions have little behavioral effect, while others cause severe deficits. A difference of only a few millimeters in the location of the lesion could make a great difference in the intercortical routes affected and the successive regions deprived of input.

Though the mapping studies are far from complete, our concept of association cortex is changing rapidly. It can even be regarded as additional sensory cortex, reached by layer-to-layer connections leading progressively toward the frontal or limbic cortex from the primary cortical sensory areas, branching here and there along different paths over the cortical surface. Clearly, the routes of sensory processing in the cerebral cortex are longer and more varied than we thought. But the term "association cortex" is still indispensable, since the sensory deficits that may result from damage are overshadowed by losses in comprehension of written and spoken words; in recognition of things, places, or faces; in speech — in short, in associative functions.

Laterality and Cerebral Dominance

Although the two cerebral hemispheres look very much alike, there are functional differences. Recently, it has been found that even the gross anatomy of the two hemispheres is dissimilar, particularly in the upper part of the temporal lobe (supratemporal plane). The hemispheres are definitely not "mirror images." Even though both hemispheres get the same sensory information (largely from the opposite side of the body), process it in the same way, and exchange information via the commissures, they make different contributions to the whole.

It has long been known that one hemisphere is dominant over the other in certain higher functions, notably speech and less definitely handedness. The general points are that:

1. Dominance seems to be a matter of the degree of difference between the hemispheres, not an absolute difference in hemispheric contribution to brain function.
2. Speech and handedness do not necessarily go together, as far as lateralization goes.
3. The left hemisphere is dominant for speech in most adults.
4. Most clinicians ascribe speech and handedness to the dominant hemisphere.

5. The degree of dominance may vary widely in people and for different functions.
6. Dominance probably has a genetic basis that is modifiable in development.

In 1851, Paul Broca, a French physician, noticed deterioration of brain tissue in the left hemisphere in a postmortem examination of two patients who had been paralyzed only on the right side and had suffered from a severe aphasia that made them speechless. He concluded that speech is mediated by a frontal region of the left side of the brain which has come to be called the anterior speech cortex, or Broca's area (see Fig. 13-7).

Studies of split-brain animals and of patient after commissurotomy to control seizures suggest the following division of labor between hemispheres:

1. The dominant or major hemisphere is mainly responsible for language, calculation, and speech — for verbal, numerical, and graphic symbolism.

2. The nondominant or minor hemisphere is important for the appreciation of spatial dimensions and the totality of a scene (including the recognition of faces). It seems to play an essential role in creative acts — in music, poetry, etc., that is, in nonverbal symbolism. The minor hemisphere is the one in which a large parietal lesion may lead to amorphosynthesis, or denial of the existence of the contralateral half of the body. It would appear that spatial summation of all the bodily afferent data coming in from the opposite side cannot be achieved, due to destruction of the neural machinery for somatic sensory synthesis.

General Concepts

A cerebral hemisphere is divided into six lobes. The occipital lobe deals with visual processing. The temporal lobe is involved in analyzing sounds, vestibular messages, and smells and in setting affective tone; it also appears to store, or at least have access to, memories. The parietal lobe is the domain of the primary and secondary somatosensory cortex and the gustatory area. In it, sensory information is integrated with somatic sensation to create a "body schema" — an awareness of the body in relation to the environment. Aphasias (speech defects) and agnosias (perceptual deficits) may result from unilateral injury or malfunction of parts of the parietal and temporal lobes. The often overlooked central lobe seems important to viscerosomatic interactions. In the frontal lobe lie the motor cortex and Broca's speech area. The more rostral parts of these lobes, including the frontal poles, are perhaps the most characteristic features of the human brain. Severe injury or loss of these lobes bilaterally has profound behavioral effects, as does damage to the sixth, or limbic, pair of lobes.

Cortical neurons are organized horizontally, in six planes or layers, and vertically, in about 500 million small, vertical columns. Each column contains some 100–300 pyramidal and stellate neurons heavily interconnected in the vertical axis. The cellular structure of a column is similar throughout the cortex, but the inputs and outputs vary depending on their location and function. The major cortical inputs arise from specific thalamic nuclei, cortical association fibers, and cortical commissural fibers. The numerous association fibers are organized in a stepwise and extremely complex manner. The "cascade concept" is an attempt to describe this sequential pattern of intercortical communication. The cortical outputs arise primarily from the pyramidal cells of layers V and VI, axons of which project throughout the brain and spinal cord.

Some of the cortical activity triggered by sensation is channeled to motor cortex, then to spinal cord via the massive high-velocity pyramidal tracts, and finally to muscles via motor neurons. But cortical influence is pervasive and irreplaceable. Cortical efferents project to nearly all subcortical gray masses, giving it sway (if not command) over the entire brain. Cortical processing is exhaustive, progressive, and bidirectional, and it results in formulation of specific addressed outputs. These directives are being drawn up almost everywhere in the intact, awake, and alert cortex: primary sensory, secondary sensory, association, prelimbic, motor, or whatever we choose to call it. Despite a tradition of mapping and labeling cortical areas — numerically, alphabetically, descriptively, functionally, now even chemically — it is the unity of sensorimotor and associative activities within the cerebral cortex that is impressive.

Glossary

Agranular cortex: regions of the cerebral cortex that depart from the usual pattern by showing a paucity of stellate (granule) cells, and consequently less distinct layers.

Allocortex: the "other" cortex, regions of the cerebral cortex that have other than a six-layered pattern (such as the hippocampus, subiculum, entorhinal area, etc.). *Note:* The terms "archicortex" and "paleocortex" have been used to designate presumed phylogenetic relationships of the *Allocortex*, but such names enjoy very limited use today; it is perhaps better to think of the allocortex as being "different" in its specialized designs, rather than in varying states of resemblance to or evolution from the presumed primitive plan of cortical organization.

Association cortex: a vast ocean of granular, eulaminate (six-layered) cortex, occupying most of the frontal lobe and an extensive territory of the parietal, occipital, and temporal lobes, without clearly defined primary sensory or motor functions; essential to integration, cognitive functions, and unified motor control.

Association fibers: see Chap. 2.

Betz cells: giant pyramidal cells found in layer IV of primary motor cortex (Brodmann's area 4); give rise to the largest and/or longest fibers of the pyramidal tract.

Central lobe: see Chap. 2.

Commissural fibers: see Chap. 2.

Cortical columns: vertical, cylindrical modules of 100–300 cortical neurons, efferent and afferent fibers, and intrinsic connections; input/output data processing ensembles that comprise the elementary working units of the cerebral cortex.

Cortical layers: one of the two major organizing features of the cerebral cortex (the other being the cortical columns); such lamination provides for orderly circuitry, progressive analysis, and cross-integration of information between adjacent columns.

External granular layer: layer II of the cerebral cortex, containing many densely packed small pyramidal and stellate (granule) cells.

External pyramidal layer: layer III of the cerebral cortex, containing numerous medium-sized pyramidal cells; its outgoing axons form association and commissural fibers.

Frontal lobe: see Chap. 2.

Granular cortex: regions of the cerebral cortex that depart from the usual pattern by showing a plethora of stellate (granule) cells, and consequently less distinct layers.

Heterotypical cortex: cerebral cortex that differs from the usual isocortical pattern; the agranular and granular variations.

Homotypical cortex: cerebral cortex that displays a more or less uniform, six-layered pattern; association cortex is generally of this type.

Horizontal cells of Cajal: neurons of the molecular layer of the cerebral cortex with horizontally directed axons; plentiful in the neonatal brain, but infrequent in the adult.

Hypercolumn: a synonym for *macrocolumn;* a large functional unit of the cerebral cortex built up of overlapping and intermixing cortical columns (as in the case of ocular dominance and orientation columns in primary visual cortex).

Inner band of Baillarger: a prominent band of myelinated fibers in layer IV of the cerebral cortex; comprised in part of terminal arborizations of specific thalamic projection fibers. *Note:* In visual cortex (area 17), this band is known as the stripe of Gennari.

Internal granular layer: layer IV of the cerebral cortex, featuring a large population of small, densely packed stellate cells; site of termination of specific thalamic projection fibers and region of initial integration of specific thalamic input.

Internal pyramidal layer: layer V of the cerebral cortex, containing a population of medium-sized to large pyramidal cells; one of the major output layers of the cortex, its axons form projection and association fibers.

Isocortex: most of the cortex of the cerebral surface; although some 200 or more local variations in its cytoarchitecture were described by early investigators, its uniformity of six-layered, columnar design makes this term more appropriate now than ever.

Koniocortex: see *Granular cortex*.

Limbic lobe: see Chap. 2.

Macrocolumn: see *Hypercolumn*.

Martinotti cell: a neuron of the cerebral cortex, generally of stellate variety, with an upwardly directed axon, i.e., one terminating in more superficial cortical layers.

Molecular layer: layer I of the cerebral cortex, composed of a small number of stellate and horizontal cells and tangential axonal and dendritic plexuses.

Multiform layer: layer VI of the cerebral cortex, composed of fairly small polymorphic cells; one of the major output layers of the cerebral cortex.

Neocortex: an extensive region, comprising most of the cerebral cortex, considered of recent phylogenetic origin; essentially equivalent to *Isocortex*, or to *Homotypical cortex* and its heterotypical variations.

Occipital lobe: see Chap. 2.

Outer band of Baillarger: a prominent band of myelinated fibers in the lower part of layer V of the cerebral cortex; includes collaterals of entering association and commissural fibers.

Parietal lobe: see Chap. 2.

Projection fibers: see Chap. 2.

Pyramidal cells: one of the two main types of cerebral cortical neurons, their small, medium-size, or large cell bodies have the form of a pyramid with a single apical dendrite and numerous basilar dendrites; the outputs of the cortex are provided by the axons of such cells.

Stellate cells: one of the two main types of cerebral cortical neurons, their usually small cell bodies have the form of a star or polygon and are generally much smaller than those of pyramidal cells; intracortical circuits are effected by the axons of such cells.

Stripe of Gennari: see *Inner band of Baillarger.*

Temporal lobe: see Chap. 2.

The Chemical Coding of Neural Circuits

14

The organizational plan of the CNS relies on neurotransmitters to carry impulses across synapses, thus making the connections between neurons good. This chemical coding of circuits has only recently been perceived; it represents a new understanding of neuroanatomy.

There are at least twenty transmitters in the CNS and perhaps a hundred or more. Why so many? Neurons are not only turned on or off by messages arriving at their surfaces from other neurons. Their responses may also be modified by transmitters to numerous purposes, such as general arousal or sleep, etc. Recently, we have come to realize that neurotransmitters may act over different time courses and in different ways: they may influence the metabolism of neurons so as to prepare cells for coming events, perhaps, or possibly to remind them of past ones.

As a rule, each transmitter has its own characteristic action, though it may be used by different fiber projections. Norepinephrine (NE) and GABA (gamma-aminobutyric acid) are always inhibitory, but NE acts more slowly and lastingly than GABA. So it is that different transmitters have different effects on neurons.

Knowledge of neurotransmitters can help in understanding neurological diseases, the nature of drug actions, and the potential side effects of drugs. Many diseases (such as Parkinson's) affect primarily a single neural subsystem (in this case, the motor system), and many drugs (such as L-Dopa) act primarily on one subsystem (again the motor system in this example).

This chapter provides an overview of the chemical circuitry of the nervous system. It is limited to those transmitters that are well established and relatively well defined in their deployment among neural circuits, and we include their relationships to function where they can be traced. Several transmitters can already be related to specific physiological or behavioral states. Some are synthesized in well-known neuronal aggregates (such as the substantia nigra) and utilized by major projections (the nigrostriatal tract). Others are encountered in remote, seldom-described regions. (The nucleus raphe obscurus and its connections, as one might infer from the name, are not high priority items in neuroanatomy courses.)

To orient the reader, we have shown each transmitter system on the same diagram of the rat brain in sagittal and horizontal sections (Fig. 14-1). This illustration serves as a guide to all the following ones (Figs. 14-2 to 14-12) of the various transmitter systems.

ACETYLCHOLINE

We begin with acetylcholine (ACh) because it was the first neurotransmitter to be identified. It is the major transmitter of the peripheral nervous system (PNS), but is less prominent in the brain and spinal cord.

In the CNS, the evidence supporting assignment of a transmitter to a structure or pathway is rarely, if ever, as compelling as that for the PNS. Here, a big problem is that we lack decisive histochemical methods for routinely visualizing cholinergic tracts in brain. One can recognize choline acetyltransferase (ChAc), the enzyme that synthesizes ACh from choline, and its coenzyme, acetyl CoA. Since ChAc is present only in cholinergic neurons, it does serve to mark those neurons specifically. Moreover, the enzyme that breaks down ACh, acetylcholinesterase (AChE), can also be localized histochemically, and thus has served as a means to "tag" central fiber tracts. In the CNS, AChE is usually found in cholinergic tracts, but it is present in noncholinergic neurons too, and therefore by itself is not a definitive marker.

Among the major cholinergic systems that have been identified are the somatic motor innervation of skeletal muscle, along with the feedback axon collaterals from alpha motor neurons to Renshaw cells (Table 14-1). Thus, ACh is the chemical messenger that brings about contraction of all our voluntary musculature, through its release by the motor fibers of spinal nerves and of cranial nerves III–VII and IX–XII. Also cholinergic are all preganglionic neurons of the autonomic nervous system, which means that ACh is released at the endings of the parasympathetic cranial nerves III, VII, IX, and X, the sympathetic thoracolumbar nerves to the paravertebral and prevertebral ganglia, and the sacral nerves to terminal ganglia in the pelvic viscera. It thus mediates the activity of all autonomic post-

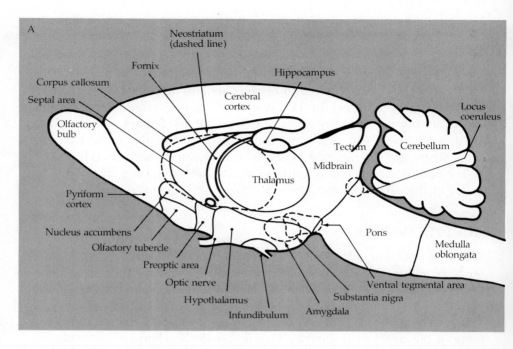

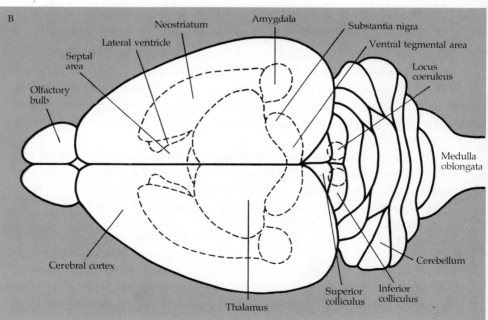

FIG. 14–1. *The rat brain in sagittal and horizontal sections.* These diagrams, in which major brain components are identified in the sagittal (A) and horizontal (B) planes, serve as reference maps for all subsequent diagrams of transmitter systems. Structures outlined with dashed lines lie away from the median plane of (A) or deep to the superior aspect of (B) at greater or lesser distances.

ganglionic neurons, wherever they may be. These postganglionic neurons are a mixed bag: nearly all the parasympathetic cells are cholinergic, but only some of the sympathetic ones are — those cells sending fibers to sweat glands. The activity of postganglionic neurons has a powerful effect on much of the smooth musculature of the body — in the iris, ciliary body, salivary glands, stomach, intestines, bladder, and sweat glands. All these structures except the last have a dual innervation, receiving noradrenergic sympathetic fibers (see below) as well as cholinergic parasympathetic ones.

ACh has a powerful inhibitory effect on heart muscle, specifically on those specialized fibers that make up the cardiac pacemaker in the sinoatrial node. And though it is not a common central transmitter, ACh does

Table 14-1. Acetylcholine Neuron Systems in the Mammalian Nervous System

System	Place of origin	Site(s) of termination
Neuromuscular junction	Spinal cord, anterior horn motor neurons	All voluntary muscles (striated)
Motor neuron–Renshaw cell	Spinal cord, anterior horn motor neurons	Renshaw cells
Preganglionic sympathetic fibers	Spinal cord, lateral horn neurons	Autonomic ganglia
Postganglionic sympathetic fibers	Certain autonomic ganglia	Sweat glands
Cranial nerves	Motor nuclei of nerves III–VII and IX–XII	
Septohippocampal tract	Septal nuclei	Hippocampal formation
Habenulointerpeduncular tract	Medial habenular nucleus	Interpeduncular nucleus
Striatal interneurons	Striatum (Caudate/putamen)	Striatum
Globus pallidus–cortical projection	Globus pallidus	Frontal, parietal cortex

turn up in certain well-defined limbic forebrain connections and in the basal ganglia.

One of the best documented cholinergic systems in the brain is the septohippocampal pathway (Fig. 14-2). Septal neurons send their axons via the fornix to the hippocampal formation, and these fibers probably modulate a number of hippocampal functions.

Certain of the basal ganglia — the caudate nucleus and putamen (neo-striatum)—contain cholinergic local-circuit neurons. These neurons, as we explained in Chapter 9, receive the nigral dopaminergic input and form synapses with striatal GABA neurons that project back to the substantia nigra, as well as effecting pallidal or striatal connections. In patients with Huntington's chorea and Alzheimer's type of presenile dementia, some of these cholinergic neurons are lost. Another cholinergic system related to the basal ganglia runs from the nucleus basalis (a cell group immediately beneath the globus pallidus) to the frontal and parietal regions of the cerebral cortex. This input accounts for about half the ChAc in these cortical regions, the remainder appearing to reside in intrinsic cortical circuitry.

The richest cholinergic innervation now identified in the brain is that of the interpeduncular nucleus of the midbrain by the habenula, a small but

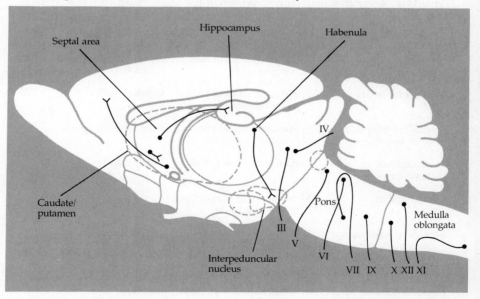

FIG. 14–2. *Cholinergic neural systems of brain.* In this figure and subsequent figures, the dots indicate positions of cell bodies and the heavy lines the projections. See also Table 14-1.

conspicuous limbic nucleus situated in the epithalamus immediately in front of the pineal gland. The interpeduncular nucleus and habenula contain the highest concentrations of ChAc in the brain, and interruption of the habenulointerpeduncular tract (fasciculus retroflexus) results in a drop in interpeduncular cholinergic properties, if not in a clearly defined functional deficit.

Monoamines

The term *monoamine* refers to an organic substance derived from a primary amine (R-NH$_2$). The most common neurotransmitter molecules of this type are dopamine, norepinephrine, epinephrine, and serotonin. Catecholamine is another term we should define: it refers to an important subgroup of monoamines (dopamine and its metabolic products, norepinephrine and epinephrine) that contains a catechol nucleus (1,2-dihydroxybenzene). Indoleamines (such as serotonin) have an indole nucleus (2,3-benzopyrrole, a 2-ring structure).

More is known about monoamine neurons and their projections in the CNS than has been learned about any other central neurotransmitter systems. The mapping of these cell clusters and pathways in brain is a direct result of an effective and beautiful technique for visualizing them: on treatment of tissue sections with formaldehyde or glyoxylic acid, monoamines fluoresce, so that the nerve cell bodies and fibers that contain them can be studied in detail with ultraviolet microscopy. The different kinds of monoamines fluoresce with a particular color, so that each class can be identified: catecholamines are green, indoleamines are yellow, and histamine (a tissue amine found throughout the animal and plant kingdoms) is blue. While differentiation of the various catecholamines is somewhat more difficult on the basis of fluorescence color alone, it can be accomplished with a variety of ancillary methods. The significant point is that histofluorescence techniques, in combination with immunohistochemistry, placement of lesions, and direct chemical analyses, have enabled investigators to describe the circuitry of particular monoamine systems, revealing networks of communication that before had been beyond the reach and even the imagination of neuroanatomists.

Monoamine cell clusters all lie in the brainstem. They have been described by name or by number. The current trend is to use conventional nomenclature wherever possible, describing the monoamine pathways in relation to known neuroanatomical structures. Originally, monoamine neuronal clusters were referred to by numerical schemes, and they sometimes still are, particularly in research papers. All dopamine (DA) and norepinephrine (NE) cell groups were assigned the prefix "A" followed by a number indicating the particular group (A1, A2, A3, etc.). Serotonin (5-HT; 5-hydroxytryptamine) cell groups were assigned the prefix "B" with a following number (B1, B2, etc.). Epinephrine (E) cell groups were designated (logically or not) by "C" (C1, C2, and so forth). In our descriptions we use classical anatomical names as much as possible. When using such terms, however, one must remember that not every neuron in a given nucleus necessarily has the same transmitter.

Dopamine Projections

The catecholamine dopamine (DA) is one of the most interesting transmitters. DA pathways seem to play a major role in cognitive, motor, and neuroendocrine functions. According to one hypothesis, excessive dopamine activity is a factor in schizophrenia.

Dopamine neurons make up a varied group of cells located principally, but not exclusively, in the upper midbrain and adjacent hypothalamus. The neurons are cytologically diverse: some are multipolar, with axons that project over considerable distances (nigral and ventral tegmental neurons are examples). Others are small cells without axons (such as the retinal and olfactory amacrine cells), whose dendrites form local circuits. Nearly all DA projections lead to specific target areas, display an orderly topography, and course unilaterally (99% of the fibers stay on one side of the brain). The major DA systems are summarized in Table 14-2.

1. *Mesotelencephalic System.* The principal DA nerve cells in the upper midbrain are found in a large ventral mass of gray matter called the substantia nigra (it contains large, melanin-pigmented neurons in its upper, compact zone) and an interposed ventral tegmental area. These two areas give rise to the mesotelencephalic axon system. The outputs are largely, though not entirely, segregated so as to make up two major subsystems: a nigrostriatal system and a mesocortical system. (Formerly, DA cells in the indistinctly separated substantia nigra-ventral tegmental area were designated as A8, A9, and A10; since these neurons do not form discrete clusters but originate instead as an embryological unit, this notation is no longer widely used.)

a. *Nigrostriatal projections.* The nigrostriatal DA projections originate from neurons in the substantia nigra and adjacent ventral tegmentum and run to the neostriatal components of the basal ganglia: the caudate nucleus and

Table 14-2. Dopamine Neuron Systems in the Mammalian Brain

System	Place of origin	Sites(s) of termination
Mesotelencephalic		
Nigrostriatal	Substantia nigra, pars compacta; ventral tegmental area	Neostriatum (caudate/putamen), globus pallidus
Mesocortical	Ventral tegmental area; substantia nigra, pars compacta	Isocortex (mesial frontal, anterior cingulate, entorhinal, perirhinal)
		Allocortex (olfactory bulb, anterior olfactory nucleus, olfactory tubercle, pyriform cortex, septal area, nucleus accumbens, amygdaloid complex)
Incertohypothalamic	Zona incerta, posterior hypothalamus	Dorsal hypothalamic area, septum
Tuberohypophysial	Arcuate and periventricular hypothalamic nuclei	Neurointermediate lobe of pituitary, median eminence
Periventricular	Medulla in area of dorsal motor vagus, nucleus tractus solitarius, periaqueductal and periventricular gray	Periventricular and periaqueductal gray, tegmentum, tectum, thalamus, hypothalamus
Retinal	Interplexiform cells of retina	Inner and outer plexiform layers of retina
Olfactory bulb	Periglomerular cells	Glomeruli (mitral cell dendrites)

From R. Y. Moore and F. E. Bloom, *Ann. Rev. Neurosci. 1*, 129–69 (1978).

putamen (Fig. 14-3). En route to these structures, the nigrostriatal bundle collects medially in the tegmentum, courses dorsally alongside the hypothalamus, and then streams abruptly upward in the internal capsule to the caudate and putamen that lie on either side. The distribution of DA axonal terminals is massive; with fluorescence techniques, these fibers make the striatum glow in ultraviolet light. This monoamine infiltration comprises about 16% of the total input to the caudate/putamen, each nigral

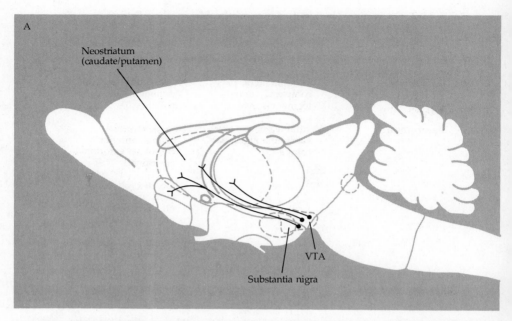

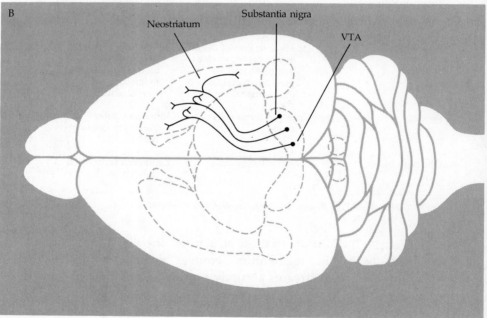

FIG. 14–3. *Nigrostriatal dopamine projections.* See also Table 14-2. VTA = ventral tegmental area.

neuron of origin liberating transmitter at about 500,000 axon terminals or beaded preterminal varicosities! Curiously, only a trickle of fibers passes into the adjacent globus pallidus, the other major basal ganglion.

While knowledge of their chemical coding greatly extends our understanding of brain tracts, the recently identified monoamine connections of the CNS do not constitute exceptions to basic organizing principles (Introduction and Chap. 1). Many of these chemically "tagged" connections represent tracts (or parts of tracts) that we knew before under some purely anatomical designation. Thus, the nigrostriatal tract has now become the nigrostriatal DA projection system, and we find that it is laid out in a highly topographic manner, just like many other central projection systems. Medial-to-lateral and anterior-to-posterior gradients of fiber distribution are evident: medial nigrotegmental neurons project to the caudate, more lateral ones to the putamen. Similar correspondences of origin and termination are noted in the longitudinal axis.

Such obvious interlocking of DA circuits in the basal ganglia suggests that there must be clinical correlates. Indeed there are. In 1955, the German anatomist Hassler noted that there are fewer neurons in the substantia nigra of parkinsonian patients. It is now known that Parkinson's disease, a progressive degenerative disorder, results primarily from a deficit of nigral DA neurons (specifically, the large, pigmented cells in the upper, compact zone) and a consequent deficiency of striatal dopamine. DA insufficiency is not the only problem in this disease: in some kinds of parkinsonism there is no absolute decrease in DA, only a DA/ACh imbalance. Even so, the characteristic signs and symptoms of "shaking palsy" and poverty of movement appear.

Parkinson's disease is associated with muscular rigidity, tremor, and poverty of movement. The patient has difficulty initiating voluntary motor activity. There is a delay in starting a movement, and if it is to continue, the movement may occupy the person's entire attention. Fortunately, the devastating motor symptoms of the disease can be alleviated (at least for many months or years) by providing the afflicted individual with large quantities of L-Dopa, the immediate precursor of DA. Unlike the transmitter itself, L-Dopa can get through the blood–brain barrier (see Chap. 15) and enter the CNS after systemic administration. The residual DA neurons in the nigra use the precursor to produce extra DA, which then restores striatal dopamine to levels commensurate with more effective motor control.

Decreases in the number of DA neurons also seem to occur during the aging process, both in humans and in animals. These decreases, and the consequent imbalance of striatal transmitters, appear related to some of the characteristic slow and irregular movements of older individuals. Thus, it is clear that the nigrostriatal pathway plays an important role in motor integration.

b. *Mesocortical projections.* As mentioned above, DA neurons in the substantia nigra and ventral tegmentum give rise to another group of projections. Because axons of this system originate in the mesencephalon and terminate (at least in part) in the cerebral cortex, it is called the mesocortical system. Some axons, however, end not in cortex but in subcortical structures such as the nucleus accumbens and amygdala.

The mesocortical system (Fig. 14-4) innervates the medial frontal, anterior cingulate, and entorhinal regions of the cortex and also the olfactory bulb and its nearby nuclear and cortical affiliates (rhinencephalon). Deeper projections lead to the amygdaloid nuclear complex, septal area, and nucleus accumbens (a large nucleus, formerly classified with the septal area, that appears to lean against the caudate nucleus and is now recognized as a striatal component with limbic connections). The density and distribution of innervation of this system vary a great deal in the different target regions, from dense and uniform in accumbens and olfactory tubercle to scattered and laminar in frontal and cingulate cortices. A curious feature of the DA projection to frontal cortex is that it seems to mimic the principal thalamofrontal projection (medial dorsal nucleus) in all those species studied to date.

The mesocortical system shows the same orderliness of projections we saw in the nigrostriatal system, although its topography is not fully worked out. For example, dorsally located neurons in the ventral tegmentum or adjacent nigra project to ventral brain structures (e.g., olfactory tubercle), while ventrally placed cells project to dorsal structures (e.g., septal nuclei).

The hallmark of the mesocortical and nigrostriatal systems is the precise arrangement of their rostrally coursing streams of axons. But, although they are wired into limbic and motor circuits, respectively, no definitive general statement can be made now about the local functional effects (excitatory, inhibitory, etc.) of these dopaminergic projections. There is strong evidence that DA neurons inhibit their target cells, but in certain terminal fields (such as the caudate) there are unanswered anatomical and physiological questions — such as the identity and action of the primary DA target interneuron.

2. *Other Dopamine Systems.* At least five other DA systems are now recognized, but no clear functional roles for them have been identified. The systems are: an incertohypothalamic or intradiencephalic system, a

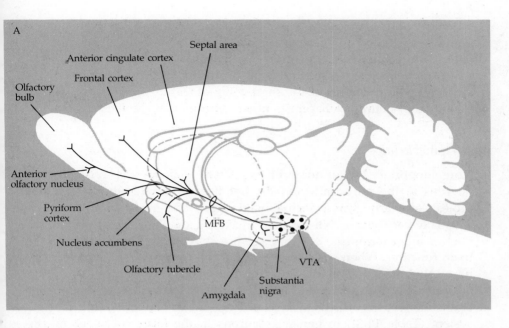

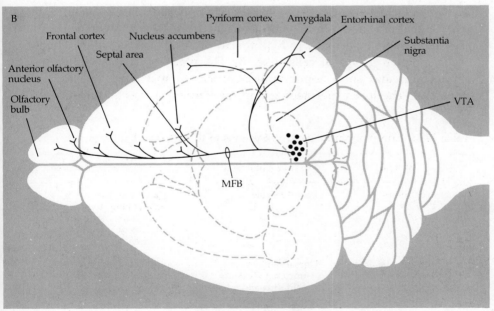

FIG. 14–4. *Mesocortical dopamine systems*. See also Table 14-2. MFB = medial fore-brain bundle.

tuberohypophysial system, a periventricular system in the brainstem, a retinal system, and an olfactory system. In the latter two systems, the DA neurons in some instances correspond to small axonless (amacrine) cells which participate in sensory integrative functions: contrast inhibition, for example, which consists of the sharpening of feature analysis by selective inhibition of neurons adjacent to other neurons that are active.

Norepinephrine

Norepinephrine (NE) or noradrenergic fibers originate from relatively few neurons in the pons and medulla, but this remarkable group of axons projects to nearly every principal brain region. The innervation, however, is usually very sparse. NE terminals make up less than one percent of the total of brain terminals, yet they seem to have a profound influence on brain function. When stimulated, virtually all noradrenergic pathways inhibit spontaneous discharge in target neurons.

There are two prominent noradrenergic systems in the mammalian brain: the locus coeruleus system and the lateral tegmental or brainstem system (Table 14-3). In general, neurons in the locus coeruleus (a pigmented cell cluster in the pons) project primarily to thalamus, telencephalon, cerebellum, and spinal cord, while neurons in the lateral tegmental area send fibers principally to hypothalamus and basal forebrain. The lateral tegmental group of cells, like the DA neurons, make well-defined connections and show topographical order. Almost all connections are unilateral. The locus coeruleus group, in contrast, projects diffusely over

Table 14–3. Norepinephrine Neuron Systems in the Mammalian Brain

System	Place of origin	Site(s) of termination
Locus coeruleus	Locus coeruleus	Spinal cord, brainstem, cerebellum, hypothalamus, thalamus, basal telencephalon, and the entire isocortex
Lateral tegmental area	Dorsal motor vagus, nucleus of tractus solitarius and adjacent tegmentum, lateral tegmentum	Spinal cord, brainstem, hypothalamus, basal telencephalon

From R. Y. Moore and F. E. Bloom, *Ann. Rev. Neurosci. 2*, 113–68 (1979).

the entire neuraxis. Its neurons show the least topographical order of all catecholaminergic neurons, and about 25% of the connections are crossed.

1. *Locus Coeruleus System.* The locus coeruleus (A6) lies in the brainstem, in the pontine reticular formation just lateral to the rostral end of the fourth ventricle. In man, it is pigmented, and its name means "blue place." In the rat, the locus coeruleus contains about 400 neurons, 43% of all NE-producing neurons in the rat brain.

Neurons of the locus coeruleus have elaborately branched axons which ramify within the entire brain (Fig. 14-5). There are three major ascending tracts — the central tegmental tract, dorsal longitudinal fasciculus, and medial forebrain bundle — as well as vascular routes to innervate the hypothalamus, thalamus, basal telencephalon, and entire isocortex.

In addition to these ascending projections, the locus coeruleus sends out two other major groups of fibers, one to the cerebellum (via the superior peduncle), the other to the spinal cord. And it also projects to sensory nuclei of the brainstem.

The terminal boutons are very distinct and generally similar in all areas: preterminal fibers break up into a highly collateralized network with fine axons which have many varicosities like beads along a string. These varicosities are loaded with synaptic vesicles in which NE is stored. Only a few (5%) of these varicosities form actual synapses, at least in the cerebral cortex. The remainder appear to secrete transmitter into the welter of fibers (neuropil) in the vicinity of neurons. In the cerebral cortex, there are even very few of these secretory varicosities relative to cortical synapses — about 1/10,000. It seems that "a little goes a long way" where norepinephrine is concerned!

The locus coeruleus has a wide domain, from olfactory bulb to spinal cord with emphasis on cortical structures, and its stimulation inhibits spontaneous neuronal discharge nearly everywhere. Yet no clear-cut behavioral effects of such stimulation have been singled out. A phrase sometimes used to describe the role of the locus is that it sets "brain tone." This generalized modulation, nevertheless, could lead to highly selective brain function. By inhibiting background activity, the locus coeruleus may depress irrelevant stimuli and allow relevant ones to stand out. Thus, by this route at least, norepinephrine may enhance the signal-to-noise ratio in brain.

2. *The Lateral Tegmental or Brainstem System.* There are two major groups of

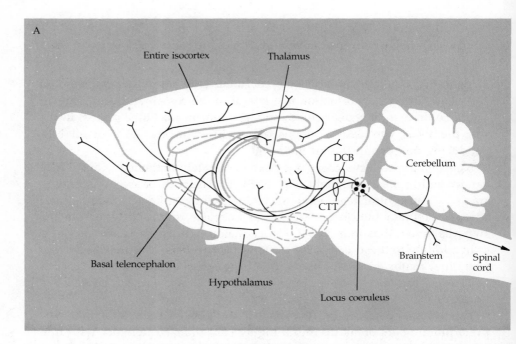

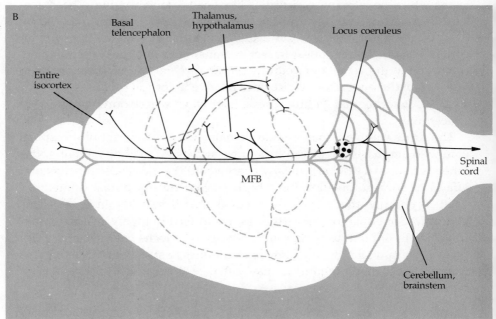

FIG. 14–5. *Locus coeruleus norepinephrine system.* See also Table 14-3. DCB = dorsal catecholamine bundle. CCT = central tegmental tract.

cell bodies in the lateral tegmental system, one in the medulla (A1, A2, and A3) and the other in the pons (A5 and A7).

The main targets of the lateral tegmental NE system are the hypothalamus, brainstem, and, to a lesser degree, the basal forebrain (see Fig. 14-6 for the pathways and targets). Axons ascending from the medullary and pontine cell groups enter the central tegmental tract, disperse among fibers of the other tegmental catecholamine radiations, and eventually run into the medial forebrain bundle. These fibers mix extensively with those from the locus coeruleus.

The NE innervation of the hypothalamus and brainstem is mostly from the lateral tegmental group, much less from the locus. In contrast to the coerulean projection, the lateral tegmental fibers reach brainstem regions other than primary sensory nuclei. In particular, some motor nuclei (trigeminal, facial, and dorsal vagal) receive a dense innervation. The pontine and medullary raphe nuclei also receive a fairly strong innervation.

The lateral tegmental system does not innervate the neocortex, and its projection to the basal forebrain is not very extensive, accounting for less NE input there than the locus coeruleus. Other projections are given in Figure 14-6.

Since the main target of this system is the hypothalamus, including the median eminence, we should expect some kind of neuroendocrine function. Indeed, this system plays an important role in regulating gonadotropin, growth hormone, and ACTH secretion. Thus, the projections of the lateral tegmental group to the hypothalamus and pituitary, the "vegetative" areas of the nervous system, give norepinephrine a role in homeostatic adaptation.

Norepinephrine neurons turn out to be cells of the reticular formation (as do the epinephrine neurons covered next). Like other core neurons, NE neurons exert widespread effects; the projections from the locus coeruleus are the most diffuse known, extending from olfactory bulb to sacral spinal cord — literally, from "nose to tail." As mentioned, this system may serve for sensory enhancement, among other things. The lateral tegmental NE system overlaps that of the locus in many places, and is also concerned with regulating hypothalamic-pituitary (vegetative) functions. Thus, the distribution of NE fibers is even more far-flung than the projections of other axons derived from the brainstem core, great though those may be (see Chap. 11). And some of the influences of NE are exerted directly (nonsynaptically) by secretion into the neuropil, while all of the effects seem to be slow-acting and long-lasting. In these respects, the norepinephrine systems appear to offer the ultimate in core mechanisms of integration.

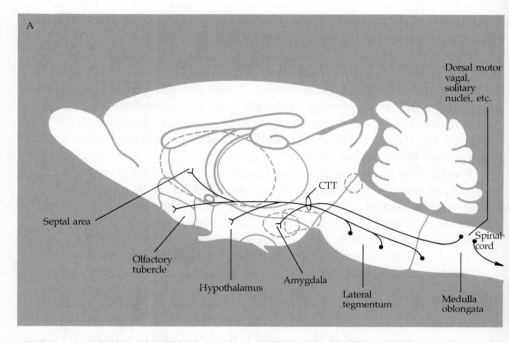

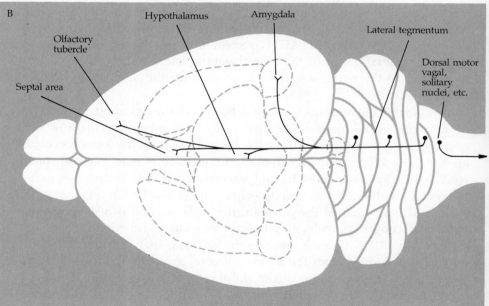

FIG. 14–6. *Brainstem norepinephrine system.* See also Table 14-3.

Table 14–4. Epinephrine Neuron System in the Mammalian Brain

System	Place of origin	Site(s) of termination
Dorsal tegmental and lateral tegmental cell groups	Caudal medulla oblongata	Spinal cord, brainstem (locus coeruleus, periaqueductal gray), hypothalamus, thalamus

From R. Y. Moore and F. E. Bloom, *Ann. Rev. Neurosci. 2*, 113–68 (1979).

Epinephrine

Epinephrine, or adrenaline, is present throughout the body, including the brain, where it is synthesized by certain brainstem neurons (Table 14-4). These neurons consist of two groups, one similar in distribution to the NE medullary lateral tegmental cell group (C1) and the other located in the rostral medulla oblongata (C2). These two cell groups give rise to an axon bundle which ascends in the reticular formation along with NE fibers from the lower brainstem (central tegmental tract; Fig. 14-7).

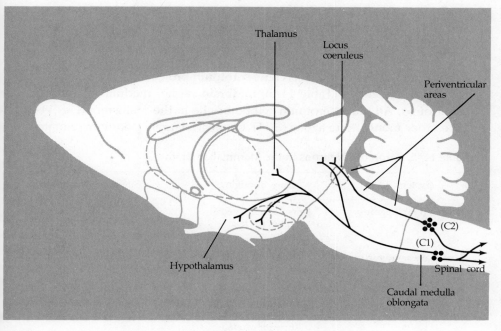

FIG. 14–7. *Epinephrine systems in the brain.* See also Table 14-4.

The epinephrine neuron system is minor relative to the NE and DA systems. Mainly it innervates parts of the spinal cord, brainstem (including the locus coeruleus and periqueductal gray), hypothalamus, and thalamus. Although dense in a few places (such as the dorsal motor nucleus of the vagus and adjoining nucleus of the tractus solitarius), its innervation is generally moderate to sparse.

Serotonin

As early as 1868 it was known that certain chemicals in the blood caused blood vessels to constrict, but it was not until 1949 that the active factor was identified as serotonin. Shortly afterward, serotonin (5-HT, 5-hydroxytryptamine) was discovered in brain tissue. It now appears that serotonin has an important role in behavioral states. Severe depression may be associated with low brain serotonin content, and, in fact, studies have indicated that brain serotonin is lower in persons who have committed suicide than in accident victims. In animals insomnia follows inhibition of 5-HT synthesis or destruction of certain 5-HT neurons. Moreover, several psychoactive drugs act on serotonin systems. Tricyclic antidepressants appear to increase its availability to receptor sites by reducing its reuptake, and LSD is a strong antagonist to serotonin receptors. Yet, while serotonin is clearly a transmitter of major importance, over 95% of it is outside the nervous system — in blood platelets and in the gastrointestinal tract.

For the progress of our overview, serotonin projections can be separated into three categories (Table 14-5): midbrain raphe, medullary, and other cell groups. All brain serotonin cell bodies lie in the brainstem (Fig. 14-8). Like other monoamine axons, 5-HT fibers are largely poorly myelinated.

Table 14–5. Serotonin Neurons in the Mammalian Brain

System	Place of origin	Site(s) of termination
Midbrain raphe group	Dorsal raphe, medial raphe, nucleus centralis	Most of the telencephalon and diencephalon
Medullary serotonin group	Medulla oblongata	Spinal cord
Other	Pontine raphe nuclei, nucleus reticularis tegmenti pontis, superior caudalis	Cerebellar and pontine areas, midbrain raphe complex

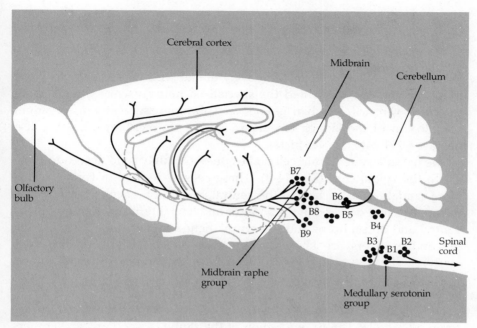

FIG. 14–8. *Serotonin systems in the brain.* See also Table 14-5.

The midbrain raphe nuclei send fibers up the brainstem to the diencephalon and telencephalon. As with the locus coeruleus projection, these fibers are very widely distributed. There are terminals in hypothalamus, thalamus, preoptic area, septum, hippocampus, olfactory bulb and tubercle, cerebral cortex, basal ganglia, and amygdala. The frontal cortex has a uniform distribution of terminals, and the entire neocortex is innervated to some extent. As is the case for norepinephrine and epinephrine, the serotonin innervation is generally sparse and lacks precise topographic organization. In the cerebral cortex, for example, serotonin boutons account for less than 0.2% of the total.

Most midbrain raphe fibers arise in three nuclei: raphe dorsalis (dorsal raphe), raphe medianus (median raphe), and centralis superior. Rostrally, these fibers enter the medial forebrain bundle. Along its course, axons or axon collaterals pass into many regions of the basal forebrain. The fibers project primarily on the same side, but a few axons cross to join the contralateral ascending bundle.

In many ways, the serotonin system is like the norepinephrine one. Both are components of the brainstem reticular formation, and both sprinkle the neuraxis with widespread and greatly overlapping projections. They differ, however, in the details of distribution and terminal innervation patterns, even though the pathways followed may be similar. Midbrain 5-HT neurons, for instance, seem more selective in their targets than cells of the locus coeruleus NE system. Moreover, unlike NE fibers, serotonin fibers innervate the ependyma and the specialized neurovascular organs about the third ventricle (median eminence, subcommissural organ, organum vasculosum of the lamina terminalis, and subfornical organ). They also liberate 5-HT into the ventricle.

The medullary serotonin cell bodies predominately send descending fibers to the spinal cord (Fig. 14-8). These cells — located in certain of the more caudal raphe nuclei and the ventral medullary reticular formation — have axons that descend in the anterior and lateral funiculi to innervate the ventral and dorsal horns and the sympathetic lateral column. Some of the descending fibers are known to synapse on spinal enkephalin interneurons. These serotonin fibers thus may provide suprasegmental control over the passage of pain signals from primary sensory neurons to secondary sensory neurons within the spinal cord (see Chap. 6).

Little is known about the projections of the other serotonin cell bodies; some seem to lead from one region of the raphe to another, while others clearly innervate the cerebellum.

The striking feature of the serotonin network is that this mere handful of cells grouped in small, discrete clusters in the brainstem apparently has prominent and powerful effects on brain function. Global swings of mood appear to follow the ebb and flow of this key transmitter — depression and insomnia, hallucinations and mania, and, no doubt, other ups and downs of our innermost selves.

Neuropeptides

In 1975, startling reports appeared: the brain contained its own endogenous opiates, peptides called enkephalins ("in the head") and endorphins ("morphinelike"). These reports followed the discovery that brain cell membranes contain highly specific receptors for opiates. Thus, it looked as if the brain had a built-in analgesia system.

But this was only the beginning of the story. Peptides, opiate and otherwise, appear to have far-reaching functions as neuroendocrine modulators and perhaps much more: an internal reward system; an ingredient of self-identity (which if altered can contribute to schizophrenia); a role in learning and memory; a mechanism in the adaptive stress response and in temperature regulation, affect, and euphoria; even a part of the elusive

"will to win" and drive of an athlete. Whatever the validity of these specu-
lations may turn out to be, they fuel the fires of investigation in this area.
And indeed, there is evidence that some of these seemingly "far-out" ideas
are correct.

These short sequences of amino acids called peptides have now become
a focal point of neurobiology. Of the many that are known to be widely
distributed in the CNS, virtually all seem to be present to some degree in
the hypothalamic nuclei. Some of these — LHRH, TRH, and somatostatin
— might be expected to be there, since they are either hypothalamic-
hypophysial releasing or inhibiting hormones. They are found in neurons
of the median eminence and are secreted into the hypothalamic-
hypophysial portal vessels; they regulate the release of anterior pituitary
hormones. Less predictable, however, have been the almost universal findings of these peptides, plus others, in the basal ganglia, brainstem, spinal
cord, and even in the cerebral cortex. In some cases the fields of innervation are very broad, in others quite small. Curiously, the cerebellum seems
devoid of peptides, at least of those so far identified.

1. *Enkephalins*

The two enkephalins are pentapeptides with opiatelike activity. They show
the following sequence of amino acids: H-tyrosine-glycine-glycine-
phenylalanine-X-OH. If the amino acid "X" is methionine, the molecule is
known as met^5-enkephalin; if it is leucine, then it is leu^5-enkephalin.

The enkephalins are the most widely distributed and abundant opiate
peptides. Their presence is detected by measuring levels in areas of dissected brain by means of immunologic techniques. At least 25 brain regions
are now known to contain enkephalins. Leu-enkephalin and met-
enkephalin are both present and their ratios differ among regions; leu-
enkephalin is generally present in higher concentrations.

The globus pallidus contains the most enkephalin, and the cerebellum
the least (Table 14-6). The distribution of opiate receptors, as would be
expected, parallels that of opiate peptides. A few long pathways for these
peptide neurons have been identified. It appears, however, that enkephalins are important primarily for interneuronal or local-circuit functions,
since the cell bodies lie mainly near their terminals. Figure 14-9 shows the
distribution of enkephalins in the brain.

Enkephalins are present almost everywhere in the CNS, and are also
found in the peripheral nervous system. Along with a series of neuroactive
peptides (neurotensin and substance P), enkephalins are encountered in

Table 14–6. Regional Distribution of Brain
Enkephalin (pmol/mg protein)

Rank order	Region	Percent
1	Globus pallidus	35.0
2	Central gray	6.5
3	Nucleus accumbens	6.3
4	Medial hypothalamus	5.0
5	Amygdala	4.5
6	Pons	3.4
7	Medulla	3.3
8	Caudate-putamen	3.1
9	Thalamus	2.6
10	Septal area	2.3
11	Lateral hypothalamus	2.1
12	Midbrain	1.5
13	Hippocampus	1.3
14	Cerebral cortex	1.3
15	Preoptic area	1.1
16	Cerebellum	none

From. Kobayashi et al., *Life Sciences 22*, 379–89, 1978.

the adrenal medulla, and enkephalin fibers appear to innervate the stomach, duodenum, ileum, and rectum. Enkephalin neurons form connections in the periphery, as one might expect from the characteristic peripheral actions of opiates (depressed respiration, decreased gastrointestinal motility, etc.).

2. Endorphins

The broader group of opiatelike molecules are the endorphins, defined as any endogenous molecule of the body with opiatelike actions. Enkephalins are endorphins, but not all endorphins are enkephalins. There are many endorphins; the most common carry the prefixes alpha, beta, and gamma, and the major type in brain is beta-endorphin. Their amino acid sequence is also found in a pituitary hormone implicated in fat metabolism, beta-lipotrophin (or lipotropin; both spellings are in use). The existence of brain enkephalins and endorphins, however, is not dependent on the pituitary, since their levels are unaffected after its removal.

The other brain endorphins (Table 14-7; Fig. 14-10) have a simpler distribution than the almost ubiquitous enkephalins. Neuronal cell bodies are all but confined to the arcuate nucleus and premammillary nuclei of the hypothalamus. Some cells form a continuous line across the floor of the

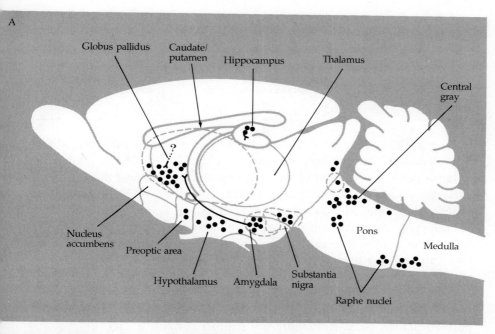

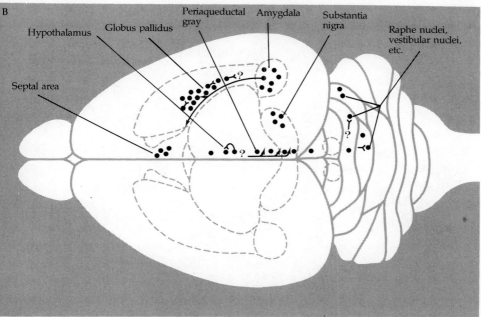

FIG. 14–9. *Enkephalin cell bodies in the brain.* See also Table 14-6.

Table 14–7. Major Endorphin System in the Mammalian Brain

System	Place of origin	Site(s) of termination
Hypothalamic diencephalic pontine system	Arcuate nucleus, premammillary nuclei	Various hypothalamic & anterior pontine tegmental nuclei

third ventricle. Very few, if any, endorphin neurons exist outside the hypothalamus. Their projections are restricted to the diencephalon and anterior pons, where their fibers occupy midline areas near the ventricular surfaces. Caudal to the level of the locus coeruleus, endorphins are very sparse, and none are present in the medulla and spinal cord.

Endorphin fibers are most dense in the anterior hypothalamus, particularly at the level of the crossing over of the anterior commissure. They extend into the stria terminalis and its bed nucleus, becoming less prominent as they approach the lateral septum and nucleus accumbens. Other hypothalamic areas that contain an abundance of these fibers are the lateral anterior hypothalamic area; the median eminence; and the supraoptic, periventricular, paraventricular, and suprachiasmatic nuclei.

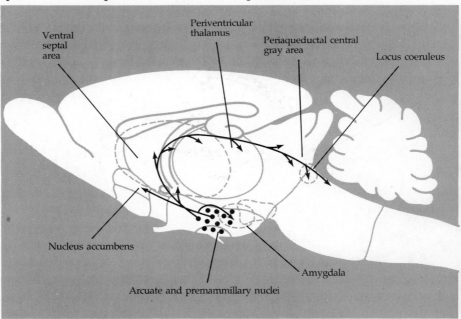

FIG. 14-10. *Endorphin cell bodies in the brain.* See also Table 14-7.

Beta-endorphin fibers enter the pons and course caudally, mostly ventral to the cerebral aqueduct in midline structures. At the level of the dorsal raphe nucleus (which is well innervated), the fibers begin to spread laterally to innervate the dorsal and lateral regions of the periaqueductal gray, and then on to supply the locus coeruleus from its medial surface.

Hypothalamic cell bodies that stain for beta-endorphin also stain for ACTH and beta-lipotrophin. Beta-endorphin and enkephalins, however, are not present in the same hypothalamic cells. High concentrations of beta-endorphin are also found in the pituitary gland, particularly in the intermediate lobe where nearly every cell stains for it. Endorphins thus appear to play a major role in neuroendocrine functions.

3. *Substance P*

In 1931, a substance was purified from horse brain and intestine and called substance P (because it was isolated as a precipitate). Substance P has ACh-like activity on smooth muscle, but unlike ACh it is not blocked by atropine. It was later found to be a peptide of ten amino acids. Substance P was the first peptide discovered in the CNS.

In general, substance P cell bodies are widely distributed (Table 14-8; Fig. 14-11). As demonstrated by immunocytochemistry, extensive networks of fibers are present in varying densities in most areas of the CNS — except in the cerebellum, hippocampus, and certain parts of the cerebral cortex. Furthermore, several neural subsystems that carry substance P fibers have been identified, and new ones are still being discovered. In all cases studied so far, substance P has a slow, long-lasting, inhibitory effect on neuron firing.

This peptide is found near the portals of the CNS. Primary sensory neurons are prominent members of this group; about 20% of the cell bodies

Table 14-8. Substance P Neuron Systems in the Mammalian Brain

System	Place of origin	Site(s) of termination
Primary sensory afferents	Dorsal root ganglia	Substantia gelatosina
Descending spinal system	Medulla oblongata	Substantia gelatosina
Striatonigral tract	Caudate nucleus	Substantia nigra
Habenulointerpeduncular tract	Medial habenular nucleus	Interpeduncular nucleus

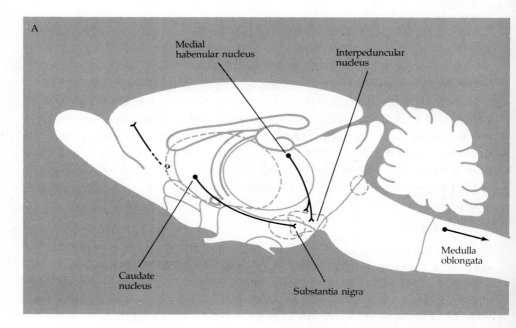

A

Medial
habenular nucleus

Interpeduncular
nucleus

Medulla
oblongata

Caudate
nucleus

Substantia nigra

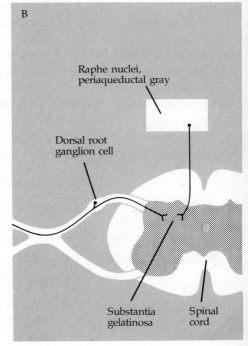

B

Raphe nuclei,
periaqueductal gray

Dorsal root
ganglion cell

Substantia
gelatinosa

Spinal
cord

FIG. 14–11. *Substance P systems in the
central nervous system.* (A) Sagittal section to show brain systems. (B) Cross
section of spinal cord to show primary
afferent and descending systems. See
also Table 14-8.

in dorsal root ganglia contain substance P. These cells, the smaller neurons in the ganglia, appear to project primarily to the substantia gelatinosa of the dorsal horn. The dendrites of these primary afferent neurons are found in the nasal mucosa, dermis, and epidermis. Moreover, most general somatic sensory nuclei in the CNS have a strong innervation from these primary sensory neurons. It thus appears that substance P is associated with somatic sensation, especially pain perception. As mentioned in Chapter 6, enkephalin fibers appear to form axoaxonic synapses with substance P fibers.

Not all primary sensory afferents use substance P as their transmitter. Some seem to use somatostatin (see below). Moreover, some substance P fibers may carry out motor functions. Sweat glands, for example, are innervated by substance P fibers.

The striatonigral tract, well known for its GABA fibers (see below), also appears to carry substance P fibers. Lesions of this tract lead to diminished substance P levels in the substantia nigra. The substance P-synthesizing cells are probably in the anterior part of the caudate nucleus. In patients with Huntington's chorea, substance P levels are decreased in the substantia nigra, along with GABA levels, as a result of the degeneration of the striatonigral tract.

Other substance P projections are now known, at least in part. Substance P fibers are present in prefrontal and limbic areas of the cerebral cortex, with a distribution very much like that of dopamine and serotonin innervation there. The cells of origin appear to lie in the brainstem. The medial habenular nucleus also contains substance P cell bodies, fibers of which travel via the habenulointerpeduncular tract to the interpeduncular nucleus of the midbrain. Lastly, substance P neurons in the medulla oblongata project downward to the substantia gelatinosa of the spinal cord. These fibers may excite enkephalin neurons there, as the serotonin fibers described earlier do.

Substance P illustrates an exciting new concept. In some neurons, it has been found to coexist with another transmitter: certain raphe cell bodies contain substance P and serotonin in various proportions. This finding is a violation of the long-standing belief (Dale's principle) that one neuron produces and releases only one transmitter. It may be that a choice of output modes is provided by combining a peptide and a monoamine.

4. Somatostatin

Somatostatin (sometimes called the growth hormone-release inhibiting hormone) is a tetradecapeptide. It was initially identified by its ability to inhibit growth hormone secretion from the pituitary. As one might expect, somatostatin cells and fibers are mainly in the hypothalamus.

The somatostatin neurons lie primarily in the periventricular region of the preoptic area and anterior hypothalamus. These cells, however, like many other hypothalamic cells, have sprawling processes that make it difficult to assign them to any single nucleus. Some periventricular cells send axons into the median eminence, and somatostatin liberated there can enter the hypophysial portal vasculature to control growth hormone and TSH release.

Additional somatostatin fibers are found elsewhere in the nervous system. Some are primary sensory afferents, originating from the dorsal root ganglia and richly innervating the substantia gelatinosa of the dorsal horn. Others are present in the spinal cord, parts of the limbic system, and the cerebral cortex. Outside the CNS, still others are encountered in the intestinal wall; and nonneuronal cell bodies containing somatostatin are present in the pancreas, thyroid gland, and gut. As with the other peptides, they are encountered in both expected and unexpected places.

Other Peptides

VIP might seem to stand for Very Important Peptide, but it is actually vasoactive intestinal polypeptide, a 28-amino acid peptide originally characterized as a gut hormone. It is also present in the CNS and is widely distributed in some hypothalamic areas, including the median eminence. Curiously, VIP neurons and terminals are present in all areas of the cerebral cortex, and 1 to 5% of all cortical neurons seem to contain this polypeptide. Most VIP neurons are in layers II–IV, and most VIP is intrinsic to cortex, since undercutting the cortical mantle does not abolish staining of it. Despite its surprising abundance, however, the function of VIP is unknown.

Cholecystokinin (CCK), an octapeptide related to the gut peptide, gastrin, is found in brain (in neuronal cell bodies and fibers) in concentrations higher than any other peptide. In the GI tract, it brings about secretion of pancreatic juice and ejection of bile. In brain, its identity as a transmitter or perhaps modulator has not been established, but there is some information suggesting a widespread distribution in the CNS.

ACTH is an interesting and unquestionably very important peptide hormone found primarily in the pituitary. Following hypophysectomy, however, ACTH concentrations in brain do not change, and in fact may even increase. How can this be? Immunocytochemical studies have shown

ACTH nerve cell bodies within and lateral to the arcuate nucleus of the hypothalamus, with typically beaded fibers scattered throughout the thalamus, amygdala, periaqueductal gray, and reticular formation. In all neurons in which its presence has been demonstrated, it seems that ACTH coexists with beta-lipotrophin, which is probably its precursor. It is well known that ACTH plays a role in stress, motivation, learning, and memory; and the above distribution in brain hints at how ACTH might participate directly in such functions.

Other peptides have been described in the CNS, including neurotensin, angiotensin II, melanocyte-stimulating hormone (alpha-MSH), thyrotrophin-releasing hormone (TRH), and luteinizing hormone-releasing hormone. The cells that contain these peptides are primarily in the hypothalamus, with sparse projections elsewhere. The alpha-MSH innervation suggests another organizing concept. Alpha-MSH fibers are seen close to the apex of the ependymal cells near the lumen of the lateral and third ventricles. This observation suggests that alpha-MSH may be released directly into the cerebrospinal fluid. Behavioral actions of alpha-MSH-like peptides are best elicited after intraventricular injections, so this finding may be significant.

In general, it seems that hypothalamic peptides have access to certain areas of the brain and spinal cord via special connections, so as to inform the CNS of neuroendocrine activity. In some cases, these connections are probably part of the general hormonal feedback on the brain, i.e., upon those brain and spinal systems involved in implementing and consolidating neuroendocrine-related activities. Exactly how these peptide neurotransmitters work is not clear; rather than a fast-acting electrical signal, they may carry a metabolic or modulatory message.

Amino Acids

A number of amino acids are known transmitters, and many more have been suggested. Well-established ones include gamma-aminobutyric acid (GABA), glycine, glutamate, and aspartate. Histamine, proline, and taurine are candidates, but the evidence is not as solid. We shall restrict our discussion to the well-established ones.

Gamma-aminobutyric Acid

The major inhibitory transmitter in brain is gamma-aminobutyric acid (GABA). Most local-circuit neurons (Golgi Type II; see Chap. 2) probably use this molecule as their transmitter, and some projection neurons do (Golgi Type I; see Table 14-9 and Fig. 14-12). GABA is produced by the removal of a carboxyl group (decarboxylation) from glutamate, a reaction catalyzed by the enzyme glutamic acid decarboxylase (GAD). This enzyme is found only in GABA neurons, so these cells can be identified by its presence. GAD has been purified, and can be localized by immunohistochemical methods or assayed directly in dissected tissues.

Prominent among GABA local-circuit neurons are the basket and stellate cells found in hippocampus, cerebral cortex, and cerebellar cortex. In addition to other connections, these modulatory interneurons receive synapses (on their cell bodies or proximal dendrites) with recurrent collaterals from projection neurons in their vicinity. Such cells suppress the firing of projection neurons, and often sharpen contrast by inhibiting nearby elements. Similar GABA interneurons are found in the spinal cord.

The first-discovered and most notable GABA projection neuron is the Purkinje cell of the cerebellar cortex. This cell, the sole output channel of the cerebellar cortex, is inhibitory, acting to suppress activity in its various targets — the lateral vestibular nucleus, the deep cerebellar nuclei, and the cortical basket cells via its recurrent collaterals. The equivalent principal projection neuron of the cerebral cortex, the pyramidal cell, does not use GABA. It is an excitatory element, which exerts inhibition only indirectly through local interneurons or by decreasing its firing rate.

The basal ganglia also feature GABA projection cells, which send fibers to the substantia nigra. Most of the nigral GABA fibers come from the globus pallidus and terminate on nigral dopamine neurons. Additional

Table 14-9. GABA Tracts and Local Circuits in the Mammalian Brain

System	Place or cells of origin	Site(s) of termination
Cerebellum	Purkinje cells	Deep cerebellar nuclei Basket cells Vestibular nuclei
Cerebellum	Basket cells	Purkinje cells
Hippocampus	Basket cells	Pyramidal and granule cells
Striatonigral tract	Basal ganglia	Substantia nigra
Cerebral cortex interneurons	Stellate neurons	Local connections

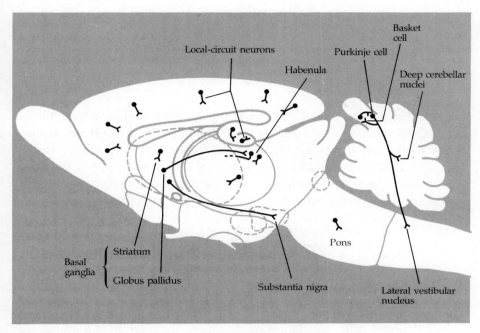

FIG. 14–12. *GABA systems in the brain.* See also Table 14-9.

nigral GABA fibers arise from the caudate and putamen. Many of the GABA neurons in the basal ganglia, however, are intrinsic, and do not project to the nigra. In Huntington's chorea, a degenerative disease associated with involuntary movements, there is a loss of GABA neurons in the caudate/putamen along with widespread atrophy of the frontal cortex. GABA is thus reduced in the nigra, which in turn (through loss of its inhibitory effect) elevates nigrostriatal dopamine. The consequent heightened DA/ACh ratio in the striatum is manifested in abnormal motor control just as the lowered DA/ACh ratio is associated with parkinsonism. Thus, different transmitters frequently work together, and imbalances in their relative contributions can lead to clinical abnormalities in brain function.

As an inhibitory messenger, GABA and its related enzyme GAD are widely distributed in the CNS, and it is certain that many neural subsystems in addition to those just described use GABA as their transmitter. For example, evidence points to the vestibulo-ocular pathway — from the vestibular nuclei to the oculomotor/trochlear motor nuclear complex — as a GABA tract. Other studies show a type of GABA amacrine cell in the retina. Thus, if inhibition can be described as a form of "sculpturing" of brain activity into meaningful patterns, GABA provides the major chemical chisel — to shape and refine neural activity throughout the brain.

Glycine

Glycine, the simplest of all amino acids, is another inhibitory transmitter. While GABA is the major inhibitory transmitter in the upper brain, glycine is the major one in the spinal cord and lower brainstem (Table 14-10). Neurophysiological studies have established this, particularly in the cord. It is difficult, however, to define the pathways that use glycine, since we do not have a good histochemical method for localizing this transmitter.

Table 14–10. Glycine System in the Mammalian CNS

System	Place of origin	Site(s) of termination
Interneurons	Ventral horn gray matter	Local circuits

In the spinal cord, glycine seems to be the transmitter of many of the innumerable small interneurons (see Chaps. 2 and 10) that inhabit the intermediate zone of gray matter between sensory and motor neurons and that appear to be most highly concentrated in the ventral horn. Glycine may also be the transmitter for some of the descending inhibitory fibers of supraspinal origin. In the pons and medulla, it has been suggested that glycine is a transmitter for certain fibers that inhibit hypoglossal motor neurons and for others that exert crossed inhibition on vestibular neurons.

Glutamate and Aspartate

Glutamate and aspartate are common amino acids present in all tissues. Yet it appears that they double as transmitters for many CNS neurons (see Table 14-11 and Fig. 14-13). Initial evidence that they might be neurotransmitters came from electrophysiological studies: the application of these acidic amino acids to neurons produced actions very similar to those expected for excitatory transmitters. Since that time, many investigators have searched the CNS for neurons and pathways that use glutamate and aspartate as transmitters. Without specific and easily applied markers for these universally occurring amino acids, the task has been difficult. Calcium-dependent release, high-affinity uptake, and pharmacological

Table 14–11. Glutamate and/or Aspartate Systems in the Mammalian CNS

System	Place or cells of origin	Target structure
Perforant path	Entorhinal cortex	Dentate gyrus
Lateral olfactory tract	Olfactory bulb	Piriform cortex
Corticostriate tract	Cerebral cortex	Caudate nucleus
Parallel fibers	Cerebellar granule cells	Purkinje cells

analysis are the best current means of identifying them. Thus, the status of glutamate and aspartate pathways is somewhat tenuous. All the same, it is widely believed that these amino acids are the major excitatory transmitters in brain.

The general rule appears to be that most cortical projection neurons utilize these two closely related amino acids as transmitters. Certainly GABA, peptides, and monoamines are not the transmitters of these major excitatory projection neurons. Among the neurons that do appear to use glutamate are the star pyramidal cells in the entorhinal (medial temporal) cortex which project to the dentate gyrus of the hippocampus and the cortical fibers which project to the caudate nucleus.

General Concepts

There is great diversity in the neural organization of various transmitter subsystems in the nervous system. Figure 14-14 gives a general overview of the innervation fields of the major chemical messengers: acetylcholine (ACh); the monoamines—dopamine (DA), norepinephrine (NE), epinephrine (C), and serotonin (5-HT); the peptides—enkephalins, endorphins, substance P, somatostatin, and others; and the amino acids — gamma-aminobutyric acid (GABA), glycine, glutamate, and aspartate. We shall summarize what we have said about all these transmitters in that order.

ACh cell bodies comprise spinal and cranial motor neurons, preganglionic autonomic neurons, postganglionic parasympathetic neurons, and certain forebrain neurons. ACh is found in numerous well-defined pathways and local circuits, and is the preeminent transmitter of the PNS and ANS.

Monoamine cell bodies are all found in the brainstem. The nigrostriatal system gives rise to a major DA input to the basal ganglia. The mesocortical system, originating in the nigral tegmental area, projects in an orderly way

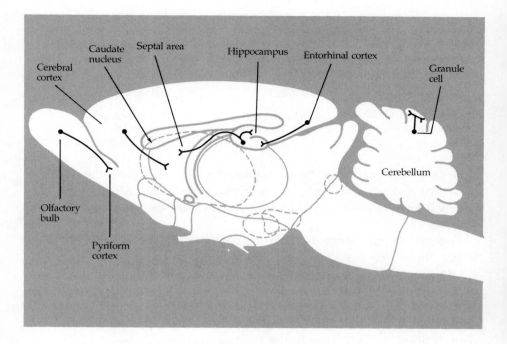

FIG. 14–13. *Glutamate systems in the brain.* See also Table 14-11.

to nearly all allocortical areas and to some subcortical structures (amygdala and nucleus accumbens). Other DA cells in the brainstem innervate the hypothalamus and periventricular areas.

Norepinephrine pathways all originate from cell groups in the pons and medulla. The locus coeruleus, a pontine nucleus, projects everywhere in the CNS with the least topographic order of any known transmitter system. By contrast, the lateral tegmental NE system projects primarily and in a more orderly manner to the hypothalamus, brainstem, and, to a lesser degree, basal forebrain. It does not innervate the neocortex.

Epinephrine is found in cell groups in the reticular formation. Projections from these cells sparsely innervate various brainstem nuclei, as well as the thalamus and spinal cord.

Serotonin neurons lie primarily in the median seam of the brainstem — the raphe nuclei of the midline. Much like neurons of the locus coeruleus, they have widespread connections over most of the CNS. Some fibers end in the ependyma and in specialized neurovascular organs about the third ventricle.

All those peptides derived from beta-lipotrophin (enkephalins, endorphins, and ACTH) are found mainly in neurons of the hypothalamus, but do turn up elsewhere in the CNS. Enkephalin cell bodies and fibers are

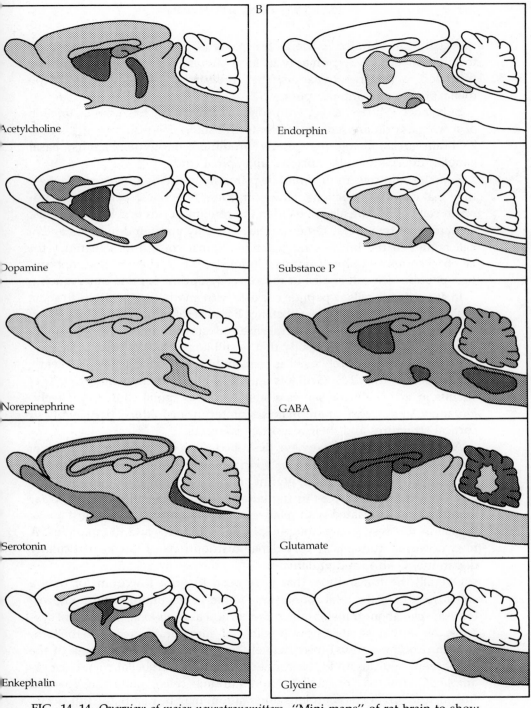

B

Acetylcholine

Dopamine

Norepinephrine

Serotonin

Enkephalin

Endorphin

Substance P

GABA

Glutamate

Glycine

FIG. 14–14. *Overview of major neurotransmitters.* "Mini-maps" of rat brain to show general domains (origins and terminations) of major chemical messengers in the CNS. Epinephrine system, which is of minor extent, has been omitted.

especially concentrated in the globus pallidus, but are also widely spread throughout the CNS, primarily in local circuits. Endorphin neurons are restricted to the hypothalamus; they project locally, as well as to the diencephalon and anterior pons.

Substance P fibers, along with somatostatin fibers, have the distinction of serving as primary sensory afferents. Substance P is also present in some 25 brain areas, being particularly prominent in hypothalamus, basal ganglia, interpeduncular nucleus, and spinal cord.

Somatostatin cells in the brain lie primarily in the hypothalamus, where they make local connections. However, these fibers, and perhaps somatostatin cell bodies, are also present in the cerebral cortex and hippocampus, to name just two areas. Other peptides usually are found in fibers and/or cell bodies in the brainstem, thalamus, spinal cord, and sometimes the cerebral cortex and hippocampus. Curiously, the cerebellum does not contain peptide-rich cell bodies or receive a significant peptide innervation.

In some nerve cells, a peptide coexists with another transmitter. In some raphe neurons, for example, substance P and serotonin are found together. If such violations of Dale's principle are widespread, dual transmitters may give neural function a flexibility that is still largely unexplored.

Amino acids are widely used as transmitters, and have cell bodies nearly everywhere in the CNS. GABA is the major inhibitory transmitter for local circuits in grain; glycine serves a similar role in spinal cord. Conversely, glutamate and aspartate are major excitatory transmitters, particularly in cortical structures and their respective efferents.

All of the transmitters we have described, with the possible exception of glutamate and aspartate, can be found in both projection neurons and local-circuit neurons. GABA, glycine, and the enkephalins, however, are best known for their roles in the latter circuits. Most transmitters so far identified are associated with relatively sparse innervations in most areas; typical in this respect are norepinephrine, serotonin, and the peptides. A few, however, turn up in very dense distributions of fibers, particularly dopamine, GABA, and glutamate.

Overall, the transmitters that have been identified account for only a small fraction of the total connections found in the brain. Little is known, for example, about transmitters in the cortical association/commissural systems. Nevertheless, it is now possible in some brain areas (cerebellum, striatum, hippocampus) to tentatively assign transmitters to most of the constituent neurons and their connections. In the cerebellar cortex, for example, GABA (basket, stellate, and Purkinje cells), glutamate (parallel fibers), and NE (locus coeruleus innervation) may be nearly the full story.

Glossary

Acetylcholine: the major transmitter of the skeletal musculature and pre-ganglionic sympathetic neurons; less prominent in the CNS, where it serves mostly local-circuit functions.

$$(CH_3)_3N^+—CH_2CH_2—O—\overset{\overset{\textstyle O}{\|}}{C}—CH_3$$

Aspartate: an acidic amino acid; one of the major excitatory neurotransmitter candidates, particularly in cortical structures.

$$HOOCCH_2\overset{\overset{\textstyle NH_2}{|}}{C}HCOOH$$

Catecholamines: a class of molecules that contains a catechol nucleus and an ethylamine group, e.g., dopamine, norepinephrine, epinephrine.

HO — ⟨ring⟩ — CH$_2$CH$_2$NH$_2$
HO

Cholecystokinin (CCK):   an octapeptide related to the gut peptide gastrin; one of the most abundant peptides; may act as a CNS moderator/transmitter.

Dopamine: a catecholamine, [2-(3,4-dihydroxyphenyl)-ethylamine]; cell bodies located mainly in the substantia nigra, ventral tegmental area, and hypothalamus; transmitter of the clinically important nigrostriatal pathway.

HO — ⟨ring⟩ — CH$_2$CH$_2$NH$_2$
HO

Endorphins: a class of endogenous polypeptides with opiatelike properties; the vast majority of cell bodies are found in the hypothalamus.

Enkephalins: two pentapeptides (leu- and met-enkephalin) with opiatelike activity; show a widespread distribution and involvement, primarily in local-circuit functions.

Epinephrine (adrenaline):   a catecholamine, [1-(3,4-dihydroxyphenyl)-2-methylaminoethanol]; apparently a very minor transmitter in the CNS, primarily found in the brainstem.

$$\underset{\text{HO}}{\underset{\text{HO}}{\bigcirc}} \quad \overset{\text{OH}}{\overset{|}{\text{CHCH}_2\text{NHCH}_3}}$$

GABA (γ-aminobutyric acid): the major inhibitory brain transmitter; found in local-circuit neurons throughout the brain.

$$\text{NH}_2\text{—CH}_2\text{—CH}_2\text{—CH}_2\text{—COOH}$$

Glutamate: an acidic amino acid; the major excitatory transmitter candidate of cortical areas.

$$\overset{\text{NH}_2}{\overset{|}{\text{HOOCCH}_2\text{CH}_2\text{CHCOOH}}}$$

Glycine: an amino acid inhibitory transmitter ; so far, found mainly in the spinal cord and lower brainstem.

$$\text{NH}_2\text{—CH}_2\text{—COOH}$$

Monoamine: any amino R—NH₂ that has one organic substituent (R) attached to the nitrogen group, e.g., dopamine, norepinephrine, serotonin.

Norepinephrine: a major catecholamine, [1-(3,4-dihydroxyphenyl)-2-aminoethanol]; cell bodies located primarily in the pons and medulla and axons projecting throughout the brain; also used as a transmitter by most postganglionic sympathetic neurons.

$$\underset{\text{HO}}{\underset{\text{HO}}{\bigcirc}} \quad \overset{\text{OH}}{\overset{|}{\text{CHCH}_2\text{NH}_2}}$$

Serotonin: a monoamine (5-hydroxytryptamine); virtually all cell bodies are located in brainstem; axonal projections to nearly all brain structures.

$$\underset{\text{N}}{\underset{\text{H}}{\text{HO}}} \quad \overset{\text{CH}_2}{\underset{\text{NH}_2}{\text{CH}_2}}$$

Somatostatin: a 14-amino-acid peptide; cell bodies primarily in the preoptic area, hypothalamus, and parts of the PNS.

Substance P: a 10-amino-acid peptide; best known as a primary afferent transmitter, but also found in limbic, motor, and brainstem areas.

Vasoactive intestinal peptide (VIP): a 28-amino-acid polypeptide; cell bodies in the hypothalamus and cerebral cortex; nearly 5% of cortical cell bodies contain VIP.

The Circulation of the Brain and the Cerebrospinal Fluid 15

The many functions of the CNS demand work by the system, and work demands energy. The nervous system obviously must have a high metabolic rate; it must produce the energy needed to maintain membrane potentials, generate action potentials, communicate across synapses through release and uptake of transmitters, move materials through its myriad cells and along their fibrous processes — and so on for a lifetime. The energy for all these efforts comes from the aerobic combustion of glucose, and the circulatory system provides these paramount raw materials, oxygen and glucose, in constant and generous amounts. In addition, the bloodstream, along with the cerebrospinal fluid that derives from it, plays the vital role of keeping the physicochemical environment of central neurons on an even keel, of insuring the homeostasis of the brain and spinal cord.

Since there is little provision for storage of oxygen and glucose in central nervous tissue, even brief failure of the cerebral circulation results in temporary or lasting loss of brain function. Clinically, such a loss may be manifested as a transient ischemic attack (TIA), in which neurologic function is briefly altered (perhaps for a day or less) by diminished blood flow for some reason, e.g., coronary insufficiency or a stenosed internal carotid artery. Or it may be a stroke, in which a brain region is deprived of blood for a time (not very long; see below). Such a shut-down might be due to the presence of vascular obstruction or leakage — from a thrombus, embolism, or hemorrhage. The resulting functional deficit may range from minor to severe, and from lengthy to permanent. The outcome depends on many factors, from the extent and duration of the deprivation to the remarkable adaptability and plasticity of the nervous system (see Chap. 5).

Normal Parameters of Cerebral Circulation and Metabolism

The facts and figures on cerebral circulation are interesting: Cerebral oxygen consumption runs somewhere around 3.3 ml/100 g brain tissue/min in a resting human. The whole brain consumes 43–49 ml/min. Of the larger body organs, only the heart and kidneys burn up oxygen at greater rates than this. This amount is about 20% of the human body's total O_2 consumption per minute under standard resting conditions.

Years ago, it was thought that the metabolic needs of the brain were small, since mental activity had no detectable effect on total body O_2 consumption. We now see that such slight fluctuations as do occur with increased or decreased function are completely overshadowed because the "resting value" is so high.

Total cerebral blood flow is another striking figure; it is estimated at 1000 ml/min under conditions of body rest. Although some brain regions (such as the inferior colliculus and the caudate nucleus) have higher flow rates (as well as higher rates of O_2 consumption) than others, average regional flow values are around 50 ml/100 g/min. This means that an "average piece" of brain is bathed by about half its total volume in blood every minute. Moreover, paralleling the ratio for brain/body O_2 consumption given above, the total cerebral blood flow accounts for 15–20% of the cardiac output. And the glucose delivered by the circulatory system to the brain as its major energy source constitutes, again, about 20% of the total body's glucose.

Normally, cerebral blood flow is autoregulated, that is, when mean arterial blood pressure is normal, it is maintained within a constant range (with fluctuations) by regional and local cellular metabolic activity. Such neural activity has a dilating effect on the cerebral vessels, an effect mediated in part (see below) by increasing extracellular pH and its dilatory influences on arteriolar resistance and diameter. Most of the time, this locally induced vasodilatation, in accord with activity, assures an adequate blood supply; only when arterial blood pressure falls to about half of its normal level does autoregulation fail and trouble begin.

Thus, in normotensive individuals, systolic systemic arterial pressure has to fall below 50–60 mm Hg to bring about inadequate cerebral blood flow. Blood pressure as low as this usually results promptly in loss of

consciousness. A similar wide margin of safety is built into the requirements for oxygen supply: arterial levels of O_2, normally at 95 mm Hg, lie
well above the values at which neuronal function is disrupted. At levels
below 40 mm Hg (a PO_2 equivalent to that of venous blood), neuronal
hypoxia will produce mental dysfunction or alteration in the state of consciousness and in changes in the electroencephalogram.

Failure of Cerebral Circulation and Thresholds of Neuronal Dysfunction

Neurons have scant capacity for anaerobic metabolism; they must have
oxygen to function normally. A variety of clinical conditions (not to mention environmental events and experimental conditions) can lead to diminished blood flow and oxygen deficits. Some terms need defining: *cerebral anoxia* (or hypoxemia) is a deprivation of oxygen from the blood (and
thus the other tissues), which continues to circulate to the brain. Typical
causes are suffocation, respiratory failure, or the greater affinity of hemo-
globin for carbon monoxide than oxygen. *Cerebral ischemia* has a different
meaning; it is a deprivation of cerebral blood flow, such as that due to
cardiac arrest or vascular occlusion (by the formation of a thrombus or the
lodging of an embolus from some other part of the circulatory system).
Clearly, the second condition is related to the first; cerebral ischemia will
bring about anoxia of the brain region that is deprived of blood, no matter
how well oxygenated that blood may have been.

Anoxic and/or ischemic failure of neuronal function appears first to
undermine neurotransmitter metabolism, and later to compromise membrane ionic pump activity. From that unhappy point on, a train of functional breakdowns follows.

Prolonged or severe anoxia or ischemia ultimately results in irreversible
loss of mitochondrial capacity for respiration, and hence neuronal death.
Such irreparable damage seems to occur when cerebral blood flow drops to
around one-fifth of its normal rate: at 10 ml/100 g/min or below (down to 20
ml/100 g/min the cells may recover, if experimental studies are any guide).
Under such a trickle of the normal flow, consciousness is lost in 10 seconds,
neuronal metabolism altered within 30 seconds, and electrical activity at an
end within a minute. After an interruption of more than four to eight
minutes' duration (as may occur in cardiac arrest), diffuse cerebral infarction (coagulation necrosis) or brain death usually results.

Short of death, however, many extremely serious consequences ensue
from cerebral anoxia or ischemia. Vascular congestion, stasis, and

hyperemia (excess of blood in a region) may result from ischemia, as they do from trauma or inflammation of the brain. Extravasation of blood or hemorrhage may also occur, due to violations of the integrity of vascular walls; in the brain, protected as it is by the skull, these walls are relatively thin and delicate (see below). Further complications include transudation of blood serum or intravascular water and the onset of brain edema, with all the ominous space-taking consequences of these events. Such seepage of fluid into the brain is caused by increased permeability of capillary endothelial cells.

To interpret the clinical expressions of these pathophysiological responses, we have to understand the anatomical and physiological features of the cerebral circulation that adjust, not only for local variations in normal metabolic demand, but also for outright disturbances in blood supply.

Anatomy of the Cerebral Circulation

Extracranial Arteries: The Dual Blood Supply to the Brain

The cephalic vessels originate at the aortic arch and ascend through the neck to enter the cranial vault through foramina in the base of the skull (Fig. 15-1). The paired carotid arteries carry 85% of the cerebral blood flow, with the remaining 15% passing through the vertebral arteries. The rate of flow through each internal carotid is rapid (350 cc/min), and the diameter of the vessel large (3.7–4.5 mm lumen). The origin of the internal carotid (at the bifurcation of the common carotid into external and internal branches) is the most common site of symptomatic arteriosclerosis in the cerebral circulation.

The other major source of blood to the brain is the pair of vertebral arteries. They vary in caliber from 0.9 to 4.1 mm, and carry flows of up to 100 ml/min each. After passing through the foramen magnum of the skull, they join on the anterior surface of the brainstem to form the basilar artery, a large, single vessel running directly upward along the midline.

Intracranial Arteries and Protective Mechanisms

The main intracranial arteries are shown in Figure 15-2. A great ring of blood vessels lies at the base of the brain: the arterial circle of Willis. This remarkable vascular loop, like a beltway encircling part of a city, provides access to many regions. In this case, the part of the brain encircled is small, but vitally important; it is principally the optic chiasm and the

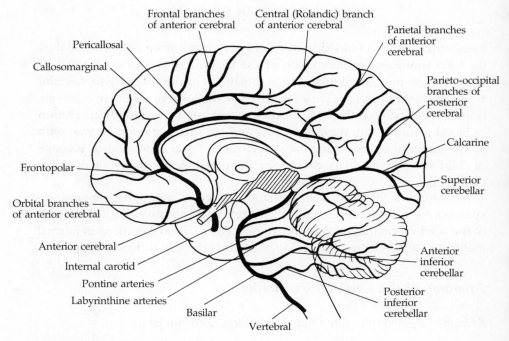

Frontal branches of anterior cerebral

Central (Rolandic) branch of anterior cerebral

Parietal branches of anterior cerebral

Pericallosal

Callosomarginal

Parieto-occipital branches of posterior cerebral

Calcarine

Frontopolar

Superior cerebellar

Orbital branches of anterior cerebral

Anterior inferior cerebellar

Anterior cerebral

Internal carotid

Pontine arteries

Labyrinthine arteries

Posterior inferior cerebellar

Basilar

Vertebral

A. Arterial supply, medial view

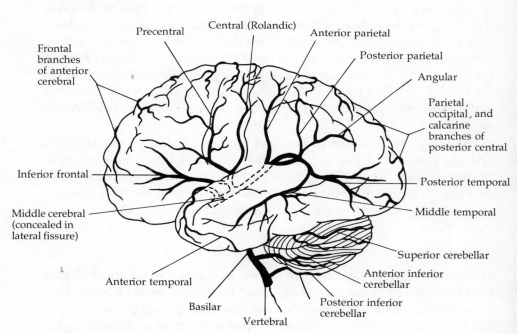

Precentral

Central (Rolandic)

Anterior parietal

Frontal branches of anterior cerebral

Posterior parietal

Angular

Parietal, occipital, and calcarine branches of posterior central

Inferior frontal

Posterior temporal

Middle cerebral (concealed in lateral fissure)

Middle temporal

Superior cerebellar

Anterior inferior cerebellar

Anterior temporal

Posterior inferior cerebellar

Basilar

Vertebral

B. Arterial supply, lateral view

FIG. 15–1. *Main arterial supply to the brain.* (A) Medial surface of the cerebrum (lateral view of brainstem below the midbrain, which has been transected as indicated by dashed lines). The brain is vascularized by two pairs of arteries, the vertebrals and internal carotids. The vertebral arteries join just caudal to the pons to form the basilar artery. Numerous branches of the vertebral-basilar axis pass into the upper cervical spinal cord, brainstem, and cerebellum. Rostrally, the basilar artery bifurcates to form the posterior cerebral arteries, which pass lateral to the midbrain, then above the tentorium to supply the medial and inferior surfaces of the temporal and occipital lobes (see also Fig. 15-3). After giving off numerous major branches, the internal carotid divides lateral to the optic chiasm into its two terminal vessels: the anterior cerebral artery and the middle cerebral artery (not visible in this view). The anterior cerebral artery curves around the corpus callosum and supplies most of the medial surface of the cerebrum through various branches. (B) Lateral surface of the entire brain. The middle cerebral artery, a direct continuation of the internal carotid, passes laterally into the (Sylvian) fissure at the base of the brain. Its numerous branches arise in a triangular region over the insula. They course upward and backward, bend around the opercula, and then fan out over the lateral convexity of the hemisphere. (Modified from M. Carpenter, *Human Neuroanatomy*, 7th Ed. Williams & Wilkins, Baltimore, 1976)

hypothalamus just behind it. The actual territory supplied by the circle of Willis, however, is much larger; trunks leading from the circle supply the entirety of the cerebral hemispheres, through numerous subsidiary vessels which nourish the cortex and the deeper white and gray matter.

The blood entering the circle of Willis comes from both the internal carotid and the vertebral-basilar systems. Anteriorly, the anterior cerebral arteries branch from the internal carotid, and are linked across the midline by a short connecting vessel, the anterior communicating artery. Posteriorly, the posterior communicating arteries lead from the internal carotid to the posterior cerebral arteries, which arise from the rostral bifurcation of the basilar. The middle cerebral artery is the largest branch of the internal carotid, essentially a direct extension of it leading anterolaterally. As Figure 15-3 shows, each of the three cerebral arteries has its own area of distribution to the cortical surface, as well as deeper individual territories that are largely beyond the scope of this overview. While the surface vessels derived from the cerebral arteries or arteries elsewhere in the brain anastomose freely, anastomoses between cortical and deeper vessels or between deeper vessels themselves are rare. In any event, union of such tiny deeper vessels is seldom adequate to sustain the CNS in its metabolic requirements if one of them is blocked.

The circle of Willis, however, is different in this respect. To some extent (at least in many individuals), it does offer collateral circulatory routes to

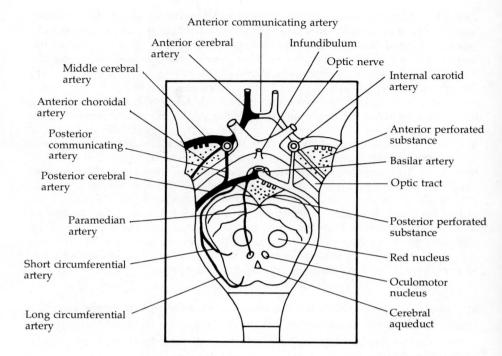

FIG. 15–2. *The arterial circle of Willis.* This view of the arteries at the base of the brain shows the wreathlike vascular circle surrounding the optic chiasm and hypothalamic/interpeduncular region. Note the positions of the basilar artery (reflected rostrally and transected to expose details of the brainstem) and internal carotids, as well as the origins and relationships of the three major cerebral arteries. The anterior perforated substance is the place where branches of the middle cerebral penetrate the brain to supply the basal ganglia and internal capsule. These so-called striate branches are very important clinically. The posterior perforated substance is a similar region of penetrating vessels in the interpeduncular fossa, in which branches of the posterior cerebral enter the brainstem tegmentum. The paramedian, short circumferential, and long circumferential branches of the posterior cerebral typify the mode of branching of most lower brainstem arteries (see Fig. 15-4); in the case of the cerebellar arteries, it is the long circumferential branch that supplies the cerebellum, with the short circumferential and paramedian vessels supplying particular mesencephalic, pontine, and medullary territories. (Redrawn from an illustration by Foix and Masson, 1923, that appeared in modified form in W. Haymaker, *Bing's Local Diagnosis in Neurological Diseases*, 15th Ed. C. V. Mosby, St. Louis, 1969)

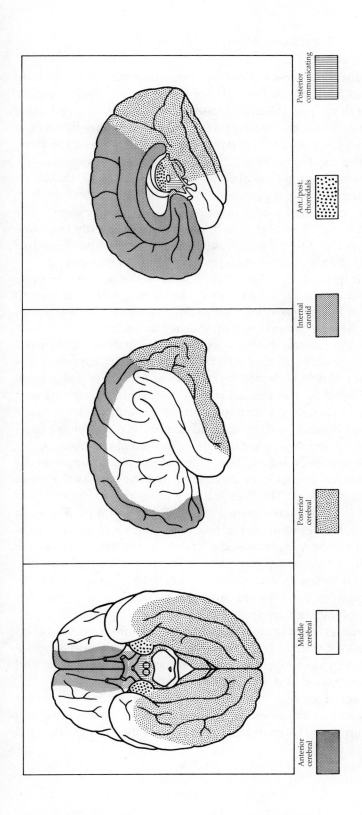

FIG. 15–3. *Cortical territories of cerebral arteries.* Each cerebral artery has its own distinctive domain of cerebral cortex, as well as a deeper realm (not shown). In general, the anterior cerebral artery nourishes most of the medial aspect of the hemisphere, while the middle cerebral supplies most of the lateral aspect. The posterior cerebral supplies a posterior basomedial region that includes the visual cortex. Smaller territories for the internal carotids, anterior and posterior choroidals, and posterior communicating artery are indicated. (Modified from Tondury, as presented in J. Sobotta, *Atlas of Human Anatomy*, 8th English Ed. by F. J. H. Figge. Hafner, New York, 1963)

Anterior cerebral

Middle cerebral

Posterior cerebral

Internal carotid

Ant./post. choroidals

Posterior communicating

safeguard the highly vulnerable brain tissue from ischemia. Normally little blood is exchanged between the two sides of the circle, due to the equality of blood pressure in the two internal carotids. If developmental variations in vessel size occur, however, the ring probably acts to equalize blood flow to various brain regions. And if the flow of blood from one of the three vessels entering the circle is occluded, then the arrangement provides obvious alternative routes and means of adjustment — depending, that is, on whether the communicating vessels are functionally adequate, which in many individuals, particularly older ones but also in young people, may not be the case. Details of arterial pattern often differ markedly from one person to another, and the communicating vessels in particular are frequently of inadequate size. Sometimes they may not even be patent.

As proof of the protective value of the circle of Willis, after bilateral common carotid occlusion in the cat, this arterial ring dilates within 10 seconds, and there is a progressive decrease in vascular resistance within the brain. Within 30 to 40 seconds, the diminished blood flow even in such a deep region as the caudate nucleus returns to normal. Such collateral circulation in the human brain may also be highly efficient, especially if it has time to develop slowly over months or years as a result of progressive stenosis (narrowing) of the extracranial vessels. Surprisingly, patients with bilateral carotid and unilateral vertebral occlusion or with basilar stenosis may have minimal ischemic symptoms and normal cerebral blood flow, due to adaptive collateral supply through extracerebral channels.

Up to now, we have been talking mainly about the blood supply to the cerebrum. We must not overlook the cerebellum and the parts of the lower brainstem which underlie it. The basilar artery gives rise to three pair of cerebellar arteries in the posterior cranial fossa, after which it terminates in the posterior cerebral arteries as mentioned. The origin and course of the vessels derived from the vertebral-basilar system are matters outside the scope of this book, but in general they fall into three main classes: paramedian, supplying an anteromedial wedge of brainstem tissue; short circumferential, supplying an adjacent anterolateral wedge; and long circumferential, supplying the remaining posterolateral region (Fig. 15-4). The cerebellar arteries represent especially long members of this third class. This scheme, of course, is a great oversimplification; microangiograms of the brainstem vasculature reveal a delicate lacework of larger and smaller arterial branches that defies brief description (Fig. 15-5).

An important set of protective mechanisms in the cerebral circulation operates in the neck, at the point of bifurcation of the common carotid artery into its external and internal branches. Here in the carotid sinus and

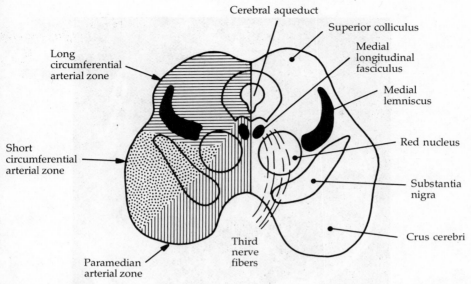

FIG. 15–4. *Arterial supply of the lower brainstem.* Arteries derived from the vertebral-basilar system fall into three main classes: paramedian, short circumferential, and long circumferential (cerebellar arteries are long members of this class). Details of vascularization vary considerably at different levels, but generally accord with this scheme, i.e., a basomedial wedge of brainstem tissue, a large basolateral region, and an equally large dorsolateral region, together with a territory of cerebellar cortex in the case of the cerebellar arteries. The pattern is illustrated here at the midbrain level; major structures are labeled for orientation and to indicate the very different functional effects that selective vascular damage can exert. (Modified from W. Haymaker, *Bing's Local Diagnosis in Neurological Disease*, 15th Ed. C. V. Mosby, St. Louis, 1969)

carotid body are found blood pressure and oxygen tension receptors, respectively. Through the sinus nerve, a small branch of the glossopharyngeal, sensory fibers pass to the nucleus of the solitary tract in the medulla oblongata, thus serving as the afferent limbs for compensatory cardiovascular reflexes that are activated by stimulation of mechanoreceptors in the sinus and chemoreceptors in the adjacent carotid body.

Intracranial arteries are unique by virtue of their thin walls. Only the largest vessels have their own intrinsic adventitial blood supply. Vasa vasorum are rarely found beyond the circle of Willis, and perivascular lymphatics and autonomic ganglion cells are absent (although autonomic fibers do accompany many of the vessels for some distance). The adventitia of even the major arteries is only 35–40 μm thick, consisting of a fine network of collagenous fibers. The tunica media contains a muscularis coat 15 cell

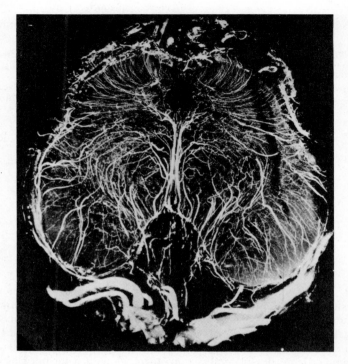

FIG. 15–5. *The pervasive vasculature of the brain.* Microangiogram of arterial supply of midbrain. Vessels are injected with radiopaque contrast medium and studied in thick (4 mm) specimens. Compare with Figs. 15-3 and 15-4 to pick out the paramedian, short, and long circumferential regions of vascularization. (From O. Hassler, *Neurology* 17:368-375, 1967)

layers thinner than that found in extracranial arteries. Circumferential smooth muscle fibers are absent, the contractile fibers running obliquely. The external elastic membrane is absent too, and the internal elastic membrane, while present in the circle of Willis, gradually decreases in thickness to become only a minor component in smaller cerebral arteries. The smallest cerebral arteries, in fact, seem to have only an endothelium surrounded by bundles of collagen, and in the fresh state look more like veins, with delicate, almost transparent walls.

Having such thin walls for their size, of course, makes our cerebral arteries somewhat vulnerable to the effects of hypertension, much as a garden hose with thin walls cannot withstand a high water pressure without weakening after a time. Degenerative changes in the walls of the smaller of these thin arteries, or injury to them from a blow to the head, can lead to the formation of a thrombus, resulting in small (lacunar) infarction of the area of brain tissue supplied. Or an aneurysm (swelling or blister) may develop on the side of an artery. Should such an aneurysm rupture, a local hemorrhage is the result.

The Microcirculation of the Brain

As indicated above, the cerebral microcirculation is ultimately responsible for regulation of cerebral blood flow. In the normal state, flow is rapid and all capillaries remain open. But the circulatory system is very sensitive to the greater or lesser needs of brain tissue from moment to moment. Changes in vascular caliber and resistance that alter blood pressure gradients and blood flow occur at the precapillary arteriolar level. Such changes reflect changes in the local concentrations of oxygen, hydrogen ions, cyclic AMP, adenosine, or cations following variations in neuronal metabolic activity.

The capillary endothelium in the brain has recently been found to be a highly selective interface between the intravascular and extravascular spaces. This relatively impermeable interface makes up what has been called the "blood-brain barrier" (BBB). It is really not a barrier, except to certain vital dyes and large molecules. It is better thought of as a controlled port of entry into brain tissue for various substances, such as amino acids, glucose, water, blood gases, and electrolytes. For these substances, it is a barrier only in the sense that certain of these substances pass through less quickly than others, in accord with various rate constants of diffusion.

During cerebral hypoxia or ischemia, the permeability of this differential filter can be rapidly increased, thus adding the insults of tissue edema and increased intracranial pressure to the injury of oxygen/glucose deprivation. A vicious cycle of brain swelling and further ischemia, due to mechanical compression of the microcirculation, may in this way propagate cerebral infarction (tissue death due to ischemia).

The older concept of a true blood-brain barrier between intravascular and extravascular spaces developed late in the 19th century. It was discovered that intravenous administration of trypan blue, a semicolloidal vital dye which binds to plasma proteins, stained the parenchyma of all tissues except the brain. If injected directly into brain substance, however, staining occurred. Although many years went by before it was understood, the anatomical basis for the BBB is now known to reside in the tight junctions between endothelial cells of the cerebral capillaries and between epithelial cells of the choroid plexus. Similar tight junctions are present between cells of the arachnoid and perineurium (peripheral nerve sheath), but not between glial, ependymal, pial, or choroid plexus capillary endothelial cells. Thus, there is no barrier between cerebrospinal fluid (CSF) and brain extracellular fluid, and there is no functional distinction to be made between the blood-brain barrier and the blood-CSF barrier.

Cerebral Veins

Venous drainage of the brain takes place though cortical, parasagittal, and basal veins that enter the dural sinuses (Fig. 15-6). Like their arterial counterparts, cerebral veins are more thin-walled than systemic veins. Three veins are of special clinical significance because of their locations in important functional regions of the cerebral hemisphere. The Rolandic vein (of Trolard) drains the sensorimotor cortex adjacent to the central sulcus. The vein of Labbé drains the posterior temporal and inferior parietal cortex, the area in the dominant hemisphere involved in speech reception, reading, and writing. The basal vein (of Rosenthal) drains the upper brainstem and lower diencephalon. The sagittal, straight, and paired lateral and sigmoid sinuses empty into the jugular veins, which carry most of the brain's venous outflow. Unilateral jugular vein occlusion is well tolerated, but bilateral surgical ligation must be performed in stages, to allow time for enlargement of collateral channels.

The dural sinuses are important to consider in evaluating patients with head injury. Skull fractures crossing a sinus may be associated with laceration of the dura and rapidly expanding subdural or epidural hematoma. Similarly, the anatomy of the middle meningeal artery (a branch of the external carotid) is relevant, since fractures crossing its branches may be associated with epidural hematoma that expands under arterial pressure.

FIG. 15–6. *Main venous drainage of the brain.* Blood drains from the brain into the dural sinuses. (A) Lateral surface of the cerebrum. Two veins serve key functional regions of the cerebral hemisphere. The superior anastomotic vein (Trolard) drains the sensorimotor strip, while the inferior anastomotic vein (Labbé) drains the temporoparietal speech cortex and its counterpart in the nondominant hemisphere.
(B) Medial surface of the cerebrum. The basal vein (Rosenthal) drains the upper brainstem. The various venous sinuses empty into the jugular veins, the major venous outlets of the brain. Various generally recognized veins are identified in the two illustrations. (Modified from M. Carpenter, *Human Neuroanatomy*, 7th Ed. Williams & Wilkins, Baltimore, 1976)

A

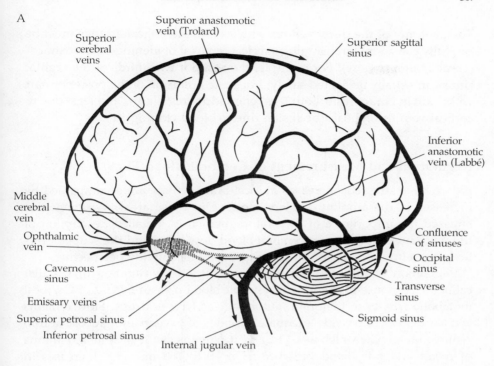

Superior anastomotic
vein (Trolard)

Superior
cerebral
veins

Superior sagittal
sinus

Inferior
anastomotic
vein (Labbé)

Middle
cerebral
vein

Ophthalmic
vein

Cavernous
sinus

Emissary veins

Superior petrosal sinus

Inferior petrosal sinus

Internal jugular vein

Confluence
of sinuses

Occipital
sinus

Transverse
sinus

Sigmoid sinus

B

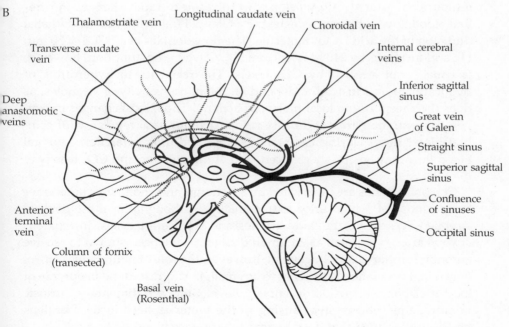

Thalamostriate vein

Longitudinal caudate vein

Choroidal vein

Transverse caudate
vein

Internal cerebral
veins

Deep
anastomotic
veins

Inferior sagittal
sinus

Great vein
of Galen

Straight sinus

Superior sagittal
sinus

Confluence
of sinuses

Occipital sinus

Anterior
terminal
vein

Column of fornix
(transected)

Basal vein
(Rosenthal)

The anatomy of the dural venous sinuses and meningeal arteries must be carefully considered in planning surgical removal of meningiomas (extracerebral benign tumors). For example, the anterior two-thirds of the sagittal sinus can usually be ligated safely, but acute occlusion of the posterior part will result in paraparesis (both legs) or quadriparesis (arms and legs) due to cortical vein thrombosis (occlusion due to blood clotting).

Regulation and Measurement of Cerebral Blood Flow

As we have stressed, increases in local brain activity are accompanied by increases in the amount of blood flowing in these areas. We have also stressed the importance of this autoregulation. A detailed description of the mechanisms regulating cerebral blood flow is beyond the scope of this text, but a brief discussion of some of them will provide perspective.

Regulation of flow is normally accomplished by variation of vascular caliber in response to changes in systemic blood pressure, PCO_2, PO_2, local metabolic activity in the brain, autonomic activity or drugs. Flow remains constant, so as to provide adequate supplies of oxygen and glucose and to remove metabolites such as CO_2, and it remains stable despite alterations of mean systemic blood pressure from 60 to 160 mm Hg. Increases in intraluminal arterial CO_2 tension (PCO_2) result in rapid changes in cerebral blood flow — by increasing extracellular pH following transendothelial diffusion of the acidic CO_2 molecule. The flow doubles at a PCO_2 of 70 mm Hg and increases by 240% at 150 mm Hg. Oxygen consumption, however, is usually not affected by CO_2 levels. The reactivity to hypercarbia or hypocarbia seems instead to depend on the pH sensitivity of arterioles, as does their response to local metabolic activity. Thus, local changes in oxygen concentration are not directly responsible for local regulation of cerebral blood flow. During cerebral ischemia and after infarction, cerebral blood flow may be grossly reduced, and autoregulation and CO_2 reactivity may fail.

Cerebral arteries are innervated by adrenergic and cholinergic autonomic fibers, most of which arise extracranially. Although the most densely supplied vessels are the large arteries and surface arterioles, intraparenchymal arteries as small as 20 μm in diameter have been shown to receive autonomic innervation. In general, however, the role of neurogenic control of cerebral circulation is thought to be small, in contrast to the major role of local metabolic factors as described above. Still, a rudimentary intrinsic noradrenergic fiber system arising in the metencephalic locus coeruleus has been identified that does appear to influence blood flow.

The Xenon Technique and Its Great Potential

At present, the most reliable technique for measuring cerebral blood flow involves the use of xenon-133, a radioactive isotope of the inert gas, xenon. Xenon-133, dissolved in a small amount of sterile saline, is injected as a bolus into one of the main cerebral arteries. The arrival and washout of the isotope are monitored over time on scintillation detectors externally placed around the head. The amount of indicator taken up by the brain is equal to the amount brought to it (arterial concentration) minus the amount carried away (venous concentration) during a given time interval. Indicators such as xenon-133 diffuse so rapidly across vessel walls and within brain tissue that measured isotope concentration depends on blood flow rather than diffusibility. Thus regional cerebral blood flow as measured by xenon-133 "washout" varies directly with local metabolic activity.

Since we know that local metabolic activity goes hand in hand with neural activity, the xenon technique gives us vivid pictures of just which areas of the brain are active from one moment to the next and of the relative amounts of that activity. Figure 15-7 shows several examples of brain activity patterns revealed by this remarkable method. The technique provides a striking validation that the circuits worked out by tracing pathways in brain sections or by electrophysiological means are operational in the awake human.

For example, voluntary movements of the mouth result in activation of cortical areas in the sensorimotor region in which the mouth, tongue, and larynx are represented. The supplementary motor area and the auditory cortex are also active. Voluntary movements of the fingers on the contralateral side of the body from the hemisphere being examined shift activity upward in sensorimotor cortex to the hand-finger area and change the pattern in supplementary motor cortex. Similarly, on the sensory side a shift from a visual task (following a moving object with the eyes) to an auditory one (listening to spoken words) will bring about a corresponding shift from visual association, frontal eye field, and supplementary motor cortex to auditory cortex and the adjacent temporal region (Wernicke's area) that contributes to understanding of speech.

The great advantage of the xenon technique is that it permits the study of the dynamics of brain function, as reflected so faithfully in local cerebral blood flow, in conscious human beings performing various tasks. The approach has already brought important insights. One has been to clarify the role of the supplementary motor area in motor activity. It turns out that this area is generally more active in dynamic motor tasks, such as the movements of speaking, writing, and typing, than in steady muscle contrac-

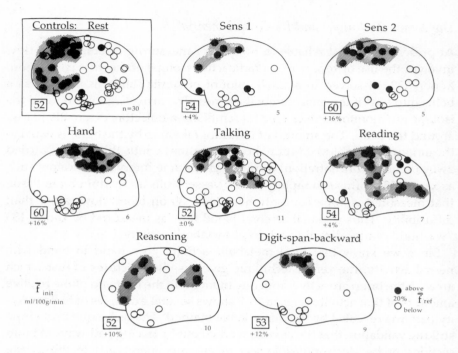

FIG. 15–7. *Regional cerebral blood flow.* Patterns determined by the radioactive xenon (^{133}Xe) technique (see text). Figure in box at upper left illustrates the regional blood flow at rest. Various tasks dramatically alter the flow according to the changing demands of brain activity. Filled circles indicate flow rate significantly higher than average, while open circles indicate below average flow.

Key: (Sens 1) electrical cutaneous stimulation of the contralateral hand with low intensity; (Sens 2) same, but with high intensity and experienced as slight pain; (Hand) voluntary hand movements; (Talking, Reading) self-explanatory, note increase in occipital region during reading and "z" pattern in both due to involvement of premotor, motor, and posterior Sylvian regions (angular gyrus and Wernicke's area; see Fig. 13-7); (Reasoning, Digit-span-backward) also self explanatory, but note differences in precentral and postcentral blood flow. Only flows 20% above and below the mean included as filled and empty circles; below each plot, absolute mean flow in ml/100 g/min is given in the small box, with the underlying smaller number indicating the mean increase during the test. (From David H. Ingvar, *Brain Research 107*: 181-191, 1976)

tions. Thus, the xenon technique has enabled us to see that the supplementary motor area is involved somehow in the planning of sequential motor tasks. The area seems to participate in programming movements, in contrast to the primary motor cortex, which plays such an important role in their execution and succession.

The Brain Ventricles and Cerebrospinal Fluid

We said in Chapter 2 that the brain is hollow, having five cavities (the paired lateral ventricles, the third ventricle, cerebral aqueduct, and fourth ventricle) that derive from the original brain vesicles during development. The ventricles form an important drainage system (refer to Fig. 2-8). Cerebrospinal fluid (CSF), actively secreted in specialized regions of these cavities, the choroid plexuses, and elsewhere within the brain, percolates down through this system, finally to escape through tiny apertures into a cleft between the brain membranes: the subarachnoid space. Once inside this space, which extends past the tip of the spinal cord, the fluid cushions and supports the heavy brain and dangling cord; the CNS floats "head-up" in this liquid like a swimmer treading water. This buoyancy reduces the effective weight of the adult brain from around 1500 to about 50 g in the living body.

But the CSF does more than contribute to the physical environment of the CNS; it ensures, in its continuity with the extracellular fluid of neurons and neuroglial cells (see Chap. 15), a more nearly constant chemical environment than could be provided by the blood plasma. Furthermore, this fluid acts as a chemical sink for removal of waste products. CSF is continually sweeping over the inner (ependymal) and outer (pial) surfaces of the CNS, washing out solutes through specialized protrusions of the subarachnoid space (the arachnoidal villi) into the bloodstream — into the superior sagittal sinus, its lateral extensions, or certain similar regions near the dorsal roots of spinal nerves. Moreover, in addition to secreting CSF, the choroid plexuses actively extract many substances, including certain neurotransmitters, from the CSF.

Thus the CSF supports and bathes the brain and spinal cord, while the choroid plexuses and arachnoidal granulations act as a kind of "kidney" of the brain.

Cerebrospinal fluid, however, can be a liability in certain situations. When CSF circulation is blocked at some point (in the third ventricle, aqueduct, or elsewhere), hydrocephalus or "water on the brain" will result. Hydrocephalus may result from congenital improper development or from acquired damage (trauma, tumors, infections, etc.) to some part of the ventriculosubarachnoid pathway. Even a slight degree of obstruction, enough to prevent absorption from keeping pace with production, may in time lead to the cardinal sign of hydrocephalus, which is enlargement of some of or all of the brain ventricles, often associated with increased intracranial pressure (see Chap. 2).

The central canal of the spinal cord, the lumen of the original neural tube, is compressed and closed by adjacent structures and accumulation of debris in the course of later development. Hence the CSF draining into the fourth ventricle does not enter it. The central canal is in a sense the "bed of a dry river," in which fluid previously did flow and exert morphogenetic effects during embryonic development. Remnants of this cavity, filled with ependymal and glial cells or other debris, may still be seen here and there. Developmental anomalies or growth of glial cell tumors (astrocytomas) in the spinal cord may result in the formation of congenital or acquired fluid-filled cavities in this vestigial central canal. This condition is called hydromyelia (water on the spinal cord). The ependymal cells lining the canal also have pathological significance in that they are responsible for a major category of intraspinal tumors, the ependymomas.

General Concepts

The brain depends on appropriate cerebral blood flow for its oxygen, glucose, and other metabolites and for the removal of CO_2 and other waste products. Each minute, even at rest, the brain is bathed by about one-half its volume of blood. Anoxia (a decrease in cerebral oxygen) or ischemia (a decrease in cerebral blood flow), if prolonged for more than a few minutes below one-fifth average values, will certainly cause brain damage.

Cerebral circulation is well designed to deliver the amount of blood required and to protect against vascular insults. Blood enters the brain through two pairs of extracranial arteries. The large carotid arteries deliver about 85% of the brain's blood supply, the somewhat smaller vertebral arteries the remainder. The internal carotids and vertebral/basilar system join the circle of Willis, a vascular loop lying at the base of the brain. Various trunks leading from the circle of Willis supply the entire cerebral hemispheres. Abundant branching takes place — arteries break up into smaller vessels, and vessels continue to branch, eventually becoming microvessels. It is through the capillary endothelium of the microvessels that the interchanges between blood and brain are made. Unlike their systemic counterparts, both cerebral arteries and cerebral veins are thin-walled. The capillary endothelium is relatively quickly penetrated by some substances, but much less so by others, accounting for the so-called "blood-brain barrier." This differential filter regulates the entry of blood-borne substances into the brain, so that any fluctuations which may occur in blood composition are not reflected in the necessarily constant milieu of the brain. Venous drainage occurs through cortical parasagittal and basilar veins which enter the dural sinuses.

The cerebral vascular system is designed to minimize many vascular insults. For example, the circle of Willis provides a means for the brain to maintain its blood supply if one of the incoming arteries is somehow injured or occluded. The remaining arteries can compensate and deliver the necessary quantity of blood. Some lesser vessels also display multiple branching, which also protects against trauma.

The circulatory system is extremely sensitive to the greater and lesser needs of the brain tissue from moment to moment. Changes in vascular caliber and resistance alter blood pressure and blood flow so as to provide adequate supplies of oxygen and glucose. Cerebral blood flow is regulated regionally through the microvasculature. The flow is sensitive to the amount of brain activity and local concentrations of oxygen, hydrogen ions, cAMP, and cations.

The use of radioactive xenon (xenon-133) has opened up a new dimension in studying the cerebral vasculature. Through the continuous detection of patterns of radioactivity, a picture is created of the constantly changing blood flow. And because blood flow is related directly to brain activity, we see in these images a shadow of brain activity. The images remind us that all those connections which seem static as we learn them are dynamic thoroughfares engaged in moment-by-moment transactions.

Glossary

Anterior cerebral artery: the smaller, more anterior of the two terminal branches of the internal carotid; supplies the medial aspect and an adjoining narrow lateral zone along the anterosuperior curvature of the cerebral hemisphere as far posteriorly as the parieto-occipital fissure.

Anterior communicating artery: a short connecting vessel, sometimes not patent (or even present), joining the two anterior cerebrals just rostral to the optic chiasm.

Basal vein (Rosenthal): a major cerebral anastomotic channel connecting the deep and superficial venous systems of the brain; originates on the medial aspect of the anterior temporal region and drains into the great vein of Galen, receiving tributaries from temporal lobe, lower diencephalon, and mesencephalon en route.

Basilar artery: a large artery, formed by union of the two vertebrals at the caudal border of the pons, running directly upward toward the circle of Willis along the midline of the anterior surface of the brainstem; through numerous side branches, normally provides the sole blood supply to the pons, superior part of the cerebellum, midbrain, posterior thalamus, occipital lobe, and basomedial temporal lobe.

Carotid body: a small, neurovascular organ at the bifurcation of the common carotid artery serving as a peripheral chemoreceptor; contains specialized nerve endings sensitive to decreases in O_2 tension and increases in CO_2 tension and H^+ ion concentration in the blood. (The carotid body, and the closely related aortic body, generally respond only to extreme conditions.)

Carotid sinus: a dilated region of the internal carotid, just above the division of the common carotid, or of the common carotid itself, containing in its wall mechanoreceptors (pressoreceptors) sensitive to changes in blood pressure.

Cerebellar arteries: three pairs of arteries, derived from the vertebral-basilar system and similar to its long circumferential branches except for longer courses, supplying the inferior and superior surfaces of the cerebellum; the posterior inferior, anterior inferior, and superior cerebellar arteries.

Circle of Willis: a wreath of arteries at the base of the brain, ringing the optic chiasm and basal hypothalamus and fed by both the internal carotid and vertebral-basilar systems; cortical and central branches supply the entire cerebral cortex and the deeper gray and white matter of the cerebrum, respectively.

Dural sinuses: large, tough endothelial-lined channels between the outer (periosteal) and inner (meningeal) layers of the dura mater; receive blood from the larger cerebral veins and drain principally into the internal jugular veins.

Emissary veins: venous outlets from the dural sinuses to various extracranial veins, such as the frontal and nasal, ophthalmic, and occipital veins.

Inferior anastomotic vein (Labbé):   anastomotic channel on the lateral surface of the temporal lobe between the superficial middle cerebral vein and transverse sinus; important tributary in the superficial venous drainage of the cerebral hemisphere and radiographic landmark.

Internal carotid arteries: a pair of distributing arteries, beginning at the bifurcations of the common carotids, running upward in the neck to enter the base of the skull and eventually the cranial vault; branching at the circle of Willis into anterior and middle cerebral arteries, supply 85% of the cerebral blood flow and thus most of the blood to the brain.

Internal jugular veins: a pair of systemic veins, continuous with the transverse sinuses at the base of the skull; major venous outlets of the brain.

Middle cerebral artery: the larger, more posterior of the two terminal branches of the internal carotid artery; supplies most of the lateral surface of the cerebral hemisphere, including the insular region, and the anteromedial part of the temporal lobe.

Middle meningeal artery: largest and most important artery of the dura mater, supplying virtually its entire calvarial (skullcap) region; an intracranial branch of the maxillary artery.

Posterior cerebral arteries: bifurcated continuations of the basilar, forming the caudal part of the circle of Willis; supply the basomedial surfaces of the occipital and temporal lobes and an adjoining narrow lateral zone along the posteroinferior curvature of the cerebral hemisphere as far anteriorly as the parieto-occipital fissure.

Posterior communicating arteries: posteriorly directed branches of the internal carotids that anastomose with the posterior cerebral arteries as they fork from the basilar; complete the circle of Willis.

Superior anastomotic vein (Trolard):   anastomotic channel on the lateral surface of the frontoparietal region between the superficial middle cerebral vein and the superior sagittal sinus; see comments for inferior anastomotic vein.

Veins of the brain: all tributaries of the internal jugular, via the dural sinuses; thin-walled, and lack valves; divided into superficial and deep groups with numerous anastomoses.

Vertebral arteries: a pair of distributing arteries, beginning as the first branch of the subclavians, running upward in the neck to enter the base of the skull through the foramen magnum; unite at the caudal border of the pons to form the basilar artery and supply blood to the medulla oblongata and inferior part of the cerebellum. Also supply the cervical cord by way of posterior and anterior spinal branches, the latter of which unites with its opposite member.

Suggested References

Bloom, W. and D. W. Fawcett *A Textbook of Histology*, 10th Ed., W. B. Saunders, Philadelphia, 1975.

Brodal, A. *Neurological Anatomy in Relation to Clinical Medicine*. Oxford University Press, New York, 1981.

Bullock, T. H., R. Orkand, and A. Grinnell *Introduction to Nervous Systems*. W. H. Freeman, San Francisco, 1977.

Carpenter, M. B. *Core Text of Neuroanatomy*. Williams and Wilkins, Baltimore, 1972.

Carpenter, M. B. *Human Neuroanatomy*, 7th Ed. Williams and Wilkins, Baltimore, 1976.

Cooper, J. R., F. E. Bloom, and R. H. Roth *The Biochemical Basis of Neuropharmacology*, 3rd Ed. Oxford University Press, New York, 1978.

Copenhaver, W. M., D. E. Kelly, and R. L. Wood *Bailey's Textbook of Histology*, 17th Ed. Williams and Wilkins, Baltimore, 1978.

Cotman, C. W. and J. L. McGaugh *Behavioral Neuroscience: An Introduction*. Academic Press, New York, 1980.

Crosby, E. C., T. Humphrey, and E. W. Lauer *Correlative Anatomy of the Nervous System*. MacMillan, New York, 1962.

Dunkerley, G. B. *A Basic Atlas of the Human Nervous System*. F. A. Davis, Philadelphia, 1975.

Eccles, J. C. (ed.) *Brain and Conscious Experience*. Springer-Verlag, Heidelberg, 1966.

Edelman, G. and V. Mountcastle *The Mindful Brain*. MIT Press, Cambridge, Mass., 1978.

Eliasson, S. G., A. L. Prensky, and W. B. Hardin, Jr. (eds.) *Neurological Pathophysiology*. Oxford University Press, New York, 1974.

Gluhbegovic, N. and T. H. Williams *The Human Brain: A Photographic Guide*. Harper and Row, Hagerstown, Md., 1980.

Granit, R. *The Purposive Brain*. MIT Press, Cambridge, Mass., 1977.

Herrick, C. J. *The Brain of the Tiger Salamander, Ambystoma trigrinum*. University of Chicago Press, Chicago, 1948.

Herrick, C. J. *Neurological Foundations of Animal Behavior*. Hafner, New York, 1962.

Herrick, C. J. *Brains of Rats and Men*. Hafner, New York, 1963.

Holmes, G. (revised by B. Matthews) *Introduction to Clinical Neurology*, 3rd Ed. Williams and Wilkins, Baltimore, 1968.

Isaacson, R. L. *The Limbic System*. Plenum Press, New York, 1974.

Jacobson, M. *Developmental Neurobiology*, 2nd Ed. Plenum Press, New York, 1978.

Krieg, W. J. *Functional Neuroanatomy*, 3rd Ed. Brain Books, Evanston, Ill., 1966.

Kuffler, S. W. and J. C. Nicholls *A Cellular Approach to the Function of the Nervous System*. Sinauer Associates, Sunderland, Mass., 1976.

Langman, J. *Medical Embryology: Human Development—Normal and Abnormal*, 3rd Ed. Williams and Wilkins, Baltimore, 1975.

Ludwig, E. and J. Klingler *Atlas Cerebri Humani*. Little, Brown, Boston, 1956.

McGeer, P., J. C. Eccles, and E. McGeer *Molecular Neurobiology of the Mammalian Brain*. Plenum Press, New York, 1978.

Merritt, H. *A Textbook of Neurology*, 5th Ed. Lea and Febiger, Philadelphia, 1973.

Mettler, F. A. *Neuroanatomy*, 2nd Ed. Mosby, St. Louis, 1948.

Moore, K. L. *Study Guide and Review Manual of Human Embryology*. Saunders, Philadelphia, 1975.

Moore, K. L. *The Developing Human: Clinically Oriented Embryology*, 2nd Ed. Saunders, Philadelphia, 1977.

Mountcastle, V. B. (ed.) *Medical Physiology*, 13th Ed., Vol. I. Mosby, St. Louis, 1974.

Noback, C. R. *The Human Nervous System: Basic Principles of Neurobiology*. McGraw-Hill, New York, 1967.

Noback, C. R. and R. J. Demarest *The Nervous System: Introduction and Review*, 2nd Ed. McGraw-Hill, New York, 1977.

Palay, S. L. and V. Chan-Palay *Cerebellar Cortex: Cytology and Organization*. Springer-Verlag, Heidelberg, 1974.

Papez, J. W. *Comparative Neurology*. Crowell, New York, 1929.

Peele, T. L. *The Neuroanatomic Basis for Clinical Neurology*, 3rd Ed. McGraw-Hill, New York, 1977.

Penfield, W. *The Mystery of the Mind*. Princeton University Press, Princeton, 1975.

Penfield, W. and H. Jasper *Epilepsy and the Functional Anatomy of the Human Brain*. Little, Brown, Boston, 1954.

Penfield, W. and T. Rasmussen *The Cerebral Cortex of Man: A Clinical Study of Localization of Function*. MacMillan, New York, 1950.

Peters, A., S. L. Palay, and H. deF. Webster *The Fine Structure of the Nervous System: The Neurons and Supporting Cells*. Saunders, Philadelphia, 1976.

Popper, K. R. and J. C. Eccles *The Self and Its Brain*. Springer-Verlag, Heidelberg, 1977.

Ranson, S. W. and S. L. Clark *The Anatomy of the Nervous System: Its Development and Function*, 10th Ed. Saunders, Philadelphia, 1959.

Romer, A. S. *The Vertebrate Body*, 3rd Ed. Saunders, Philadelphia, 1962.

Sarnat, H. B. and M. G. Netsky *Evolution of the Nervous System*. Oxford University Press, New York, 1974.

Scientific American. September 1979, Vol. 241, No. 3 (a special issue on the brain).

Shepherd, G. M. *The Synaptic Organization of the Brain: An Introduction*. Oxford University Press, New York, 1974.

Sidman, R. L. and M. Sidman *Neuroanatomy: A Programmed Text*, Vol. I. Little,
    Brown, Boston, 1965.
Weiss, P. A. *The Science of Life: The Living System—A System for Living*. Futura, Mt.
    Kisco, N.Y., 1973.
Williams, P. L. and R. Warwick *Functional Neuroanatomy of Man*. Saunders,
    Philadelphia, 1975.
Willis, W. D., Jr. and R. G. Grossman *Medical Neurobiology*. Mosby, St. Louis, 1973.
Woolridge, D. E. *The Machinery of the Brain*. McGraw-Hill, New York, 1963.
Young, J. Z. *The Life of Mammals*. Oxford University Press, Oxford, 1957.
Young, J. Z. *The Life of Vertebrates*. Oxford University Press, New York, 1962.
Young, J. Z. *Programs of the Brain*. Oxford University Press, Oxford, 1978.

Index

Abducens nerve. *See* Cranial nerves, VI
Accessory olfactory bulb, 156, 163
Accommodation response, pupillary, 108–9
Acetylcholine (ACh), 193, 315–19, 345, 347, 351
Acetylcholinesterase (AChE), 315
ACh. *See* Acetylcholine
AChE. *See* Acetylcholinesterase
ACTH, 329, 342–43, 348
Action potential, 121
Adenohypophysis, 267–68, 279
Adrenaline. *See* Epinephrine
Adventitia of intracranial arteries, 363
Afterbrain. *See* Metencephalon
Aging, 323–24
    and sense of smell, 158
Agnosias, 302, 309
Agranular cortex, 293, 310
Alerting, 240–42
Alexia, 297
Allocortex, 286, 310–11
Allodendritic neurons, 246–47, 249
All-or-none signals, 121
Alpha motor neurons, 215–16, 222–23, 227, 242, 315
Alpha-MSH. *See* Melanocyte-stimulating hormone
Alzheimer's presenile dementia, 318
Amacrine cells, 6, 90–91, 112, 154, 163
Ambiguus nucleus, 137
Amino acids, 343–47, 350. *See also* Peptides
Amorphosynthesis, 302, 309

Ampulla, 76–77, 84
Amygdala, 36–37, 48, 163, 191–92, 253, 256–57, 265
    damage to, 299
Amygdaloid nuclear complex, 151, 157–58, 163, 324
Analgesia, 139. *See also* Endorphins; Enkephalins
Anesthetics, 134
Aneurysm, 365
Angiotensin II, 343
Angular gyrus, 301
Anomia, 297
Anosmia, 158
Anoxia, cerebral. *See* Cerebral anoxia
ANS. *See* Autonomic nervous system
Ansa lenticularis, 194
Anterior cerebral artery, 358–59, 361, 373
Anterior choroidal artery, 361
Anterior commissure, 269, 279, 338
Anterior communicating artery, 359, 373
Anterior dorsal (AD) nucleus, of thalamus, 170–71, 173–74
Anterior hypothalamic area, 279
Anterior lobe of pituitary. *See* Adenohyphophysis
Anterior medial (AM) nucleus, of thalamus, 170–71, 173–74
Anterior median fissure, of spinal cord, 210–11, 227
Anterior nuclear group, of thalamus, 170–71, 173–74, 181–82, 264

Anterior olfactory nucleus, 155–56, 163
Anterior perforated substance, 360
Anterior (ventral) roots, of spinal cord, 212, 227
Anterior speech cortex. See Broca's area
Anterior ventral (AV) nucleus, of thalamus, 170–71, 173–74
Anterior white commissure, of spinal cord, 212, 227
Anterolateral system, 129, 133–34, 146, 220–21, 227, 235
Anterolateral white column, 146
Antidepressants, 332
Aphasias, 297, 301, 309
Appendicular muscles, 226
Archispinothalamic tract, 134, 138
Arcuate nucleus, 272, 279, 343, 336–37
Arousal, 240–42
Arteriosclerosis, 357
Ascending reticular activating system, 234, 249
Ascending spinal fibers, 200
Aspartate, 346–47, 350–51
Association cortex, 158, 286–87, 293, 306–8, 311
Association fibers, 37, 48, 294, 296
Association nuclei, of thalamus, 169, 174–75
Astereognosia, 302
Astrocytes, 10–11
Astrocytomas, 372
Ataxia, 198
Atopognosia, 302
Audition, 298–300
Auditory association cortex. See Wernicke's area
Auditory cortex, 65–70, 294, 299
Auditory ganglia, 7
Auditory pathway, 63–70, 100, 142
Auditory reflexes, 67–68
Auditory system, 54–72
    central circuitry, 63–67
    functional correlates, 67–69
    inner ear, 55–59
    place coding, 62–63
    relation of auditory sensations to vestibular and somatic sensations, 78–79
    tonotopy, 57–61
Autonomic ganglia, 11, 48, 216–17
Autonomic nervous system (ANS), 41–48
    hypothalamus, 278
    neurotransmitters, 315
    visceral sensations, 116
Awareness of self, 244–45
Axial muscles, 226

Axonal firing pattern, 121
Axon collaterals, 249–50
Axons, 5–7

Baillarger, bands of. See Inner band of Baillarger; Outer band of Baillarger
Basal ganglia, 18, 34, 36, 48, 191–97
    limbic system, 265, 278–79
    motor system, 185, 205–6
    neurotransmitters, 318, 320–23, 344–45
Basal vein (Rosenthal), 366–67, 373
Basilar artery, 358–60, 362, 372–74
Basilar membrane, 57, 61, 70
Basket cells, 201–4, 206, 344
Behavior, 305–6
    and autonomic nervous system, 47
    role of serotonin in, 332, 334
    thalamic lesions and, 181
Betweenbrain. See Diencephalon
Betz cells, 189, 206–7, 289, 293, 311
Bipolar neurons, 4, 7, 122, 124
    olfactory system, 151
    retinal, 40, 90–91, 112
    spiral ganglion, 63, 117
    vestibular ganglion, 117
Blind spots (scotomata), 109–10
Blood-brain barrier, 323, 365–66, 372
Blood circulation. See Circulation of the brain
Blood pressure, 355, 368. See also Hypertension
Blood pressure tension receptor, of carotid sinus, 363
Bodily sensations. See Sensations, somatic
Body movements and position, detection and sense of, 74–79, 116. See also Motor system
Body schema, 301, 309
Bony (osseous) labyrinth, 71, 74, 85
Brachium conjunctivum. See Superior cerebellar peduncle
Brachium of inferior colliculus, 170–71, 182
Brachium pontis. See Middle cerebellar peduncle
Brain. See also specific parts of the brain
    cavities, 31–34
    circulation, 354–75
    dissected, 34–39
    edema, 365
    fundamental parts, 14–20
    lateral aspect, 21–24
    sagittal aspect, 24–30
Brain death, 356
Brainstem, 27, 48–49. See also specific structures
    circulation, 358, 360, 362–63, 366

motor system, 185, 205
neurotransmitters, 319, 329, 331–34, 341,
    346
pain-transmission neurons, 141
Brainstem norepinephrine neuron system.
    See Lateral tegmental norepinephrine
    system
Brain tone, 327
Broca, Pierre Paul, 254, 309
Broca's area, 301, 309
Brodmann's areas, 287–88
    areas 1–3, 130, 300
    area 4, 300
    area 6, 305
    areas 8–12, 305
    area 17, 114, 297–98
    area 18, 297–98
    area 41, 65, 299
    area 42, 299
    areas 44–47, 305
Bulbar extensor-facilitatory area, 250
Bulbar extensor-inhibitory area, 242, 250
Bundle of Schütz. *See* Dorsal longitudinal
    fasciculus

Cajal, horizontal cells of. *See* Horizontal
    cells of Cajal
Calcarine fissure, 101–2, 112
Capillaries, 365, 372
Carbon dioxide concentration, and blood
    flow, 368
Cardiac activities, and reticular formation,
    243
Cardiac arrest, 356
Cardiac muscle, 43, 317
Cardiovascular reflexes, 363
Carotid arteries, 357, 372
Carotid body, 363, 374
Carotid sinus, 362–63, 374
Cascade concept, 306–7
Catecholamine, 276, 319, 351
Caudate nucleus, 6, 34, 36, 49, 191–93
    neurotransmitters, 318, 320–21, 336, 339,
    341, 345, 347
CCK. *See* Cholecystokinin
Celiac ganglion, 12
Cell body, neuron, 7, 24
    cerebral cortex, 26
    primary somesthetic neurons, 122
    projection neuron, 5
Central canal, of spinal cord, 10, 210, 227,
    372
Central gray substance, 257, 336
Central lobe, 49, 284, 302–3, 309–10
Central nervous system (CNS), 14–20. *See
    also specific components*

compensatory capacity, 110
dendrites, 5
distribution of receptors, 120
local-circuit neurons, 6
myelin, 6
place coding, 62–63
synapses, 6
Central sulcus (of Rolando), 21, 49, 130,
    141, 143, 284
Central tegmental tract of locus coeruleus
    system, 327, 331
Centromedian (CM) nucleus, of thalamus,
    170–71, 174, 176, 182, 194
Cerebellar arteries, 362, 374
Cerebellar cortex, 27, 197, 201–4,
    207
    GABA neurons, 344
Cerebellar peduncles, 37, 39, 49, 197. *See
    also* Inferior, Middle, and Superior
    cerebellar peduncles.
Cerebellum, 15, 19, 27, 49
    circulation, 358, 362
    damage to, 198–200
    motor system, 185, 194, 197–206
    neurotransmitters, 326–27, 332, 334, 347
    regulation of movement and posture,
    79–80
    vestibulo-ocular reflex, 83–84
Cerebral anoxia, 356, 365, 372
Cerebral aqueduct (of Sylvius), 31
Cerebral arteries, 368
Cerebral cortex, 18–19, 21, 24, 26, 34, 49,
    284–313. *See also* Auditory cortex; Gus-
    tatory cortex; Motor cortex; Olfactory
    cortex; Orbitofrontal cortex; Somes-
    thetic cortex; Visual cortex
    areas, 286–89
    cascade concept, 306–7
    columnar organization, 66, 103–105,
    143–144, 188, 293–95, 310–11
    efferent modulation, 137–38
    inputs and outputs, 294–96
    laminar organization, 291–93, 311
    laterality and dominance, 308–9
    lesions, 297, 299, 301–2, 305–6, 308–10
    and limbic system, 265–66, 278
    lobes, 296–306
    local-circuit neurons, 6
    maps, 177, 179
    motor system, 205
    neurons, 246, 289–91, 310
    neurotransmitters, 324, 333, 336, 341–42,
    344, 347
    vestibular nuclei projections, 81
Cerebral hemispheres, 18–19, 49, 308–9
Cerebral infarction, 365, 368

Cerebral ischemia, 356–57, 365, 368, 372
Cerebral veins, 366–68
Cerebrospinal fluid (CSF), 10, 31, 33–34, 343, 354, 371–72
Cerebrum, 15, 18–19, 21, 23, 49
  circulation, 355–73
  cortex. See Cerebral cortex
  lesions, 198
  lobes, 284–85
  metabolism, 355–56
  relation to cerebellum, 198
ChAc. See Choline acetyltransferase
Chemical coding of neural circuits. See Neurotransmitters
Chemoreceptors, 120
Cholecystokinin (CCK), 342, 351
Choline acetyltransferase (ChAc), 315
Cholinergic neurons, 193–95, 214, 315, 317–19
Choroid plexuses, 10, 31–33, 49, 371
Ciliary ganglion, 107–8, 112
Ciliary muscle, 109
Cingulate gyri, 27, 49, 253–54, 264, 277
Cingulum, 264–65, 279, 324
Circle of Willis, 357, 359–60, 362, 372–74
Circulation of the brain, 354–75
  anatomy of, 357–68
  failure of, and neuronal dysfunction, 356–57
  protective mechanisms, 362–63, 373
  regulation and measurement of, 368–72
Cisterna magna, 34
Climbing fibers, 201, 204, 207
CNS. See Central nervous system
Coagulation necrosis, 356
Cochlea, 56, 57–59, 71, 78
  response to sound frequencies, 61–62
Cochlear duct, 56, 57, 63
Cochlear nerve, 71
Cochlear nuclei, 63–64, 71
Columnar epithelial cells, 7
Commissural fibers, 37, 49, 296
Commissurotomy, 305, 309
Common carotid artery, 357
Conditioning, of autonomic nervous system, 47
Cones, of retina. See Rods and cones
Consciousness, disorders of, 181. See also Behavior
Consciousness, loss of, 305, 356
Cordbrain. See Myelencephalon
Cornea, 88
Corona radiata, 49–50, 189
Corpus callosum, 27, 50, 284, 305
Cortex, 11. See also Cerebellar cortex; Cerebral cortex

Corticobulbar fibers, 207
Corticopontine fibers, 37
Corticopontocerebellar pathway, 198
Corticospinal tract, 97, 189, 206–7, 220
Corticostriate tract, 347
Corticothalamic projections, 178, 296
Cranial nerves, 8, 21–22, 39–41, 50
  I (olfactory), 22, 39–40, 154, 158, 165
  II (optic), 22, 39–40, 91, 95–97, 100, 112
  III (oculomotor), 22, 40–41, 315, 317
  IV (trochlear), 22, 40, 315, 317
  V (trigeminal), 22, 40, 122–23, 135–36, 315, 317
  VI (abducens), 22, 40, 315, 317
  VII (facial), 22, 40–41, 122, 159–61, 163, 315, 317
  VIII (vestibulocochlear), 22, 56, 72, 79, 200
  IX (glossopharyngeal), 22, 40–41, 122, 159–61, 163–64, 315, 317
  X (vagus), 22, 40–41, 122, 159–61, 163, 165, 315, 317
  XI (spinal accessory), 22, 40, 315, 317
  XII (hypoglossal), 22, 40, 315, 317
Cristae ampullares, 73, 75–78, 85
Crossroads between motor and limbic systems, 265–66, 278
Crura cerebri, 30, 170–71, 189
CSF. See Cerebrospinal fluid
Cuneate nucleus, 127, 130, 137, 146
Cupula, 73, 77, 85
Cutaneous sensation. See Skin

DA. See Dopamine
Dale's principle, 341, 350
Deep sensation, 116
Deiter's nucleus, 205
Dendrites, 5–7, 246–48
Dendrodendritic synapses, 7, 154–55
Dentate gyrus, 347
Dentate nucleus, 170–72, 194–96, 198, 200, 202, 207
Dentatorubrothalamic tract, 173, 182
Dentato(rubro)thalamocortical pathway, 198
Depression, 332, 334
Dermatomes, 122–23
Descending spinal system of substance P neuron system, 339–40
Diagonal band, 265, 279
Diencephalon (betweenbrain), 18–19, 31, 50
  neurotransmitters, 332–33, 338
  venous drainage, 366
Diffuse thalamocortical activating system, 250

Dominant hemisphere, 308–9
Dopamine (DA), 193–95, 260–62, 319–26,
    345, 347, 348–51
Dopaminergic nigrostriatal system, 193
Dorsal longitudinal fasciculus, 235, 277–79,
    327
Dorsal motor vagal nucleus, 137
Dorsal root filament, 127
Dorsal root ganglia, 8, 122–23, 146
    neurotransmitters, 339, 341–42
Dorsomedial nucleus, 269–70, 280
Drinking center, 273
Dural sinuses, 366–68, 374
Dura mater, 34, 366
Dysesthesia, 116

Ear, 55–62
    tympanic membrane, 56, 72
    vestibular receptors, 73–79
Edema, brain, 357
Edinger-Westphal nucleus, 107–8, 113
Efferent modulation, 137–38, 141, 216–17,
    225–26
Efferent neurons, 214, 296, 310
Emboliform nucleus, 202
Embolism, 354, 356
Embryonic central nervous system, 14,
    16–18, 31
Emissary veins, 374
Emotions, 167–68, 173, 254, 261, 305
Encapsulated nerve endings, 118–19
Endbrain. See Telencephalon
Endolymph, 56, 57, 71, 76, 85
Endorphins, 141, 334, 336, 338–39, 384–51
Enkephalins, 141, 193, 334–37, 348–51
Entorhinal area, 158, 163, 265, 324, 347
Ependymal cells, 10–11, 334
Ependymomas, 372
Epidural hematoma, 366
Epiglottis, 159, 161
Epilepsy, 159, 305
Epinephrine (adrenaline), 319–20, 331–32,
    348, 351
Epineurium, 11
Epithelial cells, modified, 117
Equilibrium, 198
Estradiol, 277
Ethical conduct. See Behavior
Eustachian tube, 71
Evolution of nervous system, 21, 23–24, 134
Expanded-tip nerve endings, 118–19
Extensor muscles, 185–86, 198, 206, 224,
    242
External auditory meatus, 56, 71
External granular layer (layer II), of cerebral
    cortex, 291, 311

External pyramidal layer (layer III), of
    cerebral cortex, 291, 311
Exteroceptors, 120
Extrafusal fibers, 221, 227
Extraocular muscles, 214
Eye, 87–95. See also Visual system
Eye movements, 77, 79, 81, 84, 100, 105–9

Face, 135–36, 304
Facial nerve. See Cranial nerves, VII
Fasciculi proprii, 219, 227
Fasciculus, 227
Fasciculus cuneatus, 127, 218, 220, 227–28
Fasciculus gracilis, 127, 218, 220, 228
Fasciculus interfascicularis, 218
Fasciculus lenticularis, 194
Fasciculus retroflexus, 269, 280
Fastigial nucleus, 202
Fatigue, muscle, 214, 216
Feedback control, 82–83, 186, 225
Feed-forward control, 83–84, 216
Feeding center, 276
Fields of Forel, 170–71, 173, 182, 195
Fight or flight responses, 278
Filament, 127
Fila olfactoria, 154, 163
Finger movements, 304
Fissures, 21, 50, 284
Flexor motor neurons, 219–20
Flexor muscles, 185–86, 198, 206
Flocculonodular lobe of cerebellum, 80–81,
    85, 197–98, 200
Food intake, regulation of, 273, 276
Foramen of Magendie, 33
Foramina of Luschka, 33
Forebrain. See Prosencephalon
Forel's fields. See Fields of Forel
Fornix, 27, 50, 254, 261, 264, 268–69
Fourth-order somesthetic neuron, 125
Fourth ventricle, 31–34
Fovea centralis, 79, 81, 89, 113
Foveation, 73, 81, 106
Free nerve endings, 118–19
Frequency, sound, 57, 61–62, 66
Frequency of stimulus, coding of, 121
Frontal cortex, 278
Frontal gyri, 303
Frontal lobes, 28, 50, 265–66, 284–86,
    303–6, 310
Frontal pole, 305
Frontotemporal cortex, 265
Functional column of cortex, 103, 293–94

GABA (gamma-aminobutyric acid), 193,
    204, 314, 343–47, 350, 352
GAD. See Glutamic acid decarboxylase

Gage, Phineas P., 305
Gamma-aminobutyric acid. *See* GABA
Gamma loop, in stretch reflex, 222–23
Gamma motor neurons, 216, 222–23, 228, 242
Ganglion, 11–12
Ganglion cells, 40, 43, 90–92, 94–96, 102–3, 105–8, 113
Gasserian ganglion. *See* Trigeminal ganglion
Generalized thalamocortical system, 168
Generator potential, 121
Geniculate bodies, 169. *See also* Lateral geniculate nucleus; Medial geniculate nucleus
Geniculate ganglion of cranial nerve VII, 160
Geniculocalcarine tracts, 98
Gennari, stripe of. *See* Stripe of Gennari
Glial cells, 10–11, 286
Glial cell tumors, 11, 372
Global aphasia, 301
Globose nucleus, 202
Globus pallidus, 170–73, 191–93, 194–96, 207, 265
  lesions, 181
  neurotransmitters, 317, 323, 335–36, 344
Glomeruli, 154, 164, 201, 207
Glucoreceptors, 276
Glucose, 276, 354–55, 368
Glutamate, 346–49, 360, 352
Glutamic acid decarboxylase (GAD), 344–45
Glycine, 346, 350, 352
Glycoprotein, 74
Gnostic function, of parietal lobe, 300–302
Golgi, Camillo, 5
Golgi's tissue staining method, 234
Golgi tendon organs, 117, 224, 228
Golgi Type I cells, 237, 250, 344
Golgi Type II cells, 201–3, 207, 250, 343
Gonadotropin, 329
Gracile nucleus, 127, 130, 137–38, 146
Granular cortex, 289, 293, 305, 311
Granular layer, of cerebellar cortex, 202
Granule cells, 194, 201–4, 208
Gravireceptors (graviceptors), 120
Gray matter, 12, 24–27
  astrocytes, 10
  basal ganglia, 34, 36
  cerebrum, 18
  spinal cord, 210, 212, 219–20
Growth hormone, 272, 329, 341–42
Growth hormone-release inhibiting hormone. *See* Somatostatin
Gustatory cortex, 159, 162–64, 301
Gustatory hallucinations, 159, 301

Gustatory nucleus, 161–62
Gustatory receptors, 159–60
Gustatory system, 159–65
Gyri, 21, 23, 50

Habenula, 253, 256, 280, 318–19
Habenular nuclei, 265–66, 339, 341
Habenulointerpeduncular tract, 317, 319, 339, 341
Hair cells, 56, 57–60, 63, 67, 71, 73–74, 76–77, 84–85, 117
Hallucinations, 300
  and serotonin levels, 334
  uncinate fits, 159, 162, 299
Handedness, 308
Head injuries, 158–59, 366. *See also specific parts of the brain*
Head movements, 76–79, 81, 84, 299
Hearing. *See* Audition
Heart. *See entries under* Cardiac
Hemiataxia, 198
Hemiballismus, 193–95
Hemiparesis (hemiparalysis), 181, 198
Hemorrhage, 354, 357, 365
Heschl's gyrus, 65
Heterotypical cortex, 293, 311
Hindbrain. *See* Rhombencephalon
Hippocampus, 253–54, 256–57, 261–64, 280
  lesions, 261
  neurotransmitters, 336, 344
Histamine, 319
Histofluorescence, 319
Homeostasis, 267, 273, 279, 329
Homotypical cortex, 293, 311
Homunculus. *See* Motor homunculus; Sensory homunculus
Horizontal cells of Cajal, 291, 312
Horizontal cells of retina, 90–91
Hormones, 277, 343. *See also* Pituitary hormones; *names of specific hormones*
5-HT. *See* Serotonin
Huntington's chorea, 193–95, 318, 341, 345
Hydrocephalus, 31, 34, 371
Hydromyelia, 372
Hypercarbia, 368
Hypercolumn (macrocolumn), 103, 294, 312
Hyperemia, 357
Hyperesthesias, 181
Hypertension, 364
Hypocarbia, 368
Hypoglossal nerve. *See* Cranial nerves, XII
Hypoglossal nucleus, 12
Hypophagia, 276
Hypophysis. *See* Pituitary gland
Hypothalamic diencephalic pontine endorphin system, 338

Hypothalamohypophysial tract. *See*
    Neurohypophysial tract
Hypothalamus, 27, 29–30, 43, 50, 172–73,
    253–54, 256–57, 260–61, 263–64,
    267–83
    circulation, 359
    control of pituitary hormone release,
        270–72
    lesions, 276
    neuronal inputs, 273–74, 276
    neuronal outputs, 275–78
    neurotransmitters, 320, 326–27, 329,
        331–32, 336–38, 342–43
    taste and smell, 163
    vascular and hormonal influences on,
        273, 276–77
Hypotonia, 198

Idiodendritic neurons, 246–47, 250
Incertohypothalamic dopamine neuron
    system, 321, 324
Incus, 56, 60
Indoleamines, 319
Inferior anastomotic vein (Labbé), 366–67,
    374
Inferior cerebellar peduncle, 19, 37, 200, 235
Inferior colliculus, 30, 50, 65–66, 71, 170–71
Inferior fronto-occipital fasciculus, 265
Inferior olivary nucleus, 194, 200, 204, 208
Information storage and retrieval. *See*
    Memory
Inhibiting factor (hypothalamic hormone),
    271–72
Inhibition, in cerebellar cortex, 204
Inner band of Baillarger, 312
Inner ear, 55–62, 73–79
Insomnia, 243, 332, 334
Insula (island) of Reil. *See* Central lobe
Insulin, 276
Intermediate gray, of spinal cord, 189
Internal capsule, 36, 50, 170–71, 181, 189
Internal carotid arteries, 357–61, 372, 374
Internal elastic membrane, of cerebral
    arteries, 364
Internal granular layer (layer IV), of
    cerebral cortex, 291, 312
Internal granule cells, 154–55, 164
Internal jugular veins, 375
Internal medullary lamina, of thalamus,
    182–83
Internal pallidum, 194
Internal pyramidal layer (layer V), of
    cerebral cortex, 293, 312
Interneurons (internuncial neurons), 8, 12,
    20
    olfactory system, 155
    spinal, 210, 212, 217, 224–26, 229

striatal, 317
Interoceptors, 120
Interpeduncular nucleus, 257, 269, 280
    neurotransmitters, 317–19, 339, 341
Interthalamic adhesion, 168
Interventricular foramen (of Monro), 31
Intradiencephalic dopamine neuron
    system. *See* Incertohypothalamic
    dopamine neuron system
Intrafusal fibers, 216, 221, 228
Intralaminar nuclei, 133, 146–47, 169,
    174–76, 181, 183
Intramesencephalic ganglion, 137
Intraneural receptors, 120
Ipsilateral flexor muscle, 198
Ischemia, cerebral. *See* Cerebral ischemia
Isocortex, 286, 293, 312
    neurotransmitters, 321, 327
Isodendritic neurons, 246–48, 250

Jackson, John Hughlings, 305
Jacksonian fit, 305
Joints, 121–22, 301
Jugular veins, 366–67, 375
Juxtarestiform body, 200

Kainic acid, 195
Kinocilium, 56, 71, 73, 77, 85
Klüver-Bucy syndrome, 299
Knee-jerk test, 225
Koniocortex. *See* Granular cortex

Laminae of Rexed, 189, 212–13, 228
Lamina IX, of spinal gray, 224
Lamination, cellular, 94–95
Language functions, 297, 301, 308–9
Lateral cervical nucleus (LCN), 127, 130,
    132, 147
Lateral cervical system, 129
Lateral corticospinal tract, 189, 220
Lateral dorsal (LD) nucleus, of thalamus,
    169–71, 174–75, 183
Lateral fissure (of Sylvius), 21, 50, 284
Lateral forebrain bundle, 280
Lateral geniculate nucleus (LGN), of
    thalamus, 95, 97–98, 100–103, 108–9,
    113, 169–72, 174, 183
Lateral habenular nucleus, 265
Lateral hypothalamic area, 257, 270, 276,
    280
    enkephalin, 336
Lateral lemniscus, 65, 71, 170–71
Lateral olfactory striae, 156–59, 347
Lateral posterior (LP) nucleus, of thalamus,
    106, 169–71, 173–75, 183
Lateral reticular nucleus, 201, 232, 250–51
Lateral reticulospinal tract, 242

Lateral tegmental (brainstem)
  norepinephrine system, 326–27,
  329–30
Lateral ventricle, 27, 31, 33
Layers I–VI of cerebral cortex. *See* External
  granular layer; External pyramidal
  layer; Internal granular layer; Internal
  pyramidal layer; Molecular layer;
  Multiform layer
LCN. *See* Lateral cervical nucleus
L-dopa, 195, 314, 323
Lemniscal nuclei. *See* Relay nuclei
Lemniscal pathway, 127–31, 137, 147, 183
  evolutionary perspective, 134
Lens of eye, 88, 109, 113
Light response, pupillary, 107–9
Limbic forebrain, 257, 259–61, 278
Limbic forebrain–limbic midbrain circuit,
  258–59, 265
Limbic lobe, 27, 50, 253–57, 261, 264,
  284–85, 310
Limbic midbrain, 257–61, 278
Limbic striatum. *See* Nucleus accumbens
Limbic system, 43, 50–51, 172–73, 253–83
  components, 255–56
  function, 261–66
  interconnections, 257–61
Lobes of the brain, 296–306
Local-circuit neurons, 3, 5–7
Locus coeruleus, 202, 243, 251, 296
  neurotransmitters, 326–28, 331–32, 339
Long circumferential artery, 360, 362–63
LSD, 332
Lumbar cistern, 34
Luteinizing hormone-releasing hormone,
  343

MacLean, Paul, 254
Macrocolumn. *See* Hypercolumn
Macrosmats, 154, 158
Macula, of vestibular system, 74–75, 77–78,
  85
Macula lutea, of retina, 89, 101–2, 113
Macular sparing, 102, 297
Macular vision, 101
Malleus, 56, 60
Mammillary bodies, 170–73, 264, 267,
  269–70, 281
Mammillary peduncle, 281
Mammillotegmental tract, 277, 281
Mammillothalamic tract, 170–71, 173, 183,
  261, 277
Mandibular nerve, 123
Mania, and serotonin levels, 334
Maps, sensory. *See* Sensory maps
Martinotti cell, 291, 312

Mastication, 137
Maxillary nerve, 123
Mechanoreceptors, 120–21
Medial corticospinal tract, 189
Medial dorsal (MD) nucleus, of thalamus,
  169–71, 174–75, 181, 183
Medial forebrain bundle (MFB), 258,
  260–61, 265, 281, 327, 329
Medial geniculate (MG) nucleus, of
  thalamus, 65–66, 71, 98, 169–72, 174,
  183
Medial lemniscus, 127, 130, 147, 162,
  170–71, 183, 224, 235
Medial longitudinal fasciculus (MLF), 81,
  85, 106, 228, 235
Medial reticulospinal tract, 242
Median eminence, 272, 277, 281, 342
Medulla oblongata, 15, 20, 51
  influence on extensor muscles, 242
  neurotransmitters, 331–32, 334, 336, 339,
  341, 346
Meissner's corpuscles, 118, 147
Melanocyte-stimulating hormone, 343
Membranous labyrinth, 71, 74, 78, 85
Memory, 68, 261, 284, 298
Meningeal arteries, 366, 368
Meningiomas, surgical removal of, 368
Meningitis, 34
Merkel's discs, 118
Mesencephalic nucleus of nerve V, 137, 147
Mesencephalon (midbrain), 18, 30, 51
  embryonic, 31
  neurotransmitters, 320, 324, 332–34, 336
  pupillary responses to light, 107
Mesocortical dopamine system, 321, 324–25
Mesotelencephalic dopamine system,
  320–24
Metabolism, 355–56, 368
Metencephalon (afterbrain), 18–19, 31, 51
Meyer's loop, 98
MFB. *See* Medial forebrain bundle
Microcirculation of the brain, 365–66
Microglia, 10
Microvilli, of hair cells, 57
Midbrain. *See* Mesencephalon
Middle cerebellar peduncle, 19, 37, 200
Middle cerebral artery, 358–61, 375
Middle meningeal artery, 366, 375
Middle (tuberal) nuclear group, of
  hypothalamus, 267, 270
Middle nuclear group, of thalamus, 169,
  174–76, 181, 183
Milk ejection reflex, 271
Minor hemisphere, 309
Mitral cells, 154–55, 158, 164
MLF. *See* Medial longitudinal fasciculus

Modulation in the central nervous system, 67, 137–41, 216–17, 225–26
Molecular layer, of cerebellar cortex, 202
Molecular layer (layer I), of cerebral cortex, 291, 312
Monoamines, 319–34, 347, 352
Monosynaptic extensor reflex, 224–25
Mood swings, and serotonin levels, 334
Mossy fibers, 201, 204, 208
Motivational aspects of behavior, 261, 265
Motor aphasia, 301
Motor cortex, 141, 185–91, 194, 198, 205–6, 293, 304–5
    electrical mapping, 304
Motor homunculus, 143, 187–88, 206, 304–5
Motor neuron-Renshaw cell acetylcholine system, 317
Motor neurons, 4–5, 8, 12, 42, 51, 185, 210, 212–20, 222–26
    modulation, 67, 137
Motor system, 185–209
    basal ganglia, 191–97
    brainstem components, 205
    cerebellum, 79–80, 197–204
    limbic system, 265–66, 278
    reticular formation, 242
Motor unit, 214, 228
Movements. See Body movements; Eye movements; Head movements; Motor system; Reflexes
Multiform layer (layer VI) of cerebral cortex, 292–93, 312
Multiple representation, in central nervous system, 142
Multipolar neurons, 8–9, 42, 124–25
Muscle afferent system, 116–17
Muscle contraction, 214, 216, 222–24, 315
Muscles. See Cardiac muscle; Skeletal muscles; Smooth muscles
Muscle sense, 116
Muscle spindles, 117, 216, 221, 224, 228
Muscle tone, 214
Myelencephalon (cordbrain), 18, 20, 31, 51
Myelin, 6, 10, 26

Nasal passages, 136, 151–52
NE. See Norepinephrine
Neocortex, 286, 292–93, 312
Neoplasma, 11, 372
Neospinothalamic tract, 134
Nerve cell body. See Cell body
Neural crest cells, 137
Neural tube, 16
Neuroglial cells, 10–11
Neurohypophysial tract, 270–71, 281

Neurohypophysis, 267–68, 281
Neuromuscular junction, 214, 317
Neuron doctrine, 3, 105
Neurons, 3–9. See also specific types of neurons and specific structures
Neuropeptides. See Peptides
Neuropil, 48, 251, 329
Neurotensin, 343
Neurotransmitters, 180, 193–96, 314–53
Nigrostriatal dopamine projections, 320–24
Nissl substance, 289
Nociceptive pathway, 133, 138–41. See also Pain
Nociceptive/tactile anterolateral system, 201
Nociceptors, 120–21
Nodosal ganglion of cranial nerve X, 160
Nonlemniscal channels, 175, 183
Nonspecific thalamic nuclei, 251
Norepinephrine (noradrenaline; NE), 180, 202, 243, 314, 317, 319–20, 326–30, 348–50, 352, 368
Nosebrain. See Rhinencephalon
Nuclei with widespread connections, thalamic, 169, 174–76
Nucleus, 12
Nucleus accumbens, 254, 265–66, 281, 324, 336
Nucleus basalis, 318
Nucleus cuneiformis, 244–45
Nucleus gigantocellularis, 246, 251
Nucleus reticularis, 332
Nucleus reuniens, 176, 183
Nucleus solitarius, 159, 161–64, 265
Nystagmus, 81

Occipital cortex, 109
Occipital coup, 159
Occipital lobe, 29, 51, 95, 102, 284–85, 297, 309
Ocular dominance columns, of visual cortex, 103–4, 111, 113
Oculomotor nerve. See Cranial nerves, III
Oculomotor nuclear complex, 107–8
Olfactory brain. See Rhinencephalon
Olfactory bulb, 150–51, 154–55, 158–59, 164
    neurotransmitters, 321, 324, 326, 347
Olfactory cells, 152, 154, 164
Olfactory cortex, 151, 158–59, 164
Olfactory epithelium, 7, 152, 164
Olfactory gyri, 156, 164
Olfactory hallucinations, 159, 299
Olfactory nerve. See Cranial nerves, I
Olfactory receptors, 150–54
Olfactory rods, 151
Olfactory striae, 156–59, 165

Olfactory systems, 150–59, 162–65
  functional and clinical correlations,
    158–59
  layout of, 151–59
Olfactory tract, 39, 151, 156–58, 165
Oligodendrocytes, 10
Oligodendroglia, 6
Olivary fibers, 200–201
Olivocochlear bundle, 66–67, 71
Opercular region, of cerebral cortex, 162
Ophthalmic nerve, 123
Opiate peptides. See Endorphins;
  Enkephalins
Opiate receptors, 141
Optic chiasm, 95–98, 113, 268–69, 357
Optic nerve. See Cranial nerves, II
Optic radiation, 113
Optic tract, 96–98, 113, 170–71
Oral cavity, 136
Orbital gyri, 303
Orbitofrontal cortex, 256–57, 260, 265, 281
Organ of Corti, 57–60, 72
Orientation columns, of visual cortex,
  103–5, 111, 114
Osmoreceptors, hypothalamic, 273
Osmotic pressure, regulation of, 273
Osseous labyrinth. See Bony labyrinth
Ossicles, 56, 60, 72
Outer band of Baillarger, 291, 313
Oxygen, 354–56, 368
Oxygen tension receptor, of carotid body,
  363
Oxytocin, 268, 270–71

P (small peptide substance). See Substance
  P
Pacinian corpuscles, 118–19, 147
Pain, 116, 119–21, 133, 138–41, 145, 334,
  341. See also Endorphins; Enkephalins
Paleospinothalamic tract, 134, 138–41
Pallidum. See Globus pallidus
Papez, James Wenceslas, 254
Papez circuit, 173, 260–61, 264
Papillae, of tongue, 160, 165
Parafascicular (Pf) nucleus, of thalamus,
  174, 176, 183
Parahippocampal gyri, 27, 51, 253–54, 264
Parainsular region, of cerebral cortex, 162
Parallel fibers, 201–3, 208, 347
Parallel processing, 92, 142, 177
Paramedian artery, 360, 362–63
Parasympathetic division of autonomic
  nervous system, 4, 41, 43–44, 315, 317
Paraventricular nucleus, of hypothalamus,
  268–70, 281–82
Paresthesia, 116, 181

Parietal lobe, 51, 141, 284–86, 300–302, 309
Parkinson's disease, 193–96, 314, 323,
  245
Patellar extensor reflex, 225
Pattern recognition, 146
Pedes pedunculi. See Crura cerebri
Peptides, 334–43, 348–50
Periaqueductal gray, 141, 147, 282
  neurotransmitters, 331–32, 339
Perilymph, 57, 72, 85
Peripheral nervous system (PNS), 11,
  20–21, 115
  neurotransmitters, 315, 335–36
  regulation of sensory input, 242
Peripheral vision, 101
Periventricular dopamine neuron system,
  321, 326
Periventricular fiber system, 282
Periventricular nucleus, of hypothalamus,
  268, 270, 273, 282, 342
Petrosal ganglion of cranial nerve IX, 160
pH, extracellular, and regulation of blood
  flow, 368
Phagocytes, 10
Pheromones, 151, 156
Photoreceptors, 120
Pia mater, 32
Piriform cortex, 347
Pituitary gland (hypophysis), 257, 267, 269,
  280, 329, 339
Pituitary hormones, 267–68, 270–72, 335,
  342
Place coding
  auditory system, 62–63
  somatic sensations, 121
PNS. See Peripheral nervous system
Pons, 15, 19, 51
  extensor-facilitatory region, 242
  motor system, 189
  neurotransmitters, 332, 336, 338–39, 346
  trigeminal system, 136
Pontine fibers, 200
Pontine nuclei, 194, 198, 200, 205, 208
Pontine tegmentum, 64, 72, 332
Pontocerebellar fibers, 37
Pontomedullary reticular formation, 194
Postcentral gyrus, 177
Posterior cerebral arteries, 180, 358–61, 375
Posterior choroidal artery, 361
Posterior column/medial lemniscus
  pathway, 129–31, 147–48
Posterior columns, of spinal cord, 127, 130,
  148, 219–20, 224, 228–29
Posterior communicating arteries, 359, 361,
  375
Posterior hypothalamic nucleus, 269–70

Posterior lobe of pituitary. *See* Neurohypophysis
Posterior median sulcus, of spinal cord, 210, 229
Posterior nuclear group, of thalamus, 174–76, 184
Posterior nucleus, of mammillary group of hypothalamus, 282
Posterior perforated substance, 360
Posterior (dorsal) roots, of spinal cord, 212, 229
Postganglionic neurons, 42, 107, 317
Posture, 79, 82, 84, 181, 198
Preganglionic neurons, 315, 317
Premammillary nucleus, 269, 336–37
Preoptic area, 256–57, 267, 336, 342
Preoptic nucleus, 269
Preopticohypothalamic area, 141
Prerubral nucleus, 194
Pressure, sensation of, 116, 119
Pretectal area, 107–8, 110, 114
Primary motor cortex, 189, 194, 208, 293, 304
Primary sensory neurons, 12–13, 51, 63, 226
   generator potentials, 121
   stretch reflex, 221
   substance P neuron system, 339–40
Primary somesthetic cortex (S I), 135, 141, 140–45, 148, 300, 302
Primary somesthetic neurons, 122–26, 130
Primary visual cortex, 95, 114, 298
Principal mammillary fasciculus, 227, 282
Principal sensory nucleus of nerve V, 136, 148
Progression (gait), 198
Projection neurons, 3–7, 37, 51–52, 294
Proprioceptors, 120
Propriospinal fibers, 219, 229
Prosencephalon (forebrain), 18, 162–63
   neurotransmitters, 326, 329
Pseudounipolar neutrons, 4, 8, 122, 124
   gustatory system, 160
   trigeminal system, 136–37
Psychic blindness and deafness, 302
Pulvinar, 98, 169–71, 174–75, 184
Pupillomotor cell, 107–8
Pupil of the eye, 87–88, 107–9, 114
Pure word deafness, 68
Purkinje cell, 4–5, 195, 201–4, 208, 247–48
   neurotransmitters, 344, 347
Putamen, 34, 36, 52, 191–93, 194
   neurotransmitters, 318, 321, 336, 345
Pyramidal cell, 4–5, 103, 189, 208, 289–93, 295–96, 313
Pyramidal decussation, 189, 208

Pyramidal tract, 189–90, 209, 235, 289, 296, 310
Pyriform lobe, 158

Ramón y Cajal, S., 5
Ramp movements, 196
Ramp stimuli, 119
Raphe nuclei, 141, 148, 251, 256–57, 260–62
   serotonin neurons, 332–34
   sleep, 242–43
Receptive aphasia, 301
Receptive field, of retina, 92, 94
Receptors, sensory, 200
   auditory, 56
   gustatory, 159–60
   olfactory, 151–54
   retinal. *See* Rods and cones
   somesthetic, 117–21
Red nucleus, 30, 170–71, 194, 198, 205, 209
Reflexes, 132
   cardiovascular, 363
   pupillary, 107–9
   reticular formation, influence of, 242
   spinal, 219, 221–25
   vestibular system, 81–82
   vomiting, 244
Reissner's membrane, 57, 72
Relay nuclei, of thalamus, 172–75
Releasing factor, 271–72
Renshaw cell, 225–26, 229, 315, 317
Respiratory activities, 243
Restiform body. *See* Inferior cerebellar peduncle
Reticular formation, 30, 52, 81, 205, 230–52, 257
   functions that depend on, 241–45
   limbic system's influence on, 265
   location and basic characteristics, 232–37
   neurotransmitters, 329, 331
   plan of connectivity in, 237–40
   unspecialized neurons, 246–48
Reticular neurons, 236–40, 246–48
Reticular nucleus, of thalamus, 169–71, 174, 176, 184, 201
Reticular pathway, 127–29, 131–34, 137, 148
Reticulospinal tracts, 205–6, 232, 242, 252
Retina, 39–40, 87, 89–95, 114
   bipolar neurons, 7
   GABA, 346
Retinal dopamine neuron system, 321, 326
Retinal field, 92–94
Retinotopy, 100–2, 177
Rexed's laminae. *See* Laminae of Rexed
Rhinal fissure, 158
Rhinencephalon, 150, 163, 165, 324

Rhombencephalon (hindbrain), 18
Rhomboid fossa, 31
Righting reflexes, 81–82
Rods and cones, of retina, 89–92, 113–14
Rolandic vein (of Trolard). *See* Superior
    anastomotic vein
Rolando, sulcus of. *See* Central sulcus (of
    Rolando)
Roof nucleus neuron, 203
Rubrospinal tract, 205
Ruffini's endings, 118, 148

Saccule, 74, 78, 85
Sacral nerves, 315
Sacral sparing, 221
Sagittal venous sinus, 366, 368
Salivatory nuclei, 137
Saltatory conduction, 6
Satiety center, of hypothalamus, 276
Scala tympani, 72
Scala vestibuli, 72
Schizophrenia, 320
Schwann cells, 6, 10, 158
Sclera, 114
Scotomata. *See* Blind spots
Seam nuclei. *See* Raphe nuclei
Secondary sensory neurons, 52, 64, 125–26,
    200, 212, 221
Secondary somesthetic cortex (S II),
    142–43, 148, 301
Self-awareness. *See* Awareness of self
Self-repair, capacity for, 112
Semicircular canals, 73, 75–76, 85
Semilunar ganglion. *See* Trigeminal
    ganglion
Semioval center, of cerebral hemisphere, 52
Sensations, somatic, 115–16
    blending of, 144
    relation to auditory and vestibular
        sensations, 78–79
    reticular formation's influence on, 242
    substance P, 341
Sensorimotor strip, 300, 366
Sensory coding, 121–25
Sensory homunculus, 136, 140–42, 162,
    187, 300
Sensory integration, 166–67, 300–2
Sensory maps, 177
    auditory, 59–63
    somesthetic, 121
    visual, 100–2
Sensory neurons, 8, 63–64, 125, 130, 212,
    221. *See also* Primary sensory neurons;
    Secondary sensory neurons
    allodendritic, 246
    axon terminals, 118–19
    modulation, 67, 137–38

specific sensitivity, 119
Septal area, 27, 52, 253, 256–57
    neurotransmitters, 324, 336
Septohippocampal tract, 317–18
Septum pellucidum, 27
Serotonin, 141, 242–43, 260–62, 319–20,
    332–34, 348–50, 352
Short circumferential artery, 360, 362–63
Signal-to-noise discrimination, 66
Sinus nerve, 363
Skeletal muscles, 117, 185–86, 206, 213–16,
    315
Skilled movements, 198
Skin
    segmental innervation, 123
    sensations, 116, 301
Sleep and sleeplike states, 242–43
Smell, sense of, 151, 156. *See also* Olfactory
    system
    hallucinations, 159, 299
    loss of, 158–59
    and taste, 159
Smooth muscles, 43, 217, 317
Somatic functions, regulation of, 47
Somatic motor neurons, 213–16
Somatosensory thalamus, 127
Somatostatin, 272, 341–42, 350, 353
Somatotopy, 177, 219–21
Somesthetic cortex, 127, 130, 135–36,
    300–301
    blending of sensations, 144
    columnar organization, 143–44, 294
    movements, supervision of, 186, 206
    topography of somesthesis, 140–45
Somesthetic neurons, 144–46
Somesthetic pathways, 100, 125–34
Somesthetic system, 115–49
    cascade concept, 307
    modulation of afferent signals, 137–38, 141
    receptors, 117–21
    sensory coding, 63, 121–25
    topography of somesthesis, 140–45
    trigeminal system, 135–37
Sounds, 54–55
    detection, 56–59
    localization, 65
    tonotopy of auditory system, 59, 61–62
Spatial dimensions, appreciation of, 309
Special visceral afferent nerves, 41
Special visceral efferent nerves, 41
Specific thalamic nuclei, 252
Specific thalamocortical system, 168
Speech. *See* Language functions
Spinal accessory nerve. *See* Cranial nerves,
    XI
Spinal cord, 10, 16, 20, 52, 185, 210–29
    cellular groupings, 213–16

modulation of spinal input, 216–17
modulation of spinal output, 225–26
neurotransmitters, 326–27, 331–32, 334,
  344, 346
somesthetic pathway, 126–27
tracts, 212, 217–21
vestibular nuclei projections, 80
Spinal interneurons, 20, 210, 212, 217,
  224–26, 229
Spinal nerves, 4, 20–21, 315
Spinal nucleus of nerve V, 136, 148, 246
Spinal reflexes, 219, 221–25
Spinal tract of nerve V, 235
Spinal tracts, 212, 217–21, 235
Spines, of dendrites, 5
Spinocerebellar tracts, 209, 224
Spinocervical pathway, 129–30, 132,
  148–49
Spinomedullary junction, 189
Spinoreticular pathways, 138–41
Spinoreticulodiencephalic pathways. See
  Anterolateral system
Spinothalamic tracts, 133–34, 170–71, 184,
  218
Spiral ganglion, 63, 72
Spiral organ of Corti. See Organ of Corti
Splanchnic activity, 243
Stability, sense of, 73, 81
Stapes, 56, 60
Stellate cells, 103, 201–4, 209, 289–93,
  295–96, 313, 344
Stenosis of extracranial vessels, 362
Stereocilia, 57–60, 72–73, 77, 85
Stretch receptors, 117, 216, 221–24
Stretch reflex, 221–25
Stria medullaris/fasciculus retroflexus
  route, of limbic system, 258, 260–61
Stria medullaris thalami, 269, 282
Striatal interneurons, 317
Stria terminalis, 282, 338
Striatonigral tract, 339, 341, 344
Striatum, 193, 209, 265
Stripe of Gennari, 291
Stroke, 354
Subarachnoid space, 33–34, 371
Subdural hematoma, 366
Substance P, 193, 339–41, 350, 353
Substantia gelatinosa, 246, 339, 341–42
Substantia nigra, 30, 170–71, 191, 193–94,
  209, 320, 339, 344–45
Subthalamic nucleus, 170–71, 191, 193,
  194, 209
Sulci, 21, 23, 52, 284
Superior anastomotic vein (Trolard), 366–67,
  375
Superior cerebellar peduncle, 19, 39,
  170–71, 194, 200, 203

Superior colliculi, 30, 52, 105–6, 108–10,
  114, 244–45
Superior frontal gyrus, 303
Superior olivary nuclei, 64–65, 67, 72
Superior temporal gyrus, 299
Superior thalamic radiation, 141
Supplementary motor cortex, 194, 369–70
Suprachiasmatic nucleus, 269
Supramammillary nucleus, 269
Supramarginal gyrus, 301
Supraoptic nuclear group, of
  hypothalamus, 267–70, 273, 282
Sweat glands, 317, 341
Sylvius, fissure of. See Lateral fissure (of
  Sylvius)
Sympathetic nervous system, 4, 43, 45, 52,
  315, 317
Synapses, 6

Tactile pathways. See Touch
Taste, 159–65
  hallucinations, 159, 301
  and olfaction, 159
Taste buds, 160, 163, 165
Tectobulbospinal tract, 106
Tectorial membrane, 57, 72
Tectum, 52, 106, 110, 142
Tegmentum, 30, 52, 64, 252, 256
  neurotransmitters, 326–27, 329–32
Tela choroidea, 31–32
Telencephalon (endbrain), 18, 31, 52, 150
  neurotransmitters, 326–27, 332–33
Temporal coding, 121–22
Temporal lobe, 52, 151, 155, 162, 265,
  284–86, 298–300, 309, 366
Temperature receptors, 116, 119, 134
Tendons, tension-sensing devices of, 117
Texture discrimination, 145
"Thalamic hand", 181
Thalamic radiation, 179, 264, 277
Thalamic syndrome (of Dejerine-Roussy),
  181
Thalamocortical activating system, 168,
  241–42
Thalamocortical data processing, 166–68
Thalamocortical fibers, 176–80, 296
Thalamus, 19, 29–30, 53, 166–84
  functional characteristics of
    thalamocortical projections, 176–80
  gustatory system, 159, 161–63
  lesions, 68, 167–68, 177, 180–81
  limbic system, 254, 261
  motor system, 194–95, 205–6
  muscle/tendon afferent data, 224
  neurotransmitters, 180, 326–27, 331–32,
    336
  nuclei, 168–76, 180–81

Thalamus (*continued*)
  somesthetic system, 125–27, 141
  spinothalamic tracts, 133–34
  thalamocortical data processing, 166–68
  vasculature, 180
Thermoreceptors, 120
Third-order somesthetic neuron, 125–26
Third ventricle, 29, 31, 32, 334
Thirst, 273
Thoracolumbar nerves, 315
Thrombus, 354, 356, 365
Thumb movements, 304
Thyroid-stimulating hormone, 272
Thyrotrophin-releasing hormone, 272, 343
TIA. *See* Transient ischemic attack
Tongue, 159–61
Tonotopy of auditory system, 57, 61–62,
  64, 66, 177
Touch, 116, 119, 133
Tract, 13
Tractus solitarius, 165
Transduction of stimuli, 57, 58, 87–95, 117,
  121
Transient ischemic attack (TIA), 354
Transmitters. *See* Neurotransmitters
Trapezoid nuclei, 64–65, 72
Trigeminal ganglion, 12, 136
Trigeminal lemniscus, 136, 149
Trigeminal nerve. *See* Cranial nerves, V
Trigeminal sensory fibers, 136, 149
Trigeminal system, 135–37
Trigeminothalamic fibers, 170–71
Trigeminothalamic tract, 184
Trochlear nerve. *See* Cranial nerves, IV
Tuberal nuclei group, of hypothalamus. *See*
  Middle nuclei group
Tuber cinereum, 270, 282–83
Tuberohypophysial dopamine neuron
  system, 321, 326
Tuberoinfundibular tract, 270–72, 277, 283
Tufted cells, 155, 165
Tunica media, of intracranial arteries,
  363–64
'Tweenbrain. *See* Diencephalon
Tympanic membrane, 56, 72
Type I, II, and III cells, of taste buds, 160

Uncinate fasciculus, 265, 283
Uncinate fit, 159, 162, 299
Uncommitted cortex. *See* Association cortex
Unconventional synapses, 155
Uncus, 155, 157–59, 162, 165, 299
Unipolar neurons, 8, 124
Utricle, 74, 78, 86
Uvea, 114

VA. *See* Ventral anterior thalamic nucleus
Vagas nerve. *See* Cranial nerve, X
Vasa vasorum, 363
Vascular occlusion, 356
Vascular walls, 357, 363–64, 372
Vasoactive intestinal peptide (VIP), 342, 353
Vasodilation, 355
Vasomotor activities, control of, 243
Vasopressin, 268, 270–71, 273
VB complex. *See* Ventrobasal complex
Veins of the brain, 366–68, 375
Ventral anterior (VA) thalamic nucleus,
  169–71, 173–74, 181, 184, 194, 205
Ventral lateral (VL) thalamic nucleus,
  169–71, 173–74, 181, 184, 194, 198, 205
Ventral posterior inferior (VPi) thalamic
  nucleus, 81, 86
Ventral posterior (VP) thalamic nucleus,
  184, 296
Ventral posterolateral (VPl) thalamic
  nucleus, 130, 132, 149, 169–72, 174
Ventral posteromedial (VPm) thalamic
  nucleus, 135–36, 149, 161–62, 165,
  169–72, 174
Ventral tegmental area (VTA), 257, 260–62,
  283, 320
Ventricles of the brain, 31–34, 53, 371
  ependymal cells, 10
Ventricular fluid, 277
Ventrobasal (VB) complex, of the thalamus,
  130, 141, 145, 149, 172, 177, 224
Ventromedial hypothalamic nucleus,
  269–70, 273, 276, 283
Vermis, 19, 80, 197, 200
Vertebral arteries, 357–59, 372, 375
Vestibular cortex, 86, 299
Vestibular fibers, 200
Vestibular ganglia, 7
Vestibular nerve, 79–80, 86
Vestibular nuclei, 79–81, 86, 200, 202, 205,
  235
Vestibular organ, 86
Vestibular system, 73–86, 299
  central circuitry, 79–82
  feedback control, 82–83
  feed-forward control, 83–84
  inner ear and vestibular receptors, 73–79
  relation of vestibular, auditory, and
    somatic sensations, 78–79
Vestibule, of bony labyrinth, 86
Vestibulocochlear nerve. *See* Cranial
  nerves, VIII
Vestibulo-ocular pathway, 345
Vestibulo-ocular reflex (VOR), 81, 83–84,
  106

Vestibulospinal reflex, 81–83
Vestibulospinal tracts, 80, 86, 205–6, 209
VIP. *See* Vasoactive intestinal peptide
Visceral activities, control of, 47, 265, 278
Visceral brain, 254
Visceral motor neurons, 41, 43, 216–17, 229
Visceral motor system. *See* Autonomic
    nervous system
Visceral sensations, 43, 116
Viscerosomatic integration, 162, 302–3
Visual cortex, 29, 95, 100–102, 110, 142,
    297–98
  columnar organization, 103–5, 294
  developmental plasticity, 111
  lesions, 109–10
  place coding, 63
  and pupillary response in
    accommodation, 108–9
Visual field, 92–93, 96, 99–100, 102
Visual pathway, 95–103
Visual system, 87–114
  adaptability and plasticity, 109–12
  cascade concept, 307
  central circuitry, 95–105
  eye movements, 105–9
  multiple representation of visual signals,
    142

relation to vestibular system, 79
transduction of stimuli, 87–95
Visual radiation, 37
VL. *See* Ventral lateral thalamic nucleus
Vomiting, 243–44
VOR. *See* Vestibulo-ocular reflex
VP. *See* Ventral posterior thalamic nucleus
VPi. *See* Ventral posterior inferior thalamic
    nucleus
VPl. *See* Ventral posterolateral thalamic
    nucleus
VPm. *See* Ventral posteromedial thalamic
    nucleus
VTA. *See* Ventral tegmental area

Water balance, 273
Weight regulation, 273, 276
Wernicke's area, 297, 301
White matter, 13, 18, 24–27, 34
  astrocytes, 10
  internal capsule, 36
  spinal cord, 210, 212, 219
Willis, circle of. *See* Circle of Willis
Willis, Thomas, 254

Xenon technique, for cerebral blood flow
    measurement, 369–70, 373